AF334635

# Recent Results
# in Cancer Research

# 160

Managing Editors
P.M. Schlag, Berlin · H.-J. Senn, St. Gallen

Associate Editors
P. Kleihues, Lyon · F. Stiefel, Lausanne
B. Groner, Frankfurt · A. Wallgren, Göteborg

Founding Editor
P. Rentchnik, Geneva

Springer

*Berlin*
*Heidelberg*
*New York*
*Barcelona*
*Hong Kong*
*London*
*Milan*
*Paris*
*Tokyo*

R. Dummer  F. O. Nestle  G. Burg  (Eds.)

# Cancers of the Skin

Proceedings of the
8th World Congress

With 41 Figures and 27 Tables

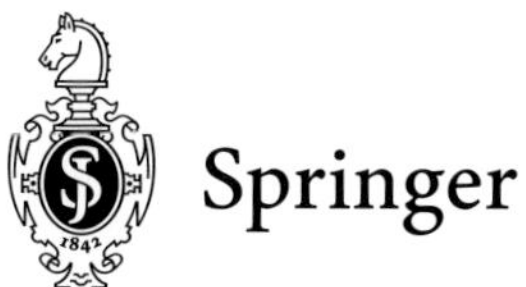 Springer

*Prof. Dr. Reinhard Dummer*
*PD Dr. Frank O. Nestle*
*Prof. Dr. Günter Burg*

University of Zurich
Department of Dermatology
Gloriastr. 31
8091 Zürich, Switzerland

---

Indexed in Current Contents and Index Medicus

---

ISBN 3-540-43005-9 Springer-Verlag Berlin Heidelberg New York
ISSN 0080-0015

Library of Congress Cataloging-in-Publication Data
Die Deutsche Bibliothek – CIP-Einheitsaufnahme
Cancers of the skin: proceedings of the 8th world congress; with 25 tables / [The Eight
World Congress on Cancers of the Skin, July 18–21, 2001, Zurich, Switzerland]. R. Dum-
mer ... (ed.). – Berlin; Heidelberg; New York; Barcelona; Hong Kong; London; Milan;
Paris; Tokyo: Springer, 2002
    (Recent results in cancer research; 160)
    ISBN 3-540-43005-9



Springer-Verlag Berlin Heidelberg New York
a member of BertelsmannSpringer Science+Business Media GmbH

http://www.springer.de



Production: PRO EDIT GmbH, 69126 Heidelberg, Germany
Typesetting: K+V Fotosatz GmbH, 64743 Beerfelden, Germany
Cover design: design & production GmbH, 69121 Heidelberg, Germany

Printed on acid-free paper   SPIN 10893447   21/3111   5 4 3 2 1

# Contents


## 1 Prevention

Public Education in Skin Cancer World-Wide . . . . . . . . . . . . . . . . . 3
  G. Burg

UV Protection and Skin Cancer . . . . . . . . . . . . . . . . . . . . . . . . 7
  R. Dummer, T. Maier

## 2 UV Protection by Clothes

Role of Clothes in Sun Protection . . . . . . . . . . . . . . . . . . . . . . 15
  T. Gambichler, P. Altmeyer, K. Hoffmann

Sun Protective Clothing: 5 Years of Experience in Australia . . . . . . . . 26
  C. R. Roy, P. H. Gies, A. McLennan

European Standards for Protective Apparel Against UV Radiation . . . . 35
  J. Laperre, F. Foubert

American Standards for UV-Protective Textiles . . . . . . . . . . . . . . . 42
  K. L. Hatch

Activities of CIE DIV-6 (Photobiology and Photochemistry)
in UV Protection and Clothing . . . . . . . . . . . . . . . . . . . . . . . . 48
  J. P. Césarini

Comparison of Methods:
Determination of UV Protection of Clothing . . . . . . . . . . . . . . . . 55
  T. Gambichler, P. Altmeyer, K. Hoffmann

Improving UV Protection by Clothing – Recent Developments . . . . . . 62
  U. Osterwalder, H. Rohwer

Dress up for Sun Protection/Creation of Public Awareness . . . . . . . . 70
  P. Césarini


## 3 Melanoma

### Pathogenesis


The Precursors of Malignant Melanoma . . . . . . . . . . . . . . . . . . . 75
  A. N. Crowson, C. M. Magro, I. Sanchez-Carpintero,
  M. C. Mihm Jr.

Interferon-$\alpha$ Sensitivity in Melanoma Cells:
Detection of Potential Response Marker Genes . . . . . . . . . . 85
  U. Certa, M. Seiler, E. Padovan, G. C. Spagnoli

Molecular Cytogenetics as a Diagnostic Tool
for Typing Melanocytic Tumors . . . . . . . . . . . . . . . . . . . . . . . 92
  B. C. Bastian

Loss of Heterozygosity and Microsatellite Instability
in Acquired Melanocytic Nevi: Towards a Molecular Definition
of the Dysplastic Nevus . . . . . . . . . . . . . . . . . . . . . . . . . . . 100
  A. Rübben, I. Bogdan, E. I. Grußendorf-Conen,
  G. Burg, R. Böni


### Epidemiology


The Changing Incidence and Mortality of Melanoma in Australia . . . . 113
  R. Marks


### Diagnostic


Why Is Epiluminescence Microscopy Important? . . . . . . . . . . . . . . 125
  K. Wolff

Sentinel Node Biopsy: Not Only a Staging Tool? . . . . . . . . . . . . . 133
  R. Essner, A. J. Cochran


### Therapy


The Impact of Surgery on the Course of Melanoma . . . . . . . . . . . . 151
  F. J. Lejeune

Perspectives of Pegylated Interferon Use in Dermatological Oncology  .  158
  H. Pehamberger

Dendritic Cell Vaccination for the Treatment of Skin Cancer  . . . . . . .  165
  F. O. Nestle

Gene-based Immunotherapy of Skin Cancers . . . . . . . . . . . . . . . . .  170
  Y. Sun, D. Schadendorf

Cytokine-Fusion-Protein-Treatment  . . . . . . . . . . . . . . . . . . . . .  185
  D. Schrama, P. thor Straten, E.-B. Bröcker,
  R. A. Reisfeld, J. C. Becker

Cytotoxic T-cell Induction in Metastatic Melanoma Patients
Undergoing Recombinant Vaccinia Virus-based
Immuno-gene Therapy . . . . . . . . . . . . . . . . . . . . . . . . . . . . .  195
  G. C. Spagnoli, P. Zajac, W. R. Marti, D. Oertli,
  E. Padovan, C. Noppen, T. Kocher, M. Adamina,
  M. Heberer

## Follow-up

A Rational Approach to the Follow-up of Melanoma Patients  . . . . . .  205
  C. Garbe

## 4 Epithelial Skin Tumors

### Therapy

Micrographic Surgery of Basal Cell Carcinomas of the Head  . . . . . . .  219
  B. Woerle, M. Heckmann, B. Konz

Repair of Cutaneous Defects After Skin Cancer Surgery  . . . . . . . . . .  225
  M. Hess Schmid, C. Meuli-Simmen, J. Hafner

Radiotherapy of Skin Tumors . . . . . . . . . . . . . . . . . . . . . . . . .  234
  R. Panizzon

Photodynamic Therapy and Fluorescence Diagnosis of Skin Cancers  . .  240
  R. M. Szeimies, M. Landthaler

Intralesional Interferon in Basal Cell Carcinoma: How Does It Work?  . .  246
  S. Büchner, M. Wernli, F. Bachmann, T. Harr, P. Erb

Epithelial Malignancies in Organ Transplant Patients:
Clinical Presentation and New Methods of Treatment ............ 251
    E. Stockfleth, C. Ulrich, T. Meyer, E. Christophers

New Treatment Modalities for Basal Cell Carcinoma ............ 259
    E. Stockfleth, W. Sterry

## 5 Lymphoma

### Pathogenesis

From Inflammation to Neoplasia: New Concepts in the Pathogenesis
of Cutaneous Lymphomas ................................. 271
    G. Burg, W. Kempf, A. Haeffner, U. Döbbeling,
    F. O. Nestle, R. Böni, M. Kadin, R. Dummer

### Clinical Presentations

Cutaneous Lymphomas and Pseudolymphomas:
Newly Described Entities ............................... 283
    D. Kazakov, G. Burg, R. Dummer, W. Kempf

Clinical Aspects and Pathology of Primary Cutaneous B-Cell
Lymphomas ............................................ 294
    H. Kerl, R. Fink-Puches, L. Cerroni

### Diagnosis

Modern Diagnosis of Cutaneous Lymphoma ................. 303
    B. Giannotti, N. Pimpinelli

### Therapy

Treatment of Cutaneous T Cell Lymphoma: 2001 .............. 309
    E.C. Vonderheid

New Biologic Agents for the Treatment
of Cutaneous T-Cell Lymphoma ......................... 321
    C. C. Vittorio, J. M. Junkins-Hopkins, M. Shapiro,
    M. Wysocka, M. H. Zaki, L. E. French, A. H. Rook

# 6 Mesenchymal Tumors

Etiology and Pathogenesis of Kaposi's Sarcoma . . . . . . . . . . . . . . . 331
B. Nickoloff, K. E. Foreman

Connective Tissue Tumors . . . . . . . . . . . . . . . . . . . . . . . . . . . . 343
B. Zelger

# 7 Psychosocial Aspects

How to Identify Patients in Need of Psychological Intervention . . . . . 351
G. Strittmatter, M. Tilkorn, R. Mawick

Psychotherapeutic Interventions in Melanoma Patients . . . . . . . . . . 362
W. Söllner, R. Gross, S. Maislinger

**Subject Index** . . . . . . . . . . . . . . . . . . . . . . . . . . . . . . . . . 371

# Principal Authors

Boris C. Bastian, MD
Comprehensive Cancer Center
and Department
of Dermatology
and Pathology
University of California
2340 Sutter Street
San Francisco, CA 94115, USA

Jürgen C. Becker, MD
Department of Dermatology
Julius Maximilians University
Josef-Schneider-Str. 2
97080 Würzburg, Germany

Stanislaw Büchner, MD
Department of Dermatology
University of Basel
Kantonsspital
Petersgraben 4
4031 Basel, Switzerland

Günter Burg, MD
Department of Dermatology
University Hospital of Zurich
Gloriastr. 31
8091 Zürich, Switzerland

Ulrich Certa, MD
F. Hoffmann-La Roche Ltd.
Pharmaceuticals Division
Bldg. 93/610
4070 Basel, Switzerland

Jean-Pierre Césarini, MD
CIE Division 6
Laboratoire de Recherche
sur les Tumeurs
de la Peau Humaine
Fondation Adolphe
de Rothschild
25, rue Manin
75019 Paris, France

Pierre Césarini
Association Sécurité Solaire
(WHO Collaborating Center)
25, rue Manin
75019 Paris, France

Reinhard Dummer, MD
Department of Dermatology
University Hospital of Zurich
Gloriastr. 31
8091 Zürich, Switzerland

zers: the Argentine Society of Dermatology (ASD) and the Fundación del Càncer de Piel (FCP).

The Skin Cancer Prevention Week – the 3rd week in November – is a yearly campaign at a national level, held since 1995 and organized by the ASD. It has National Health Ministry sponsorship but not governmental financial backing. Skin examination clinics are held at public and private institutions staffed by volunteer dermatologists across the nation, and printed material on skin self-examination, skin cancer and prevention guidelines are distributed at these clinics. From an initial number of 5364 consultations in 1994, the campaign has grown to 11313 examinations in 1999. During the summer months, brochure material and dermatological examinations have also been offered in public day-camp centers.

The FCP co-organized the 1995 World Congress of Cancers of the Skin in Buenos Aires and co-organized an Atmospheric-Sun Radiation Congress in 1997. At both meetings the emphasis was on prevention. Publications include the Spanish edition of the *"Guidelines for the Management of Cutaneous Melanoma"* from the original version published by the Australian Cancer Network, and the children's booklet *"Your Skin and the Sun"*, written for children 8–10 years old, to be released in November 2001.

The FCP has a "speaker", Mr. Solmáforo (*"sol"* is sun and *"máforo"* comes from stop light in Spanish). He is illustrated as a traffic light in the form of a face with the red, yellow or green light flashing according to the message presented. He has been presented in lighted bus stops in Buenos Aires and in national newspaper magazines during the late spring and summer months.

A sun-prevention stamp has been designed for the postal service in Argentina.


## John Hawk, M.D. (United Kingdom)

An intensifying campaign over the last 20 years to educate the public in the United Kingdom concerning skin cancer has now reached a level where all members of the public are likely to hear regularly about the dangers of inappropriate sun exposure and sunbed use.

The government-sponsored Health Education Authority has a department dedicated to the promulgation of information on ultraviolet radiation exposure. A regular Sun Awareness Week is held at the beginning of June each year. Promotional material is circulated to schools, with appropriate advice to teachers on how to protect children from sunlight damage. The sunburning risk is given daily during the summer on television and radio weather forecast programs.

## Luigi Rusciani, M.D. (Giorgio Landi, M.D.) (Italy)

The Italian Skin Cancer Foundation has been involved for about 12 years in a large number of activities. It organizes three meetings every year in different Italian cities for dermatologists and general practitioners to promote strategies on prevention and therapy of skin cancer. The Foundation also promotes collaboration between different Italian dermatologic centers interested in skin cancers to improve cooperation and to supply professional clinical services.

The Italian Skin Cancer Foundation promotes information campaigns for the public on TV and in the newspapers. The announcement "Neo" in one of the prevention campaigns in the Italian newspapers, realized by the advertising agency "Roncaglia & Wijkander", has obtained public recognition.

## Mitzi Moulds (USA)

For more than 20 years, the Skin Cancer Foundation has carried out public education programs, first in the United States, and then reaching out internationally. The many activities include elaboration and distribution of information material on prevention of skin cancer. The Foundation's public education programs are exceptional. A nationwide campaign is launched every year featuring the melanoma week, a program in which many dermatologists all over the country are involved.

The Skin Cancer Foundation is the sponsor and promoter of the World Congress on Cancers of the Skin, which takes place every 3 years.

## Jean-Pierre Césarini, M.D. (France)

In France, Sécurité Solaire has become a collaborating center for the World Health Organization's Intersun Program. The UV index is disseminated via national TV, weather service reports and newspapers. A pedagogical kit, "Living with the Sun", has been produced and given to several hundred thousand children aged 3–6 years. A Skin Cancer Day with free access to public hospitals and participating private practitioners was started in 1998 under the auspices of the French Syndicate of Dermatologists.

## Hubert Pehamberger, M.D. (Austria)

The Austrian Society for Dermatology and the Austrian Cancer League have been conducting public education campaigns since 1988. They provide information via the print media and television and broadcasting, and also distribute booklets, brochures, folders, and posters. These are given out at special information events, and at schools and public institutions, as well as on request. Skin checks take place at public baths and beaches, at special events, and on "Melanoma Days" announced in advance.

## Claus Garbe, M.D. (Germany)

Public education campaigns in Germany have been instituted for the past few years, supported by the *Deutsche Krebshilfe* and other organizations. There are special campaigns on primary and secondary prevention of skin cancer, organized on a regular basis every year, supported by TV, newspapers and radio broadcasting. A campaign on sun protection was carried out at several German airports during the summer. Access to free skin checks and advice from dermatologists on sensible skin exposure practices and avoidance of sunburn is given in many cities.

## Francisco Camacho-Martinez, M.D. (Spain)

The Spanish Association for Cutaneous Cancer has been founded. Campaigns providing information about skin cancer have been launched in schools. Regular campaigns for public education, targeting especially children and younger adults, have been organized during the past years.

## Günter Burg, M.D. (Switzerland)

Based on a model developed by the WHO, the Swiss Federal Office of Public Health (BAG) and the Swiss League Against Cancer (SKL) have initiated four national cancer control programs of particular importance in terms of health policy. One of these programs focuses on combating skin cancer. This particular group (led by G. Burg) has been appointed by the BAG and the SKL to consider the following topics:
- Health promotion and primary prevention
- Early detection, diagnosis and secondary prevention
- Therapy
- Follow-up care, support
- Epidemiology

The main emphasis of the campaign programs in past years has been on providing target group-oriented (in line with profession, age, leisure activities) and seasonally oriented (summer/winter holidaymakers) information about the following topics in particular:
- Assessment of skin type and associated risk
- Sunbathing and exposure to UV radiation
- Effective protection against UV radiation
- Early detection of skin cancer

There are many more activities going on throughout the world which hopefully in the future will reduce morbidity and mortality from skin cancer.

# UV Protection and Skin Cancer

Reinhard Dummer and Tanja Maier

## Abstract

In discussions amongst the public and the scientific community, doubts are repeatedly raised concerning the efficacy of sunscreens in preventing cutaneous malignancy. This article summarizes the most reliable references on UV protection and epithelial skin cancer and discusses the role of UV protection in melanoma prevention. We conclude that there is substantial evidence that UV protection is able to reduce the risk of actinic keratosis, squamous cell carcinoma and probably also the risk of melanoma.

## Introduction

Sunlight is the ultimate source for the development and existence of life on earth. The sun's infrared rays warm the atmosphere. We see with eyes that respond to the visible part of the sun's spectrum. Visible light is essential for photosynthesis, the biochemical process necessary for plants to produce energy and thus, serving as the basis source of food.

However, ultraviolet (UV) irradiation that comprises approximately 50% of the total solar energy arriving on the earth's surface, is largely responsible for the health problems associated with sun exposure (Dummer et al. 2001). The spectrum and the intensity of UV irradiation depends on a number of factors including season, height of the sun in the sky, time of day, geographical latitude, attenuation by atmospheric gases, particularly stratospheric ozone and pollution in the lower atmosphere, amount of cloud, reflection from different ground surfaces (e.g. water or sand) and altitude above sea level. The amount of UV exposure of humans is further influenced by behavior (amount of outdoor activity, choice of holiday destination) and the use of UV protection including protective behavior, clothing and sunscreens (Dummer and Osterwalder 2000; Frei et al. 1999).

Recent Results in Cancer Research, Vol. 160
© Springer-Verlag Berlin Heidelberg 2002

In this context it is important to recall that UVA (wavelengths 320–400 nm) and UVB (wavelengths 320–280 nm) are differently affected by the above mentioned factors. In general, UVB irradiation is more intensively reduced by the above mentioned factors. As an example, Fig. 1 shows the variation in UVB and UVA during a day in summer and winter in the Swiss mountains (Davos) (Frei et al. 1999).

In contrast, UVB includes the major wavelengths that induce a delayed erythema (sunburn) that begins about 4 h and peeks around 12 h after UVB exposure. The sunburn reaction is caused by direct and indirect damage to epidermal cells which includes alterations to DNA and the activation of inflammatory cascades including cytokine and prostaglandin pathways. There is a clear linkage between erythema and DNA damage. A rough correlation has been noted between pyrimidine dimer formation and susceptibility to erythema. Wavelengths that are most efficient in producing erythema are also the most efficient in producing pyrimidine dimers (Eller et al. 1996, 1997). This linkage has also been confirmed by mutational analysis of human skin tumors demonstrating that UV-induced pyrimidine dimers and related photoproducts are the major type of DNA damage in these malignancies.

In mouse skin, UVB irradiation has been shown to be able to initiate the multistep process of skin tumor formation. This initiation implies the acquisition of permanent genetic alterations that subsequently predispose daughter cells to become malignant. In UV-damaged human skin this alteration frequently results in inactivation of a principle tumor suppressor gene such as p53. Promotion is now the process that provides the additional mutations that are necessary to develop a fully malignant phenotype. Like complete chemical carcinogens, UVB radiation can initiate and promote cancer development. This explains the potent relationship between erythematous UV exposures and skin cancer (Naylor 1997).

Because sunburn is primarily caused by UVB irradiation and UVB is strongly absorbed by DNA resulting in the typical genetic alterations, it has been suggested that UVB is the important part of the solar UV spectrum that is also the major factor for the induction of human melanoma (Naylor

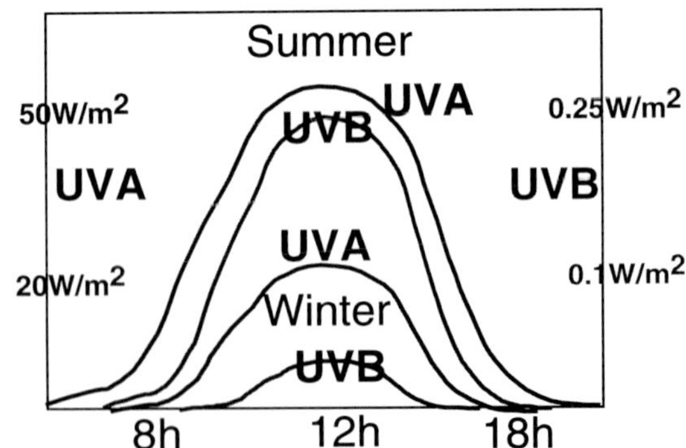


**Fig. 1.** Daily profile of comparison of the relative solar irradiation transmitted by UVA and UVB in summer and winter time during the day (Frei et al. 1999)

1997). However, UVA might also be important since up to 95% of the solar UV irradiation energy that reaches the surface of the earth is UVA. UVA includes longer wavelengths than UVB and penetrates more deeply into the skin. Although UVA is about 1000 times less effective than UVB in inducing erythema, it can induce other biological effects such as immediate pigment darkening and persistent pigment darkening. This phenomenon can be observed mainly in dark-skinned persons (Wang et al. 2001).

The possibility that UVA particularly can cause melanoma in humans was first suggested several years ago (Gilchrest et al. 1999). Garland suggested that the rising incidence of melanoma might be in part related to the widespread use of sunscreens providing only UVB protection (Garland et al. 1993). These sunscreens allow a more prolonged exposure to solar irradiation and therefore contribute to the acquisition of a larger UVA dose. A special role for UVA in the induction of melanoma is also suggested by the observation that UVA is capable of inducing melanoma in the xiphophorus hybrid fish. UVA exposure can also induce melanoma precursors in another animal model, the opossum, after prolonged exposure. Besides these animal models, there are a series of observations from cell culture models indicating that UVA damages DNA (Wang et al. 2001). UVA-induced DNA damage has also been detected in human skin by the assessment of p53 protein expression and the presence of pyrimidine dimers after UVA irradiation as well as after UVB irradiation (Burren et al. 1998). This study provided in vivo evidence that DNA damage in human skin is caused not only by UVB but also by UVA (Applegate et al. 1999).

## UV Protection and Skin Cancers

The skin is the organ that is affected by cancers most frequently. There is direct and indirect evidence that UV irradiation is involved in the pathogenesis of epithelial skin cancers such as squamous cell carcinoma and basal cell carcinoma and melanoma. With an incidence rate of approximately 100 per 100 000 inhabitants per year, epithelial skin cancers are extremely common, especially in the elderly with skin type 1 or 2 (Boni et al. 1995).

The best evidence for the efficacy of UV protection is provided by prospective randomized controlled trials.

## Reduction of Solar Keratosis (Actinic Keratosis, In Situ Squamous Cell Carcinoma) by Regular Sunscreen Use

Actinic keratoses are found commonly on sun-damaged skin. They are risk factors for basal cell carcinoma and melanoma and are precursors of squamous cell carcinoma, although the rate of malignant transformation is probably only around 10%. Thompson et al. (1993) studied the effect of regular use of sunscreens on the appearance of new solar keratosis and the disappearance of preexisting lesions. Included in this study were 588 subjects, 40 years of age or older. The subjects applied either a sunscreen cream with a sun protection factor (SPF) of 17 or the identical cream without UV filters. There was an increase in the number of solar keratosis in the group of subjects treated with placebo and a decrease in the group treated with the sunscreen. The number of remissions was higher in the subjects treated with sunscreens and there was a clear dose response relationship. This study very convincingly shows that the regular use of sunscreen prevents the development of solar keratosis and by implication probably reduces the risk of squamous cell cancer on the long term. However, this study cannot give any information on the effect of sunscreen use on the development of melanoma or basal cell carcinoma.

Naylor et al. conducted a prospective double-blind controlled trial of daily application of sunscreens versus placebo over a 2-year period. Included in the study were 53 volunteers. One half applied a sunscreen with a SPF of 29 and the other half placebo. A 36% reduction in the annual rate of actinic keratosis was found. This was statistically significant (Naylor et al. 1995).

## UV Protection by Sunscreen Reduces the Incidence of Squamous Cell Carcinomas

Green et al. (1999) performed a prospective randomized trial in 1621 individuals. One group applied a sunscreen daily with a SPF factor of 15 or more and betacarotene supplementation, another group sunscreen plus placebo tablets, betacarotene only or placebo only. After a follow-up of 4.5 years the incidences of basal cell carcinomas and squamous cell carcinomas were recorded. Betacarotene did not have any impact on the incidence rate. None of the treatments reduced the incidence of basal cell carcinomas, but the incidence of squamous cell carcinoma was significantly lower in the sunscreen group than in the no-sunscreen group.

## Sunscreen Use and Melanoma

There is no prospective randomized study that has analyzed the efficacy of sunscreen use or UVB protection on the incidence of melanoma, and it is doubtful whether such a study will be ever done. The absence of this direct proof has initiated intensive discussion (Rigel et al. 2000) and it has even been suggested that sunscreen use might actually increase the risk of melanoma (Garland et al. 1993). It is known that intense UV irradiation, especially in childhood, is reflected by a high number of melanocytic nevi and that the number of melanocytic nevi is associated with an increased risk of malignant melanoma. Therefore, it seems reasonable to study the effect of sunscreen use on the development of benign melanocytic lesions. Autier et al. (1999) have performed a study asking parents of children aged 6–7 years how frequently the children use sunscreens. They counted the nevi and compared this with the information on sunscreen use given by the parents. However, no data were collected regarding the behavior of the same children when they were younger. The authors reported that the sunscreen-using children had a higher nevus count, but this was only true in fair-skinned children with high sunscreen use.

A more recent study, however, found the opposite. Gallagher et al. (2000) have reported that regular sun exposure reduces the number of melanocytic lesions. They studied 309 school children and counted the nevi at the start and at the end of an observation period. The children were randomized to receive a SPF 30 broad-spectrum sunscreen or not to receive sunscreen and no advice concerning sunscreen use. The number of new nevi during the 3 years of the study were compared between the treatment and the control groups. There was a significant difference. Children in the sunscreen group developed fewer nevi than children in the control group. Interestingly, there was an interaction between freckling and study group: freckled children (mostly skin types 1 and 2) receiving sunscreen would develop 30–40% fewer nevi than freckled children without UV protection (Gallagher et al. 2000).

This observation is also supported by the follow-up of patients treated with psoralen and UVA (PUVA). PUVA-treated individuals regularly develop lentiginous pigmented skin lesions and in addition, have an increased risk of developing a melanoma (Wang et al. 2001). The role of UVA in the induction of melanoma is also indicated by the results of studies in animal models (Ley 1997; Setlow et al. 1993).

## Conclusion

Summarizing the above data from in vitro experiments, animal models, and prospective randomized trials in patients with actinic keratosis, squamous cell carcinoma or multiple nevi, we conclude that UV protection including the regular use of broad-spectrum sunscreens has proven benefits in reducing the risk of development of squamous cell carcinoma and its precursor actinic keratosis. Extensive investigations concerning the effects of sunscreens on the development of melanocytic nevi indicate that the incidence of melanoma may also be reduced (Lim et al. 2001). This optimism is supported by epidemiological observations such as the decreasing melanoma incidence in Australia where 75% of the population regularly use sunscreens, and the situation in the Caucasian population in Hawaii which has the highest per capita sunscreen use in the United States (Rigel et al. 2000).

## References


Applegate LA, Scaletta C, Panizzon R, Niggli H, Frenk E (1999) In vivo induction of pyrimidine dimers in human skin by UVA radiation: initiation of cell damage and/or intercellular communication? Int J Mol Med 3:467–472

Autier P, Dor JF, Ng S, Linard D, Panizzon R, Lejeune FJ, Guggisberg D, Eggermont AM (1999) Sunscreen use and duration of sun exposure: a double-blind, randomized trial (see comments). J Natl Cancer Inst 91:1304–1309

Boni R, Dummer R, Burg G (1995) Nehmen Hauttumoren zu? Schweiz Med Wochenschr 125:1619–1624

Burren, R, Scaletta C, Frenk E, Panizzon RG, Applegate LA (1998) Sunlight and carcinogenesis: expression of p53 and pyrimidine dimers in human skin following UVA I, UVA I + II and solar simulating radiations. Int J Cancer 76:201–206

Dummer R, Osterwalder U (2000) UV transmission of summer clothing in Switzerland and Germany (letter). Dermatology 200:81–82

Dummer R, Maier T, Bloch PH, Burg G (2001) Photoprotektion: Lichtschutzmaßnahmen zum Schutz vor akuten und chronischen Hautschäden. Swiss Med Forum 14:364–368

Eller MS, Ostrom K, Gilchrest BA (1996) DNA damage enhances melanogenesis. Proc Natl Acad Sci USA 93:1087–1092

Eller MS, Maeda T, Magnoni C, Atwal D, Gilchrest BA (1997) Enhancement of DNA repair in human skin cells by thymidine dinucleotides: evidence for a p53-mediated mammalian SOS response. Proc Natl Acad Sci USA 94:12627–12632

Frei T, Dummer R, Gehrig R (1999) Die UV-Belastung in der Schweiz: Abhängigkeit von Ort und Zeit und ihre Bedeutung für die Haut. Praxis 88:1023–1029

Gallagher RP, Rivers JK, Lee TK, Bajdik CD, McLean DI, Coldman AJ (2000) Broad-spectrum sunscreen use and the development of new nevi in white children: a randomized controlled trial. JAMA 283:2955–2960

Garland CF, Garland FC, Gorham ED (1993) Rising trends in melanoma. An hypothesis concerning sunscreen effectiveness (see comments). Ann Epidemiol 3:103–110

Gilchrest BA, Eller MS, Geller AC, Yaar M (1999) The pathogenesis of melanoma induced by ultraviolet radiation. N Engl J Med 340:1341–1348

Green A, Williams G, Neale R, Hart V, Leslie D, Parsons P, Marks GC, Gaffney P, Battistutta D, Frost C, Lang C, Russell A (1999) Daily sunscreen application and betacarotene supplementation in prevention of basal-cell and squamous-cell carcinomas of the skin: a randomised controlled trial (see comments). Lancet 354:723–729

Ley RD (1997) Ultraviolet radiation A-induced precursors of cutaneous melanoma in *Monodelphis domestica*. Cancer Res 57:3682–3684

Lim HW, Naylor M, Honigsmann H, Gilchrest BA, Cooper K, Morison W, Deleo VA, Scherschun L (2001) American Academy of Dermatology Consensus Conference on UVA Protection of Sunscreens: summary and recommendations. Washington, DC, 4 February 2000. J Am Acad Dermatol 44:505–508

Naylor MF (1997) Erythema, skin cancer risk, and sunscreens. Arch Dermatol 133:373–375

Naylor MF, Boyd A, Smith DW, Cameron GS, Hubbard D, Neldner KH (1995) High sun protection factor sunscreens in the suppression of actinic neoplasia. Arch Dermatol 131:170–175

Rigel DS, Naylor M, Robinson J (2000) What is the evidence for a sunscreen and melanoma controversy? Arch Dermatol 136:1447–1449

Setlow RB, Grist E, Thompson K, Woodhead AD (1993) Wavelengths effective in induction of malignant melanoma. Proc Natl Acad Sci USA 90:6666–6670

Thompson SC, Jolley D, Marks R (1993) Reduction of solar keratoses by regular sunscreen use (see comments). N Engl J Med 329:1147–1151

Wang SQ, Setlow R, Berwick M, Polsky D, Marghoob AA, Kopf AW, Bart RS (2001) Ultraviolet A and melanoma: a review. J Am Acad Dermatol 44:837–846

# UV Protection by Clothes   2

# Role of Clothes in Sun Protection


Thilo Gambichler, Peter Altmeyer, and Klaus Hoffmann


## Abstract


Ultraviolet (UV) radiation is the carcinogenic factor in sunlight. Damage to skin cells from repeated UV exposure can lead to the development of skin cancer. Apart from avoidance of the sun, the most frequently used form of UV protection has been the application of sunscreens. The use of textiles as a means of sun protection has been underrated in previous educational campaigns, even though suitable clothing offers usually simple and effective broadband protection against the sun. Apart from skin cancer formation, exacerbation of photosensitive disorders and premature skin aging could be prevented by suitable UV-protective clothing. Nevertheless, several studies have recently shown that, contrary to popular opinion, some textiles provide only limited UV protection. It has been found that one-third of commercial summer clothing items provide a UV protection factor (UPF) less than 15. Given the increasing interest in sun protection, recreationally and occupationally, test methods and a rating scheme for clothing were needed that would ensure sufficient UV protection. Various textile parameters have an influence on the UPF of a finished garment. Important parameters are the fabric porosity, type, color, weight and thickness. The application of UV absorbers into the yarns significantly improves the UPF of a garment. Under the conditions of wear and use several factors can alter the UV-protective properties of a textile, e.g., stretch, wetness and laundering. The use of UV-blocking cloths can provide excellent protection against the hazards of sunlight; this is especially true for garments manufactured as UV-protective clothing. However, further educational efforts are necessary to change people's sun behavior and raise awareness for the use of adequate sun-protective clothing.



Recent Results in Cancer Research, Vol. 160
© Springer-Verlag Berlin Heidelberg 2002

## Introduction

The incidence of skin cancer has been increasing at an alarming rate over the past several decades. In Europe, there are nearly 100 cases per 100 000 people per year of basal cell carcinoma, 25 cases of squamous cell carcinoma, and about 10 cases of malignant melanoma. Australia has the highest incidence of skin cancer in the world (non-melanoma skin cancer 1000 cases; malignant melanoma 26 cases). While there are many factors involved in the onset of skin cancers, the cumulative ultraviolet (UV) exposure of the patient has clearly been identified as an important factor. Epidemiological studies have shown that increased recreational or occupational exposure to the sun has been a major contributory factor in the rising incidence of skin cancer (Altmeyer et al. 1997; Brash and Pontén 1998; Soehnge et al. 1997). Nevertheless, there are several biopositive effects of UVR (e.g., increase in vitamin $D_3$ and HDL cholesterol levels, reduction in blood pressure), and it is well known that total avoidance of UV exposure causes substantial impairment of vitamin $D_3$ metabolism and osteogenesis (Barth et al. 1994; Holick and Jung 1999; Matsuoka et al. 1992).

Apart from avoidance of the sun, especially in peak hours, the most frequently used form of UV protection is the application of sunscreens. The use of textiles as a means of sun protection has been underrated in previous educational campaigns, even though suitable clothing offers usually simple and effective broadband protection against the sun (Altmeyer et al. 1997). However, following comments over some years by patients, usually from fairskinned men, that they suffered sunburn or developed photosensitive disorders through their clothing, it was decided first of all in Australia, to undertake investigations to study UV-protective properties of clothing. Especially in Australia, cancer educational campaigns have long urged the use of clothing in conjunction with hats, sun glasses, and sunscreens as UV protection. A number of studies have recently shown that, contrary to popular opinion, some textiles provide insufficient UV protection (Fig. 1). Thus, it has been shown that more than one-third of commercial summer garments give less than a UV protection factor (UPF) of 15 (Gambichler et al. 2001a; Dummer and Osterwalder 2000; Gies et al. 1999). Analogous to the sun protection factor (SPF) of sunscreens, the UPF is a multiplying factor which permits calculation of one's extended time in the sun, when protected by clothes.

Apart from skin cancer formation and photoaging, exacerbation of photosensitive disorders, e.g., polymorphous light eruption, lupus erythematosus, porphyrias, solar urticaria, and phototoxic/photoallergic reactions, can be prevented by UV-protective clothing (O'Quinn and Wagner 1998; Roelandts 2000). Consequently, the use of suitable textiles which block UVB as well as UVA radiation has been recommended for photosensitive patients. Most of the photosensitive diseases are predominantly provoked by wavelengths in the UVA range, and in some of these disorders even extremely small UV doses can lead to exacerbation, especially in solar urticaria. The latter can also be triggered by visible light. Interestingly, the use of optical whiteners in

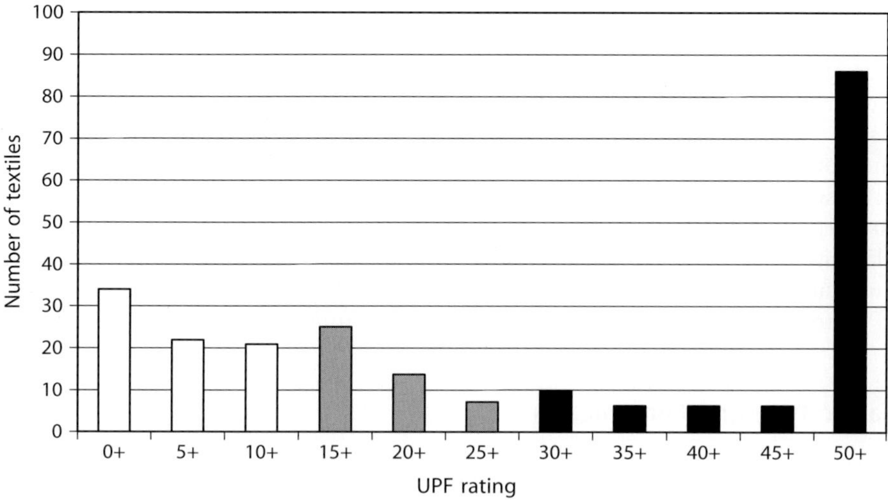

**Fig. 1.** UPF rating of 236 commercial summer clothes (spring/summer collection 2000/2001) of different fabric types, construction, and color. Of the textiles, 33% had UPF < 15 (*open bars*), 19% had UPF 15–30 (*light gray bars*), and 48% had UPF ≥ 30 (*dark gray bars*)

clothing potentially transform UVA radiation into visible light, so that in particular cases solar urticaria may even be enhanced through clothing (Gardeazabel et al. 1998).

In addition to the human suffering caused by skin cancer diseases, there is a significant economic burden due to the costs of preventive efforts, diagnosis, treatment, and care of terminally ill patients. Despite public education campaigns skin cancer rates are still on the increase. Although people are aware of the hazards of sunlight, underprotection because of inadequate application of sunscreen (e.g., amount < 2 mg/cm$^2$; no reapply; skipping ears, neck etc.) and insufficient textile photoprotection, coupled with overexposure to the sun (prolonging duration of sun exposure by using inadequate UV-protective tools) may partially explain why skin cancer incidences still increase. The results of several studies indicate that some aspects of sun protection are being practiced consistently, while others, such as the use of UV-protective clothing, are not (Barankin et al. 2001; Robinson et al. 2000). As recommended by the American Academy of Dermatology and other organizations, avoiding deliberate tanning with indoor and outdoor light, seeking shade, and limiting exposure during peak hours need to be included in sunprotective strategies (Goldsmith et al. 1996).

Given the increasing interest in sun protection, both recreationally and occupationally, a test method and a rating scheme for clothing were required, which guarantee sufficient UV protection. There are different test methods for the determination of the UPF (e.g., in vivo method analogous to SPF testing, UV dosimetry). However, spectrophotometric measurement of UV transmission through the fabric (in vitro method) is the most established test method (Gambichler et al. 2001b; Gies et al. 1997; Laperre et al. 2001; Menzies et al. 1991; Moehrle and Garbe 2000; Ravishankar and Diffey 1997). The Australian/New Zealand standard, AS/NZS 4399 (Standards Australia/Standards New Zealand 1996), was the first normative publication on the test methods to be used to determine the in vitro UPF and a classification scheme. UV-rated clothing has been on sale in Australia for some years now, in particular recreational wear such as beachwear, rash vests for surfing, and elastane body suits for small children. Apart from Australia, other countries and multinational groups (e.g., Europe, USA) have also engaged in writing UV-protective textile standard documents (Hoffmann 1998).

## Fabric Type and Construction

For undyed fabrics there are differences in the UV-absorbing properties of the fiber. Summer clothing is usually made of cotton, viscose, rayon, linen and polyester or their combinations. Other types of materials such as nylon or elastane are also found in special applications such as bathing suits and nylon stockings. In general, consumers consider light-weight nonsynthetic fabrics, e.g., cotton, viscose, and linen, the most comfortable for summer textiles. Comparison of the different types of material in relation to the UPF is difficult and only possible in a limited number of cases. This is because certain production steps (dying, finishing) depend on the material and results in a comparison of the "material-color-finish" combination and not of the material alone.

In the case of synthetic fibers (e.g., polyester, polyamide) the analysis is even more difficult because the UV protection of these materials will depend on the type and amount of additives, such as antioxidants or UV stabilizers, to the fiber. Polyester in particular usually has good UV-blocking properties, as it provides relative low UVB transmission probably due to a large conjugated system in the polymer chains (Crews et al. 1999; Davis et al. 1997). Polyester or polyester blends may be the most suitable fabric type for UV-protective garments (Fig. 2). However, its permeability to wavelengths in the UVA range is frequently higher in comparison to other fiber types; this could be of significance for many wearers suffering from photosensitive disorders.

Bleached cotton and viscose rayon provide relatively low UV protection and are thus transparent to UV radiation. This was recently confirmed by a study by Crews et al. (1999) who found that bleached cotton print cloth had a UV transmission of 23.7%, whereas unbleached cotton print cloth had a UV transmission of only 14.4%. The influence of bleaching was also evident among the silk fabrics in their study. In comparison to bleached textiles unbleached fabrics such as cotton and silk have better UV-protective properties due to UV-absorbing natural pigments and other impurities.

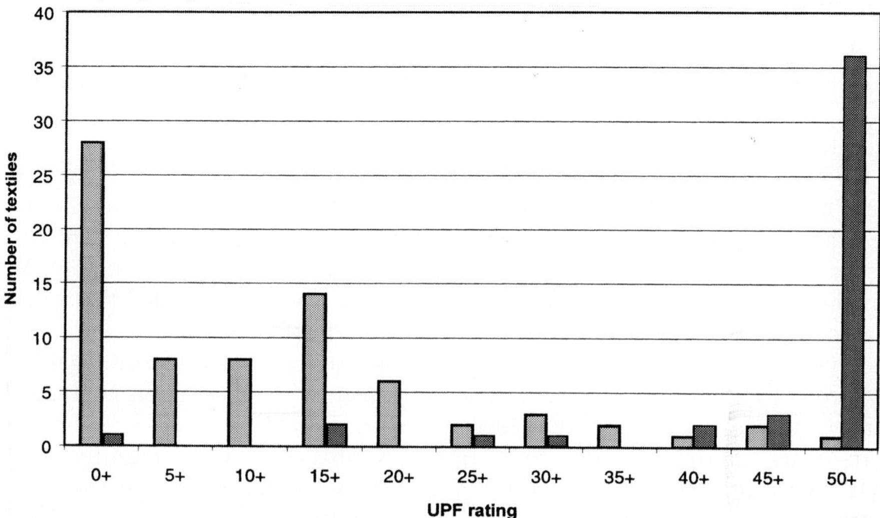


**Fig. 2.** UPF rating of 74 viscose (*light gray bars*) and 46 polyester (*dark gray bars*) summer textiles of different construction and color

The fabric construction is a primary determinant of fabric porosity followed by fabric weight and thickness of the textile (Crews et al. 1999). The closer the weave or knitting (smaller yarn-to-yarn spaces), the less the fabric's porosity – consequently, less UV radiation is transmitted. Spaces between the yarns are generally larger in a knit than in a woven textile. Further, plain woven textiles have a lower porosity than textiles woven using other weaves (Capjack et al. 1994). For an "ideal" fabric (fibers opaque to UV light) of a particular fiber content and fabric construction, an increase in weight per unit area is associated with a decrease in fabric porosity – the spaces between the yarns will be smaller in a heavier textile, therefore less UV radiation is transmitted. However, yarns are usually not opaque to UV radiation and the UPFs of "real" fabrics are therefore lower than the "ideal" fabric. In most of the studies thickness measurements for the fabrics were not undertaken or reported. However, thickness is a useful parameter for understanding differences in UV protection between fabrics. Crews et al. (1999) reported that thicker, denser fabrics transmit less UV radiation and they concluded that thickness is most useful in explaining differences in UV transmission when differences in percentage cover are also accounted for (Pailthorpe 1994).

## Fabric Color and UV Absorbers

The color of a fabric may influence the UPF as some dyes have an absorption spectrum extending into the UV spectrum. Enhanced UV protection of dyed textiles depends on the position and intensity of the absorption bands of the dyes in the UV wavelength and the concentration of the dye in the textile. The absorbance of UV radiation can influence many substrate attributes, e.g., fluorescence, photodegradation and UV protection. Generally, dark colors provide better UV protection due to increased UV absorption (Fig. 3). This holds true only for the same UV absorbent dye and provided that other characteristics of the textile, e.g., fabric type, and construction, are the same. However, dyes within particular hue types can vary considerably in degree of UV protectiveness due to their individual transmission/absorption characteristics (Srinivasan and Gatewood 2000).

In order to improve UV protection, UV absorbers have recently been added with different techniques. UV absorbers are colorless compounds that absorb in the wavelength range 280–400 nm. Hilfiker et al. (1996) found the cover factor to be useful in predicting the maximum UPF that could be achieved by treating the yarns with UV absorbers. Thus, fabrics could be made opaque to UV radiation with a sufficient level of UV absorber impregnation, and the corresponding UPFs approached the theoretically predicted levels based on the cover factor. Titan dioxide is frequently used as a UV-blocking substance in fabrics. However, the absorptive and scattering properties of titan dioxide particles in the UVA wavelength range are different and

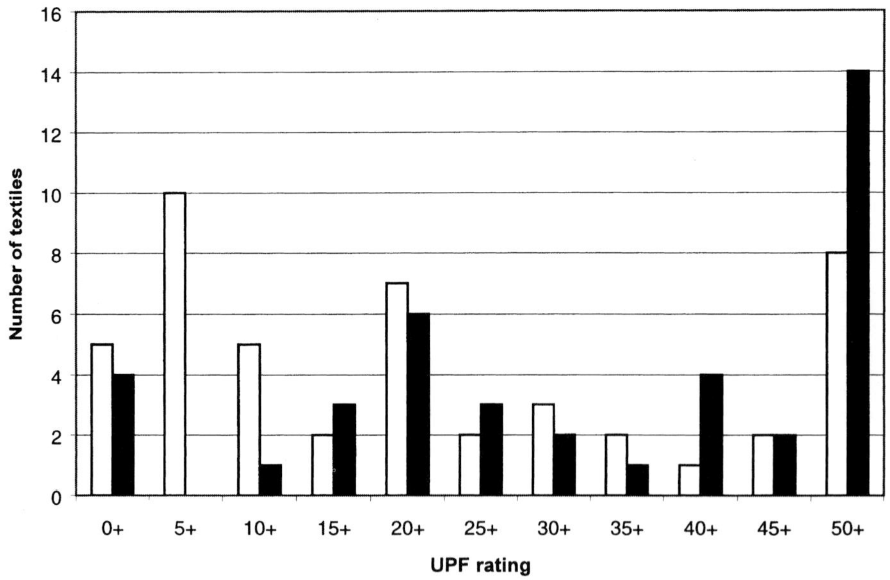

**Fig. 3.** UPF rating of white ($n = 40$) and black ($n = 44$) summer textiles of different fiber type and construction

depend mainly on the particle size and geometry. Other manufactured UV absorbers also provide less protection from UVA radiation, which should be considered when counseling patients with photosensitive disorders. Nevertheless, UV absorbers are suitable for significantly increasing UPF, especially that of nondyed lightweight summer fabrics, such as cotton and viscose (Hilfiker et al. 1996; Hoffmann et al. 1998; Eckhardt and Rohwer 2000).

## Stretch and Hydration

Woven textiles do not stretch significantly, but knitted textiles are prone to stretch causing an increase in fabric porosity with a consequent decrease in UPF. Moon and Pailthorpe (1995) have shown that stretching elastane-based garments by about 10% in both the machine and the cross-machine directions causes a dramatic decrease in the measured UPF of a textile. Their consumer survey also showed that on average about 15% stretch is achieved when these textiles are worn. However, the 15% is for power-stretch, which is only a small segment of the clothing market, and elastane-based textiles for "tight-fitting" should not be considered as defined UV-protective clothing. Kimlin et al. (1999) have reported that the UPF of 50 denier stockings decreases by 868% when stretched 30% from their original size. Notably, the most popular type of stockings (15 denier) provides a UPF of less than 2 (Sinclair and Diffey 1997). The maximum stretch point on the body for tight-fitting garments is the upper back, where textiles can be stretched up to 15%. However, realistically, the effect of stretch on the UPF of a textile may be of significance only for garments with a nonstretched UPF of less than 30, particularly leggings, women's stockings, and swimsuits.

When textiles become wet, by air hydration, perspiration, or water, UV transmission through the fabric can significantly change. A marked reduction in the UPF has been observed for textiles made from cotton and cotton blends. In a field-based study, it has recently been shown that significant UV exposures may occur beneath the garments, particularly for white cotton fabrics in the wet state (Parisi et al. 2000). Similar results have also been found for in vivo measurements of cotton and polyester blends (Gambichler et al. 2002; Jevtic 1990; Moon and Pailthorpe 1995). One explanation for this is that the presence of water in the interstices of a fabric reduces optical scattering effects and, hence, increases the UV transmission of the textile. The analogy in the visible spectral range is that T-shirts become see-through when wet. In case of fabrics made of viscose or silk, or in fabrics that have been treated with broadband UV absorbers, the UPF frequently increases when the textile becomes wet. This has also been observed in a recent study of modal fabrics treated with titan dioxide (Gambichler et al. 2002; Hoffmann et al. 1998). Thus, UV protection of wet garments is not necessarily poor.

## Durability of UPF

Most of the fabrics will undergo a combination of relaxation shrinkage and consolidation shrinkage when washed. Thus the spaces between the yarns will decrease and UV protection increases. The effect of laundering on the UPF puts into perspective other fabric parameters and factors which decrease the UPF. Stanford et al. (1995 a) conducted laundering trials using cotton T-shirts. They showed that UPFs increase after the first washing and do not change significantly with subsequent washing. For example, the original UPF rating of a new cotton T-shirt was 15 and increased to UPF 35 after the first laundering. These UPFs were also obtained when participants were instructed to wear their T-shirt for 4–8 h per week and to wash their T-shirt once per week for 10 wash-and-wear cycles (Stanford et al. 1995 b). Wang et al. (2001) have observed only a moderate increase in the UPF of cotton fabrics after laundering. They have found that adding UV-absorbing agents during laundering substantially enhances the UPF (Osterwalder et al. 2000; Wang et al. 2001).

Recently, Zhou and Crews (1998) have reported that UPF of cotton cotton/ polyester blend fabrics can be significantly enhanced by repeated laundering of the garment in a detergent containing optical brightening agent. This is not true for fabrics comprised entirely of polyester or nylon (Zhou and Crews 1998). Prolonged wear and tear beyond the "standard" lifetime of a garment may eventually cause thinning of the individual fibers and so alter the UPF. Photostability of a textile and its UV protectiveness is an important requirement for sun-protective clothing. Unfortunately, there are only limited data on the stability of the UV protectiveness of a textile against UV radiation or infrared. Below a particular wavelength, photolytic processes of fibers have been observed in various fabrics (linen $< 360$ nm, cotton $< 350$ nm, viscose $< 340$ nm; silk and polyester $< 310$ nm), independent of other factors, such as temperature, oxygen, and hydration. Photo-oxidation of fibers can occur above these wavelengths in association with oxidative and hydrolytic processes. For most of the fabrics, durability against thermic effects decreases above $80\,^{\circ}$C (Bobeth 1993). In durability tests, long-term UV exposure of 12 samples did not dramatically decrease the UPF (J. Laperre 2000, personal communication).


## Conclusions and Outlook

Defined UV-blocking clothes are not only an important element in the campaign against skin cancer, but also in prevention of photosensitive disorders and photoaging. A lot of work has been done around the world on the test methods for the UPF and factors that affect the UV protection provided by clothing. Because parameters are rarely independent, systematic research to quantify the effect of various manufacturing methods is difficult. The UPF of a garment depends on a number of factors, including fabric construction, type, color, weight, thickness, finishing processes, and presence of additives such as UV-absorbing substances (e.g., titan dioxide, brightening agents). Moreover, the UV protectiveness of a garment during use depends on wash and wear, including stretch and hydration. Thus, the UPF of a textile is influenced by fabric properties and so complex is the interaction of these properties that it is not possible to predict the UPF or to make generalizations concerning, for example, cotton vs polyester, nor is it sufficient to hold a fabric to the light and assess the amount of light seen through the spaces (Gambichler et al. 2001a). Apparel textiles assigned for UV-protective clothing should therefore be measured and labeled in accordance with a standard document (AATCC 1998; CEN 1999; Standards Australia/Standards New Zealand 1996).

Sun-protective clothing needs to be designed with special types of complex weaves which allow the passage of air to promote wearer comfort but block the passage of sunlight. Fabrics may include UV absorbers of various types to increase UV protection. It is of course essential to select substances that have a low potential for irritation and sensitization. Moreover, stringent requirements for the design should be complied with for garments assigned for sun-protective clothing (CEN 1999). In conclusion, UV-protective garments play a significant role in the prevention of skin cancer and photosensitive dermatoses. Consequently, further educational efforts are necessary to change people's sun behavior and raise awareness for the use of adequate sun-protective clothing. Clearly, whether there will be a market for labeled UV-protective clothing strongly depends on acceptance and inquiry by the consumer.

## References


AATCC (1998) Transmittance or blocking of erythemally weighted ultraviolet radiation through fabrics (method 183). American Association of Textile Chemists and Colorists

Altmeyer P, Hoffmann K, Stücker M (eds) (1997) Skin cancer and UV radiation. Springer, Berlin Heidelberg New York

Aubin F, Humbey O, Humbert P, Laurent R, Mougin C (2001) Melanoma: role of ultraviolet radiation: from physiology to pathology. Presse Med 30:546–551

Barankin B, Liu K, Howard J, Guenther L (2001) Effect of a sun protection program targeting elementary school children and their parents. J Cutan Med Surg 5:2–7

Barth J, Kohl V, Hanefeld M (1994) The effect of UV irradiation on lipid levels and other serum parameters and on the circulation. Hautarzt 45:702–707

Bobeth W (ed) (1993) Textile Faserstoffe: Beschaffenheit und Eigenschaften. Springer, Berlin Heidelberg New York

Brash DE, Pontén J (1998) Skin precancer. Cancer Surv 32:69–113

Capjack L, Kerr N, Fedosejevs R, Hatch KL, Markee NL (1994) Protection of humans from ultraviolet radiation through the use of textiles: a review. Fam Consum Sci Res J 23:198–218

CEN (1999) PrEN 13758. Textiles – solar UV protective properties – methods of test for apparel fabrics. European Standardization Committee, Brussels, Belgium

Crews PC, Kachmann S, Beyer AG (1999) Influences on UVR transmission of undyed woven fabrics. Textile Chemist Colorist 31:17–26

Davis S, Capjack L, Kerr N, Fedosejevs R (1997) Clothing as protection from ultraviolet radiation: which fabric is most effective? Int J Dermatol 36:374–379

Dummer R, Osterwalder U (2000) UV transmission of summer clothing in Switzerland and Germany. Dermatology 200:81–82

Eckhardt C, Rohwer H (2000) UV protector for cotton fabrics. Textile Chemist Colorist 32:21–23

Gambichler T, Rotterdam S, Altmeyer P, Hoffmann K (2001a) Protection against ultraviolet radiation by commercial summer clothing: need for standardised testing and labelling. BMC Dermatol 1:6

Gambichler T, Avermaete A, Bader A, Altmeyer P, Hoffmann K (2001b) Ultraviolet protection by summer textiles. Ultraviolet transmission measurements verified by determination of the minimal erythema dose with solar-simulated radiation. Br J Dermatol 144:484–489

Gambichler T, Hatch KL, Avermaete A, Altmeyer P, Hoffmann K (2002) Influence of wetness on the ultraviolet protection factor (UPF) of textiles: in vitro and in vivo measurements. Photodermatol Photoimmunol Photomed 18:29–35

Gardeazabal J, Gonzalez-Perez R, Bilbao I, Alvarez-Hernandez MI, Aguirre A, Diaz-Perez JL (1998) Solar urticaria enhanced through clothing. Photodermatol Photoimmunol Photomed 14:164–166

Gies HP, Roy CR, McLennan A, Diffey BL, Pailthorpe M, Driscoll C, et al (1997) UV protection by clothing: an intercomparison of measurements and methods. Health Phys 73:456–464

Gies P, Roy C, Toomey S, Tomlinson D (1999) Ambient solar UVR, personal exposure and protection. J Epidemiol 9:115–122

Goldsmith LA, Koh HK, Bewerse BA, Reilley B, Wyatt SW, Bergfeld WF, et al (1996) Full proceedings from the national conference to develop a national skin cancer agenda. J Am Acad Dermatol 35:748–756

Hilfiker R, Kaufmann W, Reinert G, Schmidt E (1996) Improving sun protection factors of fabrics by applying UV-absorbers. Textile Res J 66:61–70

Hoffmann K (1998) UV protective clothing in Europe: recommendation of European working party. J Eur Acad Dermatol Venereol 11:198–199

Hoffmann K, Hoffmann A, Hanke D, Böhringer B, Schindling G, Schön U, et al (1998) Sun protected from optimally designed fabrics. Hautarzt 49:10–16

Holick MF, Jung EG (eds) (1999) Biologic effects of light 1998. Proceedings of a symposium, Basel, Switzerland, 1–3 November 1998. Kluwer Academic, Norwell

Jevtic AP (1990) The sun protective effect of clothing, including beachwear. Austr J Dermatol 31:5–7

Kimlin MG, Parisi AV, Meldrum LR (1999) Effect of stretch on the ultraviolet spectral transmission of one type of commonly used clothing. Photodermatol Photoimmunol Photomed 15:171–174

Laperre J, Gambichler T, Driscoll C, Bohringer B, Varieras S, Osterwalder U, Rieker J, Camenzind M, Hoffmann K (2001) Determination of the ultraviolet protection factor of textile materials: measurement precision. Photodermatol Photoimmunol Photomed 17:223–229

Matsuoka LY, Wortsmann J, Dannenberg MJ, Hollis BW, Lu Z, Holick MF (1992) Clothing prevents ultraviolet-B radiation-dependent photosynthesis of vitamin D3. J Clin Endocrinol Metab 75:1099–1103

Menzies SW, Lukins PB, Greenoak GE, Walker PJ, Pailthorpe M, Martin JM, et al (1991) A comparative study of fabric protection against ultraviolet-induced erythema determined by spectrophotometric and human skin measurements. Photodermatol Photoimmunol Photomed 8:157–163

Moehrle M, Garbe C (2000) Solar UV-protective properties of textiles. Dermatology 201:82

Moon R, Pailthorpe M (1995) Effect of stretch and wetting on the UPF of elastane fabrics. Australas Textiles 15:39–42

O'Quinn RP, Wagner RF Jr (1998) Unusual patterns of chronic photodamage through clothing. Cutis 61:269–271

Osterwalder U, Schlenker W, Rohwer H, Martin E, Schuh S (2000) Facts and fiction on UV protection by clothing. Radiat Protection Dosimetry 91:255–260

Pailthorpe M (1994) Textile and sun protection: the current situation. Australas Textiles 14:54–66

Parisi AV, Kimlin MG, Mulheran L, Meldrum LR, Randall C (2000) Field-based measurements of personal erythemal ultraviolet exposure through a common summer garment. Photodermatol Photoimmunol Photomed 16:134–138

Ravishankar J, Diffey BL (1997) Laboratory testing of UV transmission through fabrics may underestimate protection. Photodermatol Photoimmunol Photomed 13:202–203

Robinson JK, Rigel DS, Amonette RA (2000) Summertime sun protection used by adults for their children. J Am Acad Dermatol 42:746–753

Roelandts R (2000) The diagnosis of photosensitivity. Arch Dermatol 136:1152–1157

Sinclair SA, Diffey BL (1997) Sun protection provided by ladies stockings. Br J Dermatol 136:239–241

Soehnge H, Ouhtit A, Ananthaswamy ON (1997) Mechanisms of induction of skin cancer by UV radiation. Front Biosci 2:D538–D551

Srinivasan M, Gatewood BM (2000) Relationship of dye characteristics to UV protection provided by cotton fabric. Textile Chemist Colorist 32:36–43

Standards Australia/Standards New Zealand (1996) AS/NZS 4399. Sun protective clothing – evaluation and classification. Sydney/Wellington

Stanford DG, Georgouras KE, Pailthorpe MT (1995a) The effect of laundering on the sun protection afforded by a summerweight garment. J Eur Acad Dermatol Venereol 5:28–39

Stanford DG, Georgous KE, Pailthorpe MT (1995b) Sun protection afforded by a summer weight garment: effect of wash and wear. Med J Austr 162:422–425

Wang SQ, Kopf AW, Marx J, Bogdan A, Polsky D, Bart RS (2001) Reduction of ultraviolet transmission through cotton T-shirt fabrics with low ultraviolet protection by various laundering methods and dyeing: clinical implications. J Am Acad Dermatol 44:767–774

Zhou Y, Crews PC (1998) Effect of OBAs and repeated launderings on UVR transmission through fabrics. Textile Chemist Colorist 30:19–24

# Sun Protective Clothing:
# 5 Years of Experience in Australia

Colin R. Roy, Peter H. Gies, and Alan McLennan

## Abstract

The Australian/New Zealand Standard AS/NZS 4399 "Sun protective clothing – evaluation and classification" was published in 1996. AS/NZS 4399 has been well accepted and most companies wishing to claim UVR protection for their products have complied with the labeling requirements. This standard is not mandatory, unlike two other Australian standards dealing with solar ultraviolet radiation (UVR) protection, namely the Sunscreen Standard (AS2604) and the Sunglass Standard (AS1067). With these standards there is the ability to impose substantial penalties for non-compliance. In Australia the standard-setting process is achieved by consensus and the development of AS/NZS 4399 was a long and involved process which took a number of years. The standard is not perfect; it was appreciated that issues such as garment lifetime and stretch and wet testing needed to be covered and it was planned to address these in a revised standard. In the 5 years since publication considerable work, in both Australia and overseas, has been carried out. Other national standards have been developed and published. This paper presents some of the rationale which the committee worked through prior to 1996. Also covered are many of the experiences and difficulties in the 5 years since the introduction of AS/NZS 4399, in particular the effect of local conditions and legal requirements on the operation of the standard.

## Introduction

Overexposure to solar ultraviolet radiation (UVR) is a considerable public health problem to, usually, light-skinned populations in countries with high ambient UVR. In Australia, for example, a majority of the population would expect to develop non-melanoma skin cancer during their lifetime. Incidence rates for malignant melanoma are also high compared with most other countries.

Recent Results in Cancer Research, Vol. 160
© Springer-Verlag Berlin Heidelberg 2002

Skin cancer, both non-melanoma and malignant melanoma, is increased in incidence in regions of high ambient solar UVR, is increased for UVR-sensitive individuals and occurs mainly on habitually exposed anatomical sites. However, studies have been unable to consistently show a relationship between incidence and accumulated UVR exposure. Kricker et al. (1995) found that for basal cell carcinoma (BCC) there is an initial rise in risk with increasing exposure, the rise peaking and falling for higher exposures. The effect is more noticeable in those with the ability to tan as a higher exposure would be required before a critical dose is received by the target cells. Earlier studies (Hunter et al. 1990; Vitasa et al. 1990) also postulated a peak in risk at higher doses. The implication of these studies, if correct, is that substantial reductions in exposure may be required before a decreased risk of BCC is achieved.

Protection measures against artificial UVR sources are fairly well developed and in some countries are widely adopted. The area of most concern and activity is with occupational and recreational exposure to solar UVR. The high cost of skin cancer and eye damage to society means that large benefits can result through campaigns that educate and modify the behavior of exposed workers and the public. UVB radiation can also alter the human immune system and the consequences for infectious disease control is still not known. However, the wearing of protective clothing, hats, sunscreens and the avoidance or minimization of sun exposure should also protect against an altered immune response.

The protection provided by clothing against solar UVR has been the subject of considerable interest since the use of clothing as the primary means of personal protection was first advocated in public educational campaigns. Much work was undertaken by the Australian Radiation Laboratory (now ARPANSA) in the late 1980s and early 1990s to develop test methods for evaluating the UVR-protective characteristics of fabrics and clothing. A rating scheme was devised using ultraviolet protection factors (UPFs). Efforts in Australia to promote uniform test and reporting protocols resulted in an agreement to develop and Australian standard.

The Australian/New Zealand Standard AS/NZS 4399 "Sun protective clothing – evaluation and classification" (Standards Australia 1996) was published in 1996. This standard is not mandatory, unlike two other standards dealing with solar UVR protection in Australia, namely the Sunscreen Standard (AS2604) and the Sunglass Standard (AS1067). With these standards there is the ability to impose substantial penalties for non-compliance. Nevertheless AS/NZS 4399 has been well accepted and most companies wishing to claim UVR protection for their products have complied with the labeling requirements.

In Australia the standard-setting process is achieved by consensus and the development of AS/NZS 4399 was a long and involved process which took a number of years. The standard is not perfect; it was appreciated that issues such as garment lifetime and stretch and wet testing needed to be covered and it was planned to address these in a revised standard. In the 5 years since publication considerable work, in both Australia and overseas, has been carried out. Other national standards have been developed and published. This paper discusses some of the difficulties encountered in devising the standard and presents some of the experiences and difficulties in the 5 years since the introduction of AS/NZS 4399, in particular the effect of local conditions and legal requirements on the operation of the standard.

## Test Methods and Results

### UPF and the Rating Scheme

Spectral transmission of the fabric samples are measured across the UVR region (280–400 nm) using a Labsphere UV1000 diode array spectrometer. All measurements are made in accordance with the requirements of AS/NZS 4399 (1996). Weighting of the spectral transmittance with the CIE erythemal response and the solar spectral irradiance allows calculation of a UPF as follows:

$$UPF = \frac{\sum_{290}^{400} E_\lambda \cdot S_\lambda \cdot \Delta_\lambda}{\sum_{290}^{400} E_\lambda \cdot S_\lambda \cdot T_\lambda \cdot \Delta_\lambda}$$

where:
- $E_\lambda$  is the relative erythemal spectral effectiveness (unitless)
- $S_\lambda$  is the solar UVR spectral irradiance (W m$^{-2}$ nm$^{-1}$)
- $T_\lambda$  is the measured spectral transmission of the fabric
- $\Delta_\lambda$  is the bandwidth in nanometers
- $\lambda$  is the wavelength in nanometers

The UPF ratings and the designated protection categories are given in Table 1.

**Table 1.** Summary of the UPF rating scheme for fabrics

| UPF range | UVR protection category | Effective UVR transmission (%) | UPF ratings |
| --- | --- | --- | --- |
| 40–50, 50+ | Excellent protection | 2.5 | 40, 45, 50, 50+ |
| 25–39 | Very good protection | 4.1–2.6 | 25, 30, 35 |
| 15–24 | Good protection | 6.7–4.2 | 15, 20 |

## In Vitro Versus In Vivo Test Methods

Although AS/NZS 4399 requires in vitro testing, there has been some debate over whether in vivo testing is more appropriate. The in vitro test method provides a repeatable and reproducible method of determining protection, but there is some concern that protection could be overestimated in comparison to in vivo ratings. Overestimation could have significant consequences to people who rely on rated sun-protective clothing. However, Ravishankar and Diffey (1997) have shown that many garments actually have higher UPFs when worn compared to laboratory test results, where worst-case conditions with the incident UVR at right angles to the garment are simulated. This worst-case situation would occur during only a small percentage of the time when garments are worn outdoors. Protection provided by fabrics worn in sunlight is on average 50% higher than obtained by conventional laboratory testing using collimated beams.

A set of 16 fabric samples were evaluated using the standard in vitro laboratory test method and an in vivo test using a modified test method from the sunscreen standard AS/NZS 2604 (Gies et al. 2000). The results are given in Table 2. There is no significant difference between the two sets of results. The results provide additional confidence in the chosen test method diminishing the need for expensive in vivo testing.

## International Comparisons

The growing awareness of the need for increased personal protection against solar UVR has meant that more countries are embarking on the evaluation of UVR-protective clothing. The first international comparison (Gies et al. 1997) was conducted between five laboratories in Australia, the UK and the USA. The results were promising with differences of the order of 10–15% in measured UPF. ARPANSA has recently coordinated a second international comparison of test methods and measurements. Ten countries (including

**Table 2.** A comparison of the measured SPFs (in vivo) and UPFs (in vitro) for the fabric samples. Values are means ± SD

| Sample number | SPF | UPF |
| --- | --- | --- |
| 3 | 14.7 ± 0.94 | 13.2 ± 0.6 |
| 5 | 22.7 ± 2.4 | 25.8 ± 2.6 |
| 7 | 42.4 ± 3.9 | 50.0 ± 4.6 |
| 17 | 28.7 ± 3.2 | 31.4 ± 0.6 |
| 18 | 22.2 ± 2.5 | 22.8 ± 0.5 |
| 19 | 10.5 ± 1.1 | 10.3 ± 0.5 |
| 20 | 15.8 ± 1.7 | 16.8 ± 2.5 |
| 22 | 46.4 ± 5.1 | 54.3 ± 6.9 |
| 25 | 39.2 ± 6.7 | 37.8 ± 5.3 |
| 26 | 50+ | 51.2 ± 1.9 |

The front of the tag has the ARPANSA UPF logo and rating plus words on protection from the Australian Cancer Society. The back has further text, the wording of which has changed over the years. However, a number of points are covered including:

- Testing is in accord with AS/NZS4399
- Rating is for the fabric and not the manufactured article
- Rating may change with stretching, wetting and wear
- The UPF rating scheme
- UPF: what it means

The impact of these messages on people's awareness of the need for sun protection is not known. A survey would provide useful information for the future direction of the programme.

## Discussion

A timetable for the revision of the standard has not yet been established. Issues that could not be resolved at the time of drafting the standard remain contentious. In particular these issues include the effects of stretch, wetting, wearing, and chemical additives on UVR-protective characteristics.

### Stretch

The stretching of both knitted and woven fabrics will cause a decrease in UPF. The actual reduction in protection is very dependent on the actual material and generally the reduction will be greater for knitted rather than woven materials. Stretching cannot be included in the standard until a reproducible stretching method can be agreed upon.

### Wetting

The wetting of fabric can result in a large increase in transmission and decrease in UPF – this is especially true for light-colored cotton fabrics. However, for elastane the effect is much smaller, and examples have been found where the UPF actually increases. There is a need for wet testing to be included in the standard, but again a uniform method has not been agreed upon.

### Wearing

The UPF standard test is for new fabric and concern has often been raised that the rating may no longer be valid for a garment after several wash and wear cycles. This issue will be addressed during the revision of the standard but most tests indicate that the protection generally improves with wearing. This is thought to be due to the matting and shrinking of the fabric.

## Chemical Additives

The treatment of fabrics to improve their UVR-protective characteristics has been advocated for a number of years. Early claims were often fraudulent, to the concern of many working in the area. Ciba Chemicals have recently developed an additive for washing detergent. Tests have shown that the protection improves with the number of wash cycles but the product is not yet commercially available.

## Conclusions

Educational programmes now operating in many countries have succeeded in creating an awareness of the dangers of overexposure to UVR. Changes in knowledge and attitudes have been accompanied by behavioral changes indicating that educational programmes are having an effect. Avoidance of the sun is not always possible or desirable. Most clothing provides good solar UVR protection. Clothing, unlike sunscreens, is not dependent on the amount and frequency of application. The rating of clothing provides the customer with confidence about the UVR-protective characteristics of the garment. Swing tags provide additional useful information on further protection strategies. UPF ratings have now been in use for about 10 years and testing standards for more than 5 years. The concept has been very successful. Standards have, and are being, developed in many countries. Hopefully the next generation of standards will successfully address many of the issues that proved to be too difficult in the first standards.

## References


Gies HP, Roy CR, McLennan A, Diffey BL, Pailthorpe M, Driscoll C, Whillock M, McKinlay AF, Grainger K, Clark KI, Sayre RM (1997) UV protection by clothing: an intercomparison of measurements and methods. Health Phys 73:456–464

Gies HP, Roy CR, Holmes G (2000) Ultraviolet radiation protection by clothing: comparison of in vivo and in vitro measurements. Radiat Protect Dosimetry 91:247–250

Hunter DJ, Colditz GA, Stampfer MJ, Rosner B, Willett WC, Speizer FE (1990) Risk factors for basal cell carcinoma in a prospective cohort of women. Ann Epidemiol 1:13–23

Kricker A, Armstrong BK, English DR, Heenan PJ (1995) A dose-response curve for sun exposure and basal cell carcinoma. Int J Cancer 60:482–488

Ravishankar J, Diffey BL (1997) Laboratory testing of UV transmission through fabrics may underestimate protection. Photodermatol Photoimmunol Photomed 13:203–203

Standards Australia (1996) AS/NZS 4399. Sun protective clothing – evaluation and classification. Standards Australia, Sydney
Vitasa BC, Taylor HR, Strickland PT, Rosenthal FS, West S, Abbey H, Ng SK, Munoz B, Emmett EA (1990) Association of nonmelanoma skin cancer and actinic keratosis with cumulative solar ultraviolet exposure in Maryland watermen. Cancer 65:2811–2817

# European Standards for Protective Apparel Against UV Radiation

Jan Laperre and Fred Foubert


## Abstract

The first European standard which describes the test procedure to determine the UV-protection factor of clothing is about to be completed. A second part of the same standard, dealing with labelling and marking aspects, is ready to be submitted to public enquiry. In this effort a group of experts from most EU member states have cooperated with a high degree of consensus. In this chapter we explain this European standard together with the standard developed in the UK.


## Introduction

In Europe, standards are an essential tool to establish free movement of products and services within the European Community. They are developed in various economical and technological fields to support European legislation. CEN, the European Committee for Standardization, is recognized in the European Community for planning, drafting and adoption of European standards in all areas of economic activity with the exception of electrotechnology (CENELEC) and telecommunication (ETSI). When a new European standard is approved, all CEN member states, which include the EU member states, the EFTA members and the Czech Republic, have to adopt this standard as a national standard and have to withdraw conflicting national standards. Therefore, the standardization process is conducted as a consensus process with all parties concerned.

In recent years several national standards for the determination of the degree of ultraviolet (UV) protection of textile materials have been developed. A standard such as AS/NZS 4399 (Standards Australia 1996) has shown the way and has been followed by other national standards such as BS 7914 in the UK (BSI 1998), AATCC method 183 (AATCC 1998) and ASTM D 6544


Recent Results in Cancer Research, Vol. 160
© Springer-Verlag Berlin Heidelberg 2002

(ASTM 2000a) in the USA. Currently, the only standard that transcends the national level is the European draft standard prEN 13758-1 (CEN 2001).

Labelling aspects have also received attention in standardization. Again the AS/NZS 4399 (Standards Australia 1996) has set the pace. The British Standards Institution (BSI) and the American Society for Testing and Materials (ASTM) have issued, respectively, BS 7949 (BSI 1999) and ASTM D 6603 (ASTM 2000b) which address labelling issues. In Europe a draft standard with reference prEN 13758-2 (CEN 2002) has been agreed at expert group level.

In this chapter we discuss the standardization activities in the field of UV-protective clothing in Europe. For historical reasons, we also discuss the standards developed in the UK. However, in the future this standard will become obsolete because the only standards on UV-protective clothing in Europe will be the standards developed by CEN.

## Standardization in Europe

CEN, the European Committee for Standardization, is the major provider of European standards and technical specifications. As has been said before, it is the only organization that is recognized for planning, drafting and adoption of European standards in all areas of economic activity with the exception of electrotechnology (CENELEC) and telecommunication (ETSI). CEN has a special relationship with European legislation in the case of "New Approach" directives. In the "New Approach" option, harmonized European standards, developed by CEN are the tool *par excellence* to prove conformity with the provisions of European legislation as laid down in European Directives. CEN member states have to integrate European standards into their national standardization and have to withdraw national standards which cover the same topic. Together with the use of harmonized standards in support of European legislation, this principle helps to remove technical barriers to trade in Europe.

Within CEN, the technical committee CEN/TC248 "Textiles and Textile Products", is in charge of standardization in the field of textiles, except for items covered by specific "end-use" committees such as CEN/TC162 "Protective Clothing" and CEN/TC205 "Medical Devices" (for e.g. bandages and surgical gowns). This technical committee has set up a working group, CEN/TC248 WG14 "UV Protective Clothing", with the mission to produce standards on the UV-protective properties of textile materials. This working group started its activities in March 1998. A first draft entitled "Textiles – Solar UV Protective Properties – Part 1: Method of Test for Apparel Fabrics" was made available in November 1998. It entered the public enquiry stage as prEN 13758-1 (CEN 2001). Public enquiry or CEN enquiry means a period during which interested parties from all CEN members can comment on the document. In November 2000 a final draft standard was made available for "formal vote". This 2-month period started on 24 March 2001 and forms the last stage in the European standardization process before the prEN can become a fully accepted EN standard.

In March 1999 CEN decided to allocate a new work item to CEN/TC248 WG14. This new work item was the development of a classification and marking system for UV-protective clothing. The group started work during the beginning of 2000 and a first document (committee draft) was available at the end of 2000. This document entitled "Textiles – Solar UV Protective Clothing – Part 2: Classification and Marking of Apparel" with reference prEN 13758-2 (CEN 2002) entered public enquiry in May 2001. It is expected that the comments generated by the CEN members will be discussed at the end of 2001 and that in the course of 2002 EN 13758-2 will be finalized and become available as an EN.

## European Standards on UV-Protective Clothing

The method described in prEN 13758-1 (CEN 2001) to determine UV protection is a spectrophotometric method using equipment with an integrating sphere. It allows the use of a $0°/d$ or a $d/0°$ geometry. The method is intended to be used for apparel fabrics which are worn in close proximity to the skin but not on the skin. The materials are in standardized temperature and humidity conditions. In the case of fluorescent materials, a suitable filter (UG11) of not more than 3 mm thickness should be used. In order to determine the ultraviolet protection factor (UPF) the following calculation is applied:

$$UPF = \frac{\sum_{290}^{400} E(\lambda)\varepsilon(\lambda)\Delta\lambda}{\sum_{290}^{400} E(\lambda)\varepsilon(\lambda)T(\lambda)\Delta\lambda}$$

where:
– $T(\lambda)$ is the spectral transmittance
– $E(\lambda)$ is the solar irradiance measured in Albuquerque
– $\varepsilon(\lambda)$ is the erythema action spectrum of McKinlay and Diffey (1987)
– $\Delta\lambda$  is the wavelength interval

Five different samples are measured from the same material and the average UPF is determined. In the CEN standard the lower confidence limit is reported:

$$UPF - t_{a/2,n-1}\frac{stdev}{\sqrt{n}}$$

In cases in which this value is larger than 50, then UPF > 50 is reported. In addition the average transmission in the UVA and UVB region is calculated.

The European standard also contains information on the precision of the new test method. For this the working group has organized an interlaboratory trial. In this trial the repeatability and reproducibility of the test method was determined (Laperre 2001). It has been shown that the repeatability varies little with the UPF level. The reproducibility, however, indicates that large differences can occur between laboratories for high UPF levels.

This result has been taken into account when drafting part two of the standard. This part addresses the labelling and marking aspects of UV-protective clothing. The working group has chosen not to use classification schemes as used, for example, in Australian and American standards. There were two main reasons for this. First, the interlaboratory results indicated that differences between laboratories, due to differences in instruments, operator, etc, could be very large, without being statistically significantly different. This could result in a different classification and all the related problems that that would entail. Second, it was felt necessary to avoid misleading comparison between different levels of UPF.

Finally, it was decided that the first requirement to call a garment UV-protective is a UPF larger than 30. A second requirement concerns broadband protection. The average transmission in the UVA region should be smaller than 5%. Further there are design requirements. The upper body and/or the lower body should be covered. The upper body is defined as the torso, from the neck to the hip and across the shoulders down as far as three-quarters of the upper arm. The lower body is understood as that part of the body from the waist to the patella. If these conditions are fulfilled then the manufacturer may mark a product with a pictogram and add a leaflet with additional information.

This forthcoming standard (prEN 13758-2) (CEN 2002) is not restricted to children as in the UK, but is applicable to any kind of cohort. The European standard also describes a pictogram which can be attached to the garment such that the user or customer immediately recognizes that the clothing complies with the standard. This pictogram is attached to the garment together with a leaflet explaining the dangers of exposure to solar radiation. In this way it is hoped that the label will not only promote the UV-protective garment but will also increase the awareness of the need for UV protection.

## International Standardization

The International Standards Organization (ISO) is a non-governmental organization in which more than 140 countries participate. As CEN, its intention is to facilitate international exchange of goods and services. In 1991 CEN and ISO decided upon technical cooperation in the development of standards, called the "Vienna Agreement". This cooperation is not limited to matching agendas and work programmes, but goes as far as jointly developing standards when they are relevant to both parties. In November 2000 at the meeting of the technical committee CEN/TC248, ISO asked to use the fast-track procedure to adopt EN 13758-1 also in the ISO system.

## Standardization in the UK

In the UK standardization in the field of UV-protective clothing was initiated in the autumn of 1996 by the BSI. The first standard was published in 1998 and is referred to as BS 7914 "Method of Test for Penetration of Erythemally Weighted Solar Ultraviolet Radiation Through Clothing Fabrics" (BSI 1998). The method described in this document makes use of a photospectrometer equipped with an integrating sphere. From the experimentally determined transmission coefficient $T(\lambda)$, the degree of penetration P is obtained as follows:

$$P = \frac{\sum_{290}^{400} E(\lambda)\varepsilon(\lambda)T(\lambda)\Delta\lambda}{\sum_{290}^{400} E(\lambda)\varepsilon(\lambda)\Delta\lambda}$$

where:
- $T(\lambda)$ is the spectral transmittance
- $E(\lambda)$ is the solar irradiance measured in Melbourne
- $\varepsilon(\lambda)$ is the erythema action spectrum (McKinlay and Diffey 1987)
- $\Delta\lambda$   is the wavelength interval

After finishing this work the BSI working group continued on the labelling aspects of UV-protective apparel for children older than 6 months. The first requirement concerns the design of the clothing. The second requirement sets a maximum UV penetration of 2.5%. Subsequently, BSI published a new British Standard with these specifications as BS 7949 "Children's clothing – Requirements for Protection Against Erythemally Weighted Solar Ultraviolet Radiation" (BSI 1999).

When European standardization comes into force, then BSI will have to replace these two standards by BS EN 13758-1 and BS EN 13758-2.

## Outlook

There are still a number of problems waiting to be discussed. The first series of standards, prEN 13758-1 and prEN 13758-2 (CEN 2001, 2002), are limited to materials tested under standard conditions. There is not yet a European or international standard for wet and/or stretched samples. Also the standard series is limited to materials worn in close proximity to the skin, and is thus not suitable for umbrellas or shade structures which offer protection at a distance. In both cases the relevance of the test method is questionable. Wet materials generally stick to the skin and are thus worn on the skin. It has been shown that in this case in vivo measurements poorly correlate with in vitro measurements (Menzies et al. 1991). Further it has been shown that the minimum erythemal dose (MED) decreases (Gambichler and Schröpl 1998) when the skin is wet and it is questionable whether the action spectrum of wet skin is identical to the action spectrum of dry skin.

For umbrellas and shade structures the albedo is not taken into account and the present standard will overestimate the protection provided by these items. Also, in occupational situations, such as among others welding activities and UV-curing processes, high levels of actinic radiation are emitted. Although encapsulation of UV sources and the use of screens are to be considered as primary safety measures, it cannot be excluded that people working in the vicinity of these sources are exposed to UV radiation. Clothing, as a part of personal protective equipment, can protect the skin in these situations. Hence, there is clearly a need to establish performance criteria for textile materials in order to offer sufficient protection to the wearer against various occupational sources of UV radiation.

## Conclusion

Standardization is an ongoing process. There is a gradual but clear evolution from national to regional (Europe's ENs) and to international (ISO) standards. The use of one single test method to determine a product's properties or the use of the same product specification in a group of countries can contribute to a higher degree of transparency in the market, as it allows better comparison between the alternatives offered. Standardization in the field of UV-protective clothing will contribute to these objectives.

## References


AATCC (1998) Transmittance or blocking of erythemally weighted ultraviolet radiation through fabrics (method 183). American Association of Textile Chemists and Colorists

ASTM (2000a) D6544. Standard practice for preparation of textiles prior to UV transmission testing. American Society for Standards and Testing, West Conshohocken, PA

ASTM (2000b) D6603. Standard guide for labelling of UV-protective textiles. American Society for Standards and Testing, West Conshohocken, PA

BSI (1998) BS 7914. Method of test for penetration of erythemally weighted solar ultraviolet radiation through clothing fabrics. British Standards Institution, London

BSI (1999) BS 7949. Children's clothing – requirements for protection against erythemally weighted solar ultraviolet radiation. British Standards Institution, London

CEN (2001) prEN 13758-1. Textiles – solar UV protective properties – part 1: method of test for apparel fabrics. European Standardization Committee, Brussels

CEN (2002) prEN 13758-2. Textiles – solar UV protective properties – part 2: classification and Marking of apparel. European Standardization Committee, Brussels

Gambichler T, Schröpl F (1998) Changes of minimal erythemal dose after water and salt baths. Photodermatol Photoimmunol Photomed 14:109–111
Laperre J, Gambichler T, Driscoll C, Bohringer B, Varieras S, Osterwalder U, Rieker J, Camenzind M, Hoffmann K (2001) Determination of the ultraviolet protection factor of textile materials: measurement precision. Photodermatol Photoimmunol Photomed 17:223–229
McKinlay AF, Diffey BL (1987) A reference action spectrum for ultraviolet induced erythema in human skin. CIE J 6:17–22
Menzies S, Lukins P, Greenoak G, Walker P, Pailthorpe M, Martin J, David S, Georgouras K (1991) A comparison study of fabric protection against ultraviolet-induced erythema determined by spectrophotometric and human skin measurements. Photodermatol Photoimmunol Photomed 8:157–163
Standards Australia (1996) AS/NZS 4399. Sun protective clothing – evaluation and classification, Standards Australia, Sydney

# American Standards for UV-Protective Textiles

Kathryn L. Hatch

## Abstract

During the last 3 years, three standard documents that pertain to the testing and labeling of UV-protective textile products have been published by the American Society for Testing and Materials (ASTM) and the American Association of Textile Chemists and Colorists (AATCC). The titles of these documents, which are available for purchase at www.astm.org and www.aatcc.org are: ASTM D 6544 "Standard Practice for the Preparation of Textiles Prior to UV Transmission Testing", AATCC 183 "Test Method for Transmittance or Blocking of Erythemally Weighted Ultraviolet Radiation Through Fabrics", and ASTM 6603 "Standard Guide to Labeling of UV-protective Textiles". This chapter summarizes the content of each document and shows how the documents are linked together to make a comprehensive plan for the testing and labeling of UV-protective textile products to be sold in the United States. It also describes the intended future work in the United States on UV-protective textile standards.

## Introduction

The development of standard documents for ultraviolet- or sun-protective clothing began in earnest in the United States with the issuing of "Draft Guidance for the Preparation of a Premarket Notification (510)K) Submission for Sun Protective Clothing". The document bears the dates of 24 September 1993 and 10 August 1994, the latter being the date a revised document was issued. The US Food and Drug Administration (Plastic and Reconstructive Surgery Devices Branch) drafted this document after receiving a request from a garment manufacturer which was seeking permission to make a claim of sun protection on its products. Because the US-FDA is the regulatory agency that regulates the labeling of sunscreen lotions Tend because the clothing manufacturer wanted to have its garments classed as medical devices, this US agency was a logical one to approach to gain the wanted approval.

Recent Results in Cancer Research, Vol. 160
© Springer-Verlag Berlin Heidelberg 2002

The document, which was never finalized, requires (a) that the textile product be fully characterized and (b) that the fabric be laundered and exposed to simulated UV radiation, simulated abrasive action, and other environmental conditions that might alter (increase) UV transmission through a fabric. It states that the protection factor of the fabric is to be determined using in vivo testing and that the capability of the fabric to protect against solar UV be stated as a sun protection factor (SPF) value on the product label. The document does not, however, outline a specific in vivo procedure to be used. The document states that an in vitro procedure is allowed only when in vivo testing would be unduly long (when a fabric has a high SPF value). This draft also calls attention to the need for testing sufficient numbers of specimens so that repeatability of the test method, variability within a bolt, and bolt-to-bolt variability, can be determined.

After a couple of years, administrators at the FDA decided that it would not be involved in formulating standards for the testing of sun- or UV-protective clothing or other textile products. The matter was turned over to the Federal Trade Commission (FTC) and the Consumer Products Safety Commission (CPSC). They, in turn, turned to the American Society of Testing and Materials (ASTM) to seek development of standard documents addressing sun- or UV-protective textiles.

A meeting was held in April 1996 at ASTM headquarters to discuss the formation of a subcommittee within the textiles section (D13) that would focus on the development of UV-protective textile standard documents. The meeting was attended by 15 people: nine representatives of fiber, fabric or apparel manufacturers, one representative of a chemical supplier to the textile industry, one representative from the FTC, two members of the American Academy of Dermatology, and two individuals associated with testing companies. Committee D13.65 called UV "Protective Fabrics and Clothing" was formed and first met in July 1996. This committee has met twice each year. Current membership is about 30.

The American Association of Textile Chemists and Colorists (AATCC) formed Technical Committee RA 106, UV Protective Textiles, in May 1996 with 22 people in attendance. Attendees included academic researchers, textile-chemical, fiber, fabric, and garment manufacturer representatives, dyestuff producer representatives, and instrument company representatives. Current membership is about 20.

The purpose of this chapter is to convey the work of these committees, highlighting the three standard documents they have published and work currently underway. The reader can obtain the documents discussed at www.astm.org and www.aatcc.org. The chapter is organized by discussing the published documents in the order in which they would be used, not the order in which they were completed and published. The combination of all three documents forms a fairly comprehensive plan for the testing and labeling of UV-protective textile products to be sold in the United States today.

## ASTM D 6544

ASTM D6544 "Standard Guide for the Preparation of Textiles Prior to UV Transmission Testing" focuses on how fabric is to be prepared prior to submission to UV transmission testing. It only focuses on the preparation of fabrics that will be used to construct garments (textile products worn next to the skin) or to the preparation of fabric taken from already constructed garments. It does not address the preparation of fabric intended for shade devices such as umbrellas, tents, and baby carrier covers. The ASTM D 13.65 committee adopted the philosophy started at the FDA that any UV protection claim made in the consumer marketplace on textile products should reflect the least amount of UV protection the fabric probably would be capable of providing during 2 years of "average/normal" use. Use conditions thought or known to alter the capability of some fabrics to protect skin from UV radiation included abrasive action, laundering (washing and drying), sun exposure, and chlorinated pool water exposure. Other factors were stretching and wetting of the fabric during wear. Of these use conditions, three were selected to be included in preparation testing. The major criterion that guided the selection was availability of a standard testing procedure. Other factors were magnitude of the exposure on the UV-protection capability of the fabric and cost to conduct the test.

The document directs that apparel fabrics:

(a) Be given 40 home launderings (washing and drying). The conditions of laundering are to be those provided on the care label instructions for the fabric. AATCC TM 135 and 172 provide specific directions for the laundering of apparel fabric with chlorine bleach and with non-chlorine bleach, respectively.

(b) Be exposed to 100 AATCC fading units of simulated sunlight using AATCC test method 16[E].

(c) Be exposed to simulated chlorinated pool water (for swimsuit/wear fabrics only) using AATCC TM 162.

Considerable discussion centered on how closely the preparation testing should simulate what happens during actual product use. For non-swimsuit fabrics this would usually be repeated cycles of exposure to UV radiation while wearing the garment and laundering to refresh the fabric. Such cycling of tests was considered to be prohibitive due to (a) differences in specimen sizes for the exposures, (b) the cost of preparation testing and (c) lack of data to show alternating laundering and UV exposure would lead to different results than laundering 40 times followed by 100 fading units of UV exposure.

Document D6544 also specifies how fabric sampling is to be accomplished. Sampling is an important feature of this document as it is necessary in making a claim to know the lot of fabric or garments to which the claim of UV protection applies.

## AATCC Test Method 183-1988

AATCC Test Method 183 "Transmittance or Blocking of Erythemally Weighted Ultraviolet Radiation Through Fabrics" is intended to be used "to determine the ultraviolet radiation blocked or transmitted by textile fabrics intended to be used for UV protection". Either a spectrophotometer or spectroradiometer equipped with an integrating sphere is needed to measure the irradiance of UV through air and that transmitted through the fabric. Appendix A of the test method provides the specifications for instruments that are suitable for use. In the AATCC test method, specimens are conditioned prior to test ($70 \pm 2\,°F$, $65 \pm 2\%$ RH), three sets of transmission data are collected per specimen (the second and third each after a $45°$ rotation), and scans are made every 2 nm. The specimen spectral transmittance is the average of the three sets of data collected per specimen. Directions are provided for using these data to calculate specimen UPF, specimen UVA transmittance, specimen UVB transmittance, specimen percent blocking, and specimen percent UVA blocking, and specimen percent UVB blocking.

AATCC 183 is similar to the transmittance method written in AZ/NZS 4399:1996, to BS 7914-1988 "Method of Test for Penetration of Erythemally Weighted Solar Ultraviolet Radiation Through Clothing Fabrics", and to CEN/TC248 WG 14-1998 "Apparel Fabrics, Solar UV Protective Properties – Method of Test". All the tests are in vitro (instrumental) and use the same formulas for calculating UPF and UVA transmission and blocking and UVB transmission and blocking. The solar spectral irradiance values used in the formulas differ. These values are either those obtained in Melbourne, Australia, on 17 January at noon, or in Albuquerque, N.M., USA, at noon on 3 July. Other differences among the tests include (a) number of specimens to be tested (two or four), (b) number of sets of data per specimen – whether the specimen is rotated or not (one or three), (c) the scanning interval (1, 2, or 5 nm), (d) whether the specimens are conditioned or not and (e) the type of instruments that can be used for the transmission testing (only instruments that illuminate directionally and collect via a sphere, or instruments that illuminate diffusely and collect directionally). No studies have been conducted using the same set of fabrics to compare UPF values collected following each of the three current transmittance methods.

To be ready to use ASTM D 6603 as a guide to labeling, the specific specimens that need to be submitted for UV transmission testing are the "prepared-for-testing" specimens (as given above), "unprepared (new or unexposed)" specimens, and "laundered-once" specimens when the fabric or garment made from it is labeled "Launder Once Before Using". The latter specimens will usually be knit fabrics that only qualify as being UV-protective following one laundering. During this laundering, the fabric shrinks sufficiently so that its UPF value increases to at least 15. Using AATCC 183, two specimens of each type would have to be submitted for transmission testing.

## ASTM D 6603

ASTM D6603 "Standard Guide for Labeling of UV-Protective Textiles" focuses on the labeling of UV-protective textiles (apparel/garments as well as shade devices). It directs the determination of the label UPF value using the specimen UPF values obtained from following AATCC 183 (see Table 1 for the series of calculations required). It also directs the determination of the label percent blocking (UVA and UVB) using specimen UPF values obtained from using AATCC 183. It gives information about the protection categories to be included on a label and specifies what may and may not be written on a UV-protection label.

The guiding principle used by the ASTM committee D13.65 in writing the labeling standard document was that the information appearing on the label of UV-protective textiles must indicate the least amount of protection that would be provided by the fabric during 2 years of use. First, the label UPF values obtained for the prepared-for-testing specimens would have to be compared to the label UPF values obtained for the unprepared specimens or to the label values obtained for the laundered-once specimens. If the preparation testing increases transmittance of UV through the fabric, then the label value for the prepared-for-testing specimens would appear on the product label. Otherwise, the value on the label would be that of the unprepared specimens or the laundered-once specimens. To obtain the potential label UPF values, the calculation described in steps 1 through 5 in Table 1 must be done. This sequence is identical to that described in AS/NZS standard document, in which it is only necessary to calculate one label UPF as only unprepared specimens are submitted for UV transmission testing.

Further, to ensure that the value on the label reflects the lowest protection to be expected during use of the fabric, it is necessary to compare the potential UPF label value to the UPF values for each specimen (step 6 in Table 1). When the calculated potential label UPF is less than the lowest specimen UPF of the sampling unit, then the lowest specimen UPF value becomes the label UPF.

**Table 1.** Schematic for determining the label UPF and protection wording for a given fabric using a) the prepared-for-testing specimen UPF values for the sampling unit and b) either the unprepared specimen UPF values for the sampling unit or the laundered – once specimen UPF values for the sampling unit

1. Calculate the mean (sample) UPF value
2. Determine the standard error (E) in the mean UPF
3. Calculate sample UPF–E
4. Round the result of step 3 to a multiple of 5 to give a potential label UPF
5. Select the lower sample UPF value as the potential UPF label value
6. Compare the potential UPF values from step 5 with the UPF of each specimen in the sampling unit. If there is a specimen UPF value less than the potential label UPF value from step 5, that specimen value becomes the label value
7. Select the correct protection category[a]

[a] UPF ≥40, excellent protection; UPF 25–39, very good protection; UPF 15–24, good protection

Then, the label UPF is used to determine how the degree of UV protection provided will be described on the product label. When the UPF is at least 15 but not greater than 24, the words to be used are "Good UV Protection", when it is between 25 and 39, the words are "Very Good UV Protection", and when it is 40 or greater, the words are "Excellent UV Protection". These protection categories are identical to those in the Australian/New Zealand standard.

ASTM D 6603 requires that three items of information appear on the consumer product label: the UPF value determined following the procedure outlined above, wording that reveals the amount of protection, and a statement that the product has been labeled following ASTM D 6603. It forbids that the label state or imply that the fabric/product prevents skin cancer, aging of the skin, and similar medical claims. The standard allows other information to be added.

## Forthcoming Documents

The American Association of Textile Chemists and Colorists (AATCC) technical committee RA 106 is undertaking research necessary to write a protocol for wetting of fabrics prior to UV transmission testing. The ASTM D13.65 Committee is beginning work on a standard guide for determining or confirming the UPF and UV-blocking values for apparel; a document that will link the three current American UV-protective textile documents. This committee is also considering a standard document to address the preparation of textiles intended for making textile shade products, as the exposures would be different from those for apparel/garment fabrics.

# Activities of CIE DIV-6
# (Photobiology and Photochemistry)
# in UV Protection and Clothing

Jean-Pierre Césarini

## Abstract

Clothing can provide substantial protection against solar ultraviolet radiation (UVR). A technical committee (TC6-29), formed by experts in the field of UVR and photoprotection, was raised and, after extensive exchanges of information on the various existing test methods, prepared a technical report. The report is circulating within the CIE national committees for approval which is expected before the end of 2001. P. Gies (Australia) was in charge of collecting all information and prepared the final document. In the report, various test methods for measurement of UVR transmittance through fabrics are discussed. The measured transmittances can be used to calculate the erythemally weighted UVR transmitted by the fabric and thus the amount of protection provided. Factors affecting the UVR transmission of fabric, i.e. the characteristics of the radiometer, weave, color, weight, stretch, water, quality (holes) and eventual UV-absorbers are also detailed. In vivo and in vitro tests were found to be in broad agreement, particularly when the test method detailed in the AS/NZS 2604 "Sunscreen products – evaluation and classification", with the fabric substituted for the sunscreen, was used. The report concludes:

*"The UVR transmission of fabrics depends on too many factors to be predicted and must be measured. Particular attention must be paid to sampling to account for variations due to weave and non-uniformity of the product. Accurate and reliable assessment of the protection factors requires spectral measurements of the total (i.e. direct and scattered) UVR transmission. A detection system, which closely matches human skin response, can be used to determine protection factors, but should always be checked against the spectral transmission measurement."*

Recent Results in Cancer Research, Vol. 160
© Springer-Verlag Berlin Heidelberg 2002

## Introduction

Clothing can provide substantial protection against solar ultraviolet radiation (UVR).

A technical committee (TC6-29) of the division 6 of the Commission Internationale de l'Eclairage (CIE) made up of experts in the field of UVR, photoprotection and radiation measurements was formed. Gies (Australia) was in charge of collecting all information and of writing the report final document (CIE 2001). A technical report has been prepared after extensive exchanges of information on the various existing test methods. The technical report is circulating within the CIE national committees for approval, which is expected before the end of 2001. The membership of the technical committee during the preparation of the document is given in Table 1.

## Content of the Report

Several authorities in countries with high levels of solar exposures have proposed various test methods for measurement of UVR transmittance through fabrics. A scheme to quantify the amount of UVR protection of materials, using ultraviolet protection factors (UPFs) was developed and is used in Australia to label many items currently on the market. Factors affecting the UVR transmission of fabric, i.e. characteristics of radiometers, weave, color, weight, stretch, water, quality (holes) and eventual UV-absorbers are taken into consideration.

In vivo and in vitro tests have been found to be in broad agreement, particularly when the test method detailed in the AS/NZS 2604 "Sunscreen products – evaluation and classification", with the fabric substituted for the sunscreen, is used (Standards Australia/Standards New Zealand 1998).

**Table 1.** Members of the CIE TC6-29 "UV-protection and clothing" technical committee

| | |
|---|---|
| Dr. F. Denner | South Africa |
| Prof. D.L. Diffey | United Kingdom |
| Dr. C. Driscoll | United Kingdom |
| Dr. K. Georgouras | Australia |
| Dr. P. Gies | Australia |
| Dr. R. Landry | USA |
| Prof. M. Pailthorpe | Australia |
| Prof. L.R. Ronchi | Italy |
| Dr. R. Sayre | USA |
| Dr. D. Sliney | USA |
| Dr. F. Wilkinson | Australia |
| Dr. C.F. Wong | Australia |

## Summary of Previous Work

Berne and Fischer (1980) examined a small number of garments worn by photosensitive patients in a medical environment. They found a wide range of protection factors using simple radiometric methods. They focused on three wavelengths: 313, 365 and 436 nm. Following this early work, Welsh and Diffey (1981) used a monochromator to irradiate a number of fabrics across the UVB region (290–320 nm). They weighted the transmission measurement by an erythemal effectiveness function in order to calculate protection factors. They found that the tightness of weave was an essential factor in determining the amount of UVR transmitted by a fabric. Robson and Diffey (1990) improved the method by incorporating a PTFE diffuser to determine the UVR spectral transmission of a large range of fabrics and then calculated the protection factors by weighting the transmitted UV with the erythemal action spectrum of the CIE (1987). Roy et al. (1988) evaluated the spectral UVR transmission of different fabric types in relation to personal protection. Jevlic (1990) compared protection factors in vitro and in vivo (testing on volunteers with a solar simulator) and found a significantly reduced photoprotection when the fabric was wet. Gies et al. (1992, 1994) compared the protection offered by fabrics using a number of test methods and suggested the UPF classification. These documents are the basis for the norm adopted in AS/NZS 4399 (Standards Australia/Standards New Zealand 1996).

## Material and Methods

The transmittance of solar UVR through a fabric sample is determined as the ratio of the erythemally weighted solar UVR irradiance measured by a detector with the fabric sample in place to that measured with no fabric present.

An effective UVR dose (ED) for unprotected skin is calculated by convoluting the incidence solar spectral power distribution with the relative spectral effectiveness function (human skin erythema) and summing over the wavelength range 290–400 nm. In order to get the effective dose for the skin when it is protected ($Ed_m$), the calculation is repeated with the spectral transmission of the protection fabric as an additional weighting factor. The PF is then defined as the ratio ED to $Ed_m$.

The results of thousands of tests indicate that clothing fabrics have UPFs from as low as 5 to a maximum well in excess of 100; most summer fabrics have UPFs around 20–50. These fabrics provide a daily protection sufficient to handle the daily total ambient solar UVR in the order of 60 standard erythema doses (SEDs) for a typical cloudless summer day.

In vivo testing results in an SPF, which is the ratio of the time necessary to produce the erythemal endpoint in human volunteers with and without fabric in position. There is generally excellent agreement between the SPF and the UPF. This is particularly true when using a xenon solar simulator filtered to obtain a good match with a mid-summer solar spectral distribution. High UPF or SPF values are at the limits of in vivo testing since above 50, few experiments have been conducted. The spectral measurements of UVR transmission can be performed by spectroradiometers, spectrophotometers or diode array spectrometers. Each technique has its limits and advantages.

## Factors Affecting the Protection Provided by Clothes

A number of factors may affect the protection provided against solar UVR by fabrics:

- Weave: this is the main factor affecting transmission.
- Color of the fibers: darker fabrics have a higher UPF than lighter shades. The dye, the selection and concentration of which determine the color, is the major factor.
- Weight: the weight of the materials varies from 80 to 300 $g/m^2$, and this greatly affects the UPF.
- Stretching: Lycra is a very stretchable material and shows a wide range of variations under significant tension. A UPF of 100 with the fabric unstretched may become 20 when the fabric is stretched.
- Porosity: this factor is dependent on the quality control of the fabric, and transmission values may show variations up to 30%. The variation in a good quality fabric are below 10% while that in a bad quality fabric may be above 30%.
- Nature of the fibers: some fabric fibers transmit UVR. A fabric made with such fibers tightly woven may have a low UPF.
- Humidity, water: when wet, fabrics transmit significantly more UVR and, as a consequence, have a reduced UPF. This change is more important with cotton than with polyester or Lycra.
- UV absorbers: these chemicals can be added during the washing or rinsing of fabrics in order to increase the UV protection.

The committee responsible for the technical report has proposed a standard test method, and the apparatus for testing UVR transmittance, the scale calibration, the sample preparation and conditioning are briefly described. Additional tests to evaluate the stretching conditions and the wet test are provided as well as the calculation of the UPF and the expression of the results.

## In Vivo/In Vitro Comparison of UVR Protection of Fabrics

Some years ago, Menzies et al. (1992) and, more recently, Hoffmann et al. (2000) and Gies et al. (2000) performed a series of experiments to validate the correlation between UPF and SPF. We performed an experiment of the same kind and evaluated the quality of the protection provided by repeated washing with UV-absorbing agent (Tinosorb$^{TM}$) adsorbed on the fibers.

## Introduction

Clothing is considered one of the most important elements in sun protection. Due to the nonuniformity of the fabric structure and variety of weave and dye of a textile, prediction of the UV-protective properties has been proven to be difficult without appropriate evaluation. In most of the previous studies the protectiveness of a textile against UV radiation has been assessed by combining the parameters of the spectral irradiance of global radiation, the erythemal action spectrum and the spectral UV transmission of a textile. The Australian/New Zealand standard (AS/NZS) on the test methods to be used to assess UV-protective properties was formulated with the intention of regulating the test methods (Standards Australia/Standards New Zealand 1996). According to AS/NZS, the determination of the UV-protection factor (UPF) of textiles has become an accepted laboratory-based method using spectrophotometric measurements (in vitro method). The UPF is classified into three categories: UPF 15–24, good protection (UPF rating 15, 20); UPF 25–39, very good protection (UPF rating 25, 30, 35); UPF 40 and more, excellent protection (UPF rating 40, 45, 50, 50+). Other normative documents also recommend spectrophotometric measurements for UPF determination (AATCC 1998; CEN 1999).

However, the validity of the in vitro UPF determined in the laboratory has been a controversial issue with regard to its significance in the field. Several studies have verified the in vitro UPF by comparing it with the in vivo test method on human skin using solar-simulated radiation for the determination of the minimal erythema dose (MED), both with fabric protection and without protection (Césarini et al. 2001; Gambichler et al. 2001, 2002; Gies et al. 2000; Greenoak and Pailthorpe 1996; Hoffmann et al. 2000; Lowe et al. 1995; Menzies et al. 1991). Furthermore, the use of UV dosimeters has been recently suggested to be a practical and valid method for the determination of the UPF (Holman et al. 1983; Moehrle and Garbe 2000; Parisi et al. 2000; Ravishankar and Diffey 1997). In this chapter we briefly review the methods of testing the UV protectiveness of apparel textiles and provide current data on the determination of UPF using biological UV dosimetry.

## In Vitro Test Methods

Direct and diffuse UV transmittance through a fabric is the crucial factor determining the UV protectiveness of a textile (Fig. 1). Simple radiometric broadband UV dosimetry is only suitable for measurements where the relative variation in the UPF is required. By contrast spectroradiometers and spectrophotometers are suitable for the assessment of spectral irradiance. These devices collect both transmitted and scattered radiation with the aid of an integrating sphere positioned behind the textile sample. Although spectrophotometers fitted with a double monochromator have a large dynamic range and high accuracy, regular scans of the UV source, e.g. deuterium or

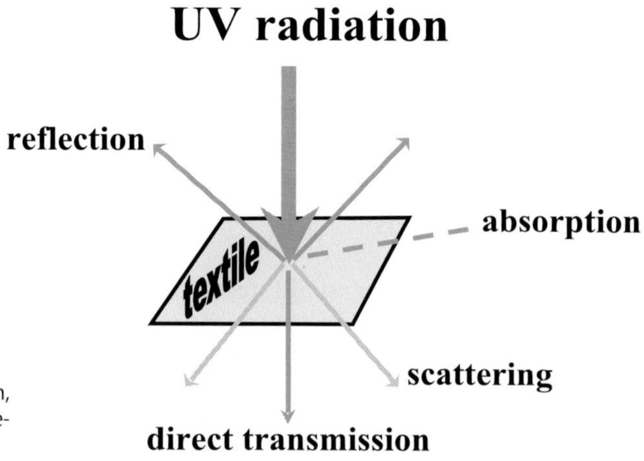

# UV radiation



**Fig. 1.** UV reflection, absorption, and transmission in textile materials

xenon arc lamps, are required to provide reference data (Capjack et al. 1994; Gies et al. 1994, 1997). As suggested by Australian, American, and European standard documents, the spectrophotometer should be fitted with a fluorescence filter, e.g. UG-11 (Schott, Mainz, Germany) to minimize errors caused by fluorescence from whitening agents (AATCC 1998; CEN 1999; Standards Australia/Standards New Zealand 1996).

The spectrophotometric measurements are usually performed in the wavelength range 290–400 nm in 5-nm steps or less. Spectrophotometric measurements of textiles are generally made under "worst-case" conditions, with collimated radiation beams at right angles to the fabric. For UPF determination, at least four textile samples must be taken from a garment – two in the machine direction and two in the cross-machine direction. To determine the in vitro UPF, the spectral irradiance (both source and transmitted spectrum) is weighted against the erythemal action spectrum (Diffey 1998), and the UPF is calculated as follows:

$$UPF = \frac{\int E_\lambda S_\lambda d_\lambda}{\int E_\lambda S_\lambda T_\lambda d_\lambda}$$

where $E_\lambda$ is the relative erythemal spectral effectiveness, $S_\lambda$ is the solar spectral irradiance in watts per meter squared (Melbourne, 37.8 °S, 17 January 1990), $T_\lambda$ is the spectral transmission of the sample, $d_\lambda$ is the bandwidth in nanometers, $\lambda$ is the wavelength in nanometers, and the integrals ($\int$) are calculated over the wavelength range 290–400 nm.

In an analogous manner to the sun-protection factor (SPF) of sunscreens, the UPF is defined as the ratio of the average effective UV radiation irradiance calculated for unprotected skin to the average effective UV radiation irradiance calculated for skin protected by the test fabric (Standards Australia/Standards New Zealand 1996). Intra- and interlaboratory comparative trials have shown that spectrophotometry is a precise test method for the determination of the UPF, in particular for samples with UPFs below 50 (Gies et al. 1994; Hoffmann et al. 2001; Laperre et al. 2001). UPFs greater than 50 are only of theoretical interest as even in Australia the maximum daily UV exposure is less than 40 MEDs.

## In Vivo Test Methods

In an analogous manner to SPF testing, in vivo measurements in human volunteers with the sun as UV source are extremely impracticable for the determination of the UPF. In general, xenon arc solar simulators with collimated radiation beams are used with filters to absorb wavelengths below 290 nm and to reduce visible and infrared radiation. Stanford et al. (1997) and Gies et al. (2000) have reported in vivo test protocols that are not based on previous in vitro testing. In most studies, however, the in vivo method has been conducted by in vivo checking of the UPF values measured in vitro (Gambichler et al. 2001, 2002a; Gies et al. 2000; Greenoak and Pailthorpe 1996; Hoffmann et al. 2000; Lowe et al. 1995; Menzies et. 1991).

Based on the skin phototype, the MED is determined with incremental UVB doses on the upper back of a subject and is read after 24 h. To measure the MED of the protected skin the textile is placed on the skin of the other side of the back (Gambichler et al. 2001). The incremental UVB doses for determination of the MED of unprotected skin are multiplied by the UPF determined in vitro resulting in incremental UVB doses for the MED testing of the protected skin. If the in vitro method is in agreement with the in vivo method, the ratio of the MED of protected skin to the MED of unprotected skin gives the original in vitro UPF. Several studies (Gambichler et al. 2001; Greenoak and Pailthorpe 1996; Hoffmann et al. 2000; Menzies et al. 1991), however, have shown that the UPFs determined using the in vivo method are significantly lower than the UPF values obtained in vitro when the fabric samples were tested "on-skin" (Table 1). In contrast, Césarini et al. (2001)

**Table 1.** Comparison between the in vitro method, the in vivo method, and biological UV dosimetry with DRL biofilms for determination of UPF. The methods were as described by Gambichler et al. (2001) and Gambichler et al. (2002b). The mean fabric weight was 117.4 g/m$^2$ (range 85–180 g/m$^2$). Four measurements for each fabric and method were performed. UPFs are given in mean values

| Fabric type | Weave | In vitro UPF using spectro-photometry | In vivo UPF (on-skin) using solar simulator | Biofilm UPF using solar simulator |
|---|---|---|---|---|
| Viscose | plain | 3.2 | 2.1 | 2.9 |
| Cotton * | single knit | 3.5 | 3.3 | 2.9 |
| Polyester | plain | 3.8 | 1.8 | 3.6 |
| Viscose | plain | 25.2 | 16.7 | 19.8 |
| Polyester | plain | 29.6 | 22.2 | 22.3 |

and Gies et al. (2000) observed no differences between the UPF values obtained by in vitro and in vivo testing.

In vivo testing has also been performed in the "off-skin" mode which corresponds better to a real wearing condition. It was shown that UPF values obtained by the in vivo "off-skin" testing differ insignificantly from UPF values obtained by the in vitro method (Gambichler et al. 2001; Menzies et al. 1991). The inconsistency in the data between these studies is certainly due to different methodology (e.g. different test protocols, UV sources, and textile materials).

## UV Dosimetry

Previously, UV dosimetry has been used to measure erythemal UV exposures beneath and above textile materials. Polysulfone films have been used in in vivo-simulated studies in the form of small portable badges monitoring UV doses on manikins and mobile subjects (Holman et al. 1983; Moehrle and Garbe 2000; Parisi et al. 2000; Ravishankar and Diffey 1997). Ravishankar and Diffey (1997) concluded that the protection provided by textiles worn in sunlight is, on average, 50% higher than obtained by conventional in vitro testing using collimated radiation beams. Thin film polymers such as polysulfone degrade after exposure to UV radiation, especially in the UVB range. The optical absorbance increases in a dose-dependent manner. The polysulfone and CR-39 films show high sensitivities compared to the MED curve between 312 and 330 nm. However, sensitivity is low at wavelengths below 305 nm and above 335 nm. In contrast, the sensitivity curve of biological UV dosimeters such as DLR biofilm (*Bacillus subtilis*) is similar to the action spectrum of UV-induced erythema in human skin. The DLR biofilm is a wavelength- and time-integrating biological UV dosimeter which weights the UV radiation according to its DNA-damaging potential (Quintern et al. 1997). Prior to measurement, UV dosimeters have to be calibrated to the UV source (e.g. sun, solar simulator). The effective UV doses are calculated using the calibration curve. The UPF is then calculated by dividing the UV dose recorded on the textile-unprotected site by the dose received through the textile at the adjacent skin site.

It has been shown that cycling jerseys have comparable UPF values when tested spectrophotometrically according to the AS/NZS or under stationary sun exposure with DLR biofilms (Moehrle and Garbe 2000; Standards Australia/Standards New Zealand 1996). However, in accordance with results reported by Ravishankar and Diffey (1997), the jerseys revealed a much higher UPF when tested under "real" conditions during cycling. We have also conducted a field-based study with biofilms and found that the UPF of a garment worn during outdoor activities is significantly higher than the UPF measured in the laboratory (Gambichler et al. 2002b). By contrast we observed in the laboratory-based part of the study that biological dosimetry performed with solar-simulated radiation produced in three of five fabrics significantly lower UPFs than spectrophotometric measurements (Table 1).

## Conclusions

In vitro tests as well as in vivo testing with solar-simulators are usually performed with collimated UV radiation beams incident orthogonally to the fabric in a worst-case scenario. In practice, clothing is worn outdoors when the wearer is exposed to both direct and diffuse rays of sunlight (Gies et al. 1994; Kimlin et al. 1999). The UPF can be assessed as a function of angle of incidence of the radiation beam by rotating the UV source in an arc around the detector. Ravishankar and Diffey (1997) reported that the UPF increases with angle of incidence from the normal due to the scattering of radiation and enhanced path length through the fabric. They found that at 45° from normal, the UPF may be a factor of three or so higher than when determined at normal incidence.

Thus, laboratory testing with collimated radiation provides "safe" UPFs which are usually lower than UPFs determined in a realistic exposure situation. Therefore, different correlations between in vitro and in vivo tests ("on-skin", "off-skin") of the UPF may be due to complex optical-geometrical properties of textiles and different amounts of direct and diffuse radiation passing through the textile. In comparison with in vivo testing the in vitro method is much more practicable and inexpensive. Thus, the in vitro test method is generally recommended for determination UPF of apparel textiles. Biological UV dosimetry with DLR biofilms is a promising alternative method for UPF testing, first because the action spectrum of the biofilm is very similar to the erythema curve of human skin (Quintern et al. 1997), second because measurements are valid and can be easily performed in real exposure situations with solar UV radiation, and third because this method is relatively inexpensive and practicable.

## References

AATCC (1998) Transmittance or blocking of erythemally weighted ultraviolet radiation through fabrics (method 183). American Association of Textile Chemists and Colorists

Capjack L, Kerr N, Fedosejevs R, Hatch KL, Markee NL (1994) Protection of humans from ultraviolet radiation through the use of textiles: a review. Fam Consum Sci Res J 23:198–218

CEN (1999) PrEN 13758. Textiles – solar UV protective properties – methods of test for apparel fabrics. European Standardization Committee, Brussels

Césarini JP, Osterwalder U, Schlenker W, Rohwer H, Baschong W (2001) In vivo/in vitro comparison of ultraviolet radiation protection of fabrics. The Eighth World Congress on Cancers of the Skin, Zurich, 18–21 July 2001, poster no. 31

Diffey BL (1998) The CIE ultraviolet action spectrum for erythema. In: Mathes R, Sliney D (eds) Measurements of optical radiation hazards. Märkl-Druck, Munich, pp 63–67

Gambichler T, Avermaete A, Bader A, Altmeyer P, Hoffmann K (2001) Ultraviolet protection by summer textiles. Ultraviolet transmission measurements verified by determination of the minimal erythema dose with solar-simulated radiation. Br J Dermatol 144:484–489

Gambichler T, Hatch KL, Avermaete A, Altmeyer P, Hoffmann K (2002a) The influence of wetness on the ultraviolet protection factor (UPF) of textiles: in vitro and in vivo measurements. Photodermatol Photoimmunol Photomed 18:29–35

Gambichler T, Hatch KL, Avermaete A, Bader A, Herde M, Altmeyer P, Hoffmann K (2002b) Ultraviolet protection factor of fabrics: comparison of laboratory and field-based measurements. Photodermatol Photoimmunol Photomed (in press)

Gies HP, Roy CR, Elliott G, Zongli W (1994) Ultraviolet radiation protection factors for clothing. Health Phys 67:131–139

Gies HP, Roy CR, McLennan A, Diffey BL, Pailthorpe M, Driscoll C, et al (1997) UV protection by clothing: an intercomparison of measurements and methods. Health Phys 73:456–464

Gies HP, Roy CR, Holmes G (2000) Ultraviolet radiation protection by clothing: comparison of in vivo and in vitro measurements. Radiat Protect Dosimetry 91:247–250

Greenoak GE, Pailthorpe M (1996) Skin protection by clothing from the damaging effects of sunlight. Australas Textiles 16:61

Hoffmann K, Kaspar K, Gambichler T, Altmeyer P (2000) In vitro and in vivo determination of the UV protection factor for lightweight cotton and viscose summer fabrics: a preliminary study. J Am Acad Dermatol 43:1009–1016

Hoffmann K, Kesners P, Bader A, Avermaete A, Altmeyer P, Gambichler T (2001) Repeatability of in vitro measurements of the ultraviolet protection factor (UPF) by spectrophotometry with automatic sampling. Skin Res Technol 7:223–226

Holman CDJ, Gibson IM, Stephanson M, Armstrong BK (1983) Ultraviolet irradiation of human body sites in relation to occupation and outdoor activity: field studies using personal UVR dosimeters. Clin Exp Dermatol 8:269–277

Kimlin MG, Parisi AV, Meldrum LR (1999) Effect of stretch on the ultraviolet spectral transmission of one type of commonly used clothing. Photodermatol Photoimmunol Photomed 15:171–174

Laperre J, Gambichler T, Driscoll C, Bohringer B, Varieras S, Osterwalder U, Rieker J, Camenzind M, Hoffmann K (2001) Determination of the ultraviolet protection factor of textile materials: measurement precision. Photodermatol Photoimmunol Photomed 17:223–229

Lowe NJ, Bourget TD, Hughes SN, Sayre RM (1995) UV protection offered by clothing: an in vitro and in vivo assessment of clothing fabrics. Skin Cancer 10:89–96

Menzies SW, Lukins PB, Greenoak GE, Walker PJ, Pailthorpe M, Martin JM, et al (1991) A comparative study of fabric protection against ultraviolet-induced erythema determined by spectrophotometric and human skin measurements. Photodermatol Photoimmunol Photomed 8:157–163

Moehrle M, Garbe C (2000) Solar UV-protective properties of textiles. Dermatology 201:82

Parisi AV, Kimlin MG, Mulheran L, Meldrum LR, Randall C (2000) Field-based measurements of personal erythemal ultraviolet exposure through a common summer garment. Photodermatol Photoimmunol Photomed 16:134–138

Quintern LE, Furusawa Y, Fukutsu K, Holtschmidt H (1997) Characterization and application of UV detector spore films: the sensitivity curve of a new detector system provides good similarity to the action spectrum for UV-induced erythema in human skin. J Photochem Photobiol B Biol 37:158–166

Ravishankar J, Diffey BL (1997) Laboratory testing of UV transmission through fabrics may underestimate protection. Photodermatol Photoimmunol Photomed 13:202–203

Standards Australia/Standards New Zealand (1996) AS/NZS 4399. Sun protective clothing – evaluation and classification. Sydney/Wellington

Stanford DG, Georgouras KE, Pailthorpe M (1997) Rating clothing for sun protection: current status in Australia. J Eur Acad Dermatol Venereol 8:12–17

# Improving UV Protection by Clothing – Recent Developments

Uli Osterwalder and Hauke Rohwer

## Abstract

The assessment of UV transmittance of clothing and the determination of the UV protection factor (UPF) are now well established and the influencing factors such as type of fiber, color, and fabric construction are known. Quick and reliable instruments to measure UV transmittance are crucial. Besides expensive scientific laboratory instruments, a low-cost UV meter is now available for this purpose. The questions arise as to what can be done about a given garment and whether there are ways to improve textiles by the consumer. The many opportunities to improve UV protection of clothing along the textile chain of manufacturing are discussed. The latest possibility for improving the UV-protective properties of clothing is now available at the fabric care stage in every household. A UV absorber can be brought into contact with a fabric during the wash or rinse cycle of a laundry operation. The high UV transmittance of 30% of a thin, bleached cotton swatch in the dry state (UPF 3), can be reduced tenfold to about 3% (UPF >30) in ten washes cycles. This is more than the effect achieved by dyestuffs. The detergent should contain about 0.1–0.3% of the special UV absorber. The same effect can be achieved as early as after one wash cycle with a higher concentration provided by a special laundry additive. Yet another form of application is via rinse cycle fabric conditioner. To make these new types of improvement of fabrics visible the Skin Cancer Foundation now provides the possibility for laundry products to qualify for the "Seal of Recommendation".

## Introduction

Wearing clothing ought to be the number one measure in sun protection after avoidance of the sun. Although clothing has always been used for sun protection long before sunscreens came on the market little was known about the degree of effective protection until recently. With fashion trends to-

Recent Results in Cancer Research, Vol. 160
© Springer-Verlag Berlin Heidelberg 2002

wards lighter and brighter summer clothing, it becomes crucial to learn more about UV protection by clothing.

The world's first standard that assesses the UV protection of clothing became official 5 years ago in Australia and New Zealand (Standards Australia/ Standards New Zealand 1996). Since then similar developments have been under way in the United States and Europe. This paper describes how simple techniques for the measurement of UV transmittance are being used to show that not all summer clothing always protect sufficiently. It is now becoming well known what the influencing factors are (Hoffmann et al. 2001). The various techniques to improve the protection by clothing are reviewed. Furthermore, it is shown that making the effect of improved UV protection visible to the consumer, e.g. via labeling, is crucial for the acceptance of such clothing.

## UV Radiation Transmittance Measurement

UV transmittance measurement has become well accepted for assessing the protection of clothing. One instrument that has proved especially useful is the UV-1000F UV transmittance analyzer produced by Labsphere (www.labsphere.com) (Fig. 1). Besides measuring the UV transmittance from 250 to 450 nm, it calculates the UV protection factor (UPF) and the rating according to the Australian standard. With the Labsphere instrument the accuracy decreases with smaller transmittance values. The relative uncertainty becomes more than ±25% at transmission levels below 2%, This corresponds

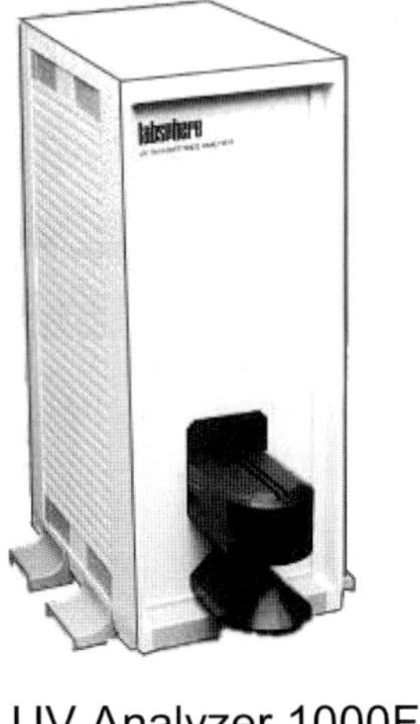


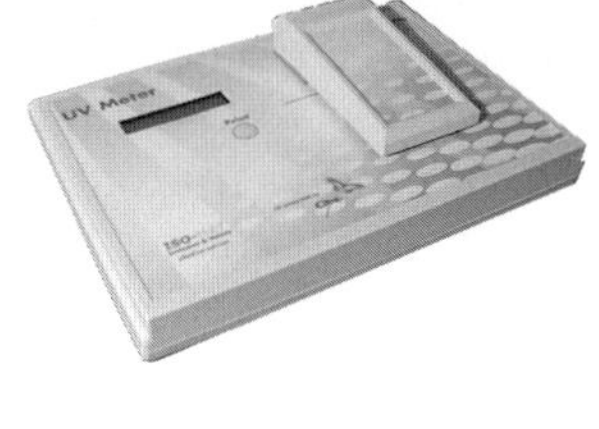


**Fig. 1.** Conventional UVR transmittance analyzer from Labsphere and low-cost UV meter from ISO-MET

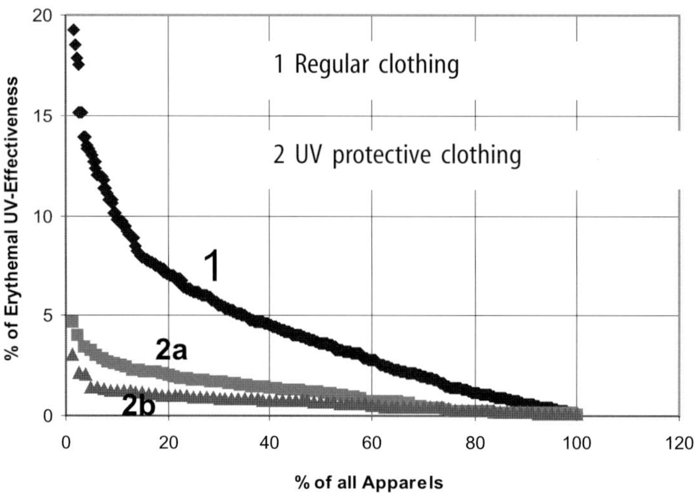


**Fig. 2.** Distribution of UVR transmittance of clothing. Potential for improvement by special treatment

to UPF values greater than 50. A better accuracy is not required at this high level of protection.

The Swiss Cancer League has used the Labsphere instrument over the last few years to demonstrate to the public how much UV radiation (UVR) is transmitted through clothing (Dummer and Osterwalder 2000). The data from such measurements are best represented as a distribution of the weighted UVR penetration, i.e. the inverse of the UPF value (BSI 1998). Figure 2 shows such a distribution together with the distribution of special UV protective garments of the "Fun in the Sun" line of Quelle/Steilmann (Quelle 1997).

About half of normal untreated clothing shows UVR penetration of greater than 3.3%, and hence a UPF below 30. About 25% of normal clothing has a transmittance greater than 7 and hence a UPF value below 15. In contrast to this normal summer clothing, specially treated UV-protective clothing transmits less than 3.3% (Fig. 2, curve 2a; UPF >30). After one season of wearing and washing protection even improves (Fig. 2, curve 2b). The gap between the transmission curves of normal and that of special UV protective-clothing represents the potential for improvement of normal clothing.

There is a general interest among manufacturers, suppliers and traders of UV-protective clothing for a transmittance analyzer. The Labsphere instrument is too expensive for smaller companies. Therefore a low-cost UV meter has been developed by ISO-MET (www.measureuv.com) with the help of Ciba Specialty Chemicals (Fig. 1). This low-cost instrument is equipped with a lamp and detector for UVA measurement and for UVB measurement. The accuracy of this UV meter is 20% for transmittance values above 2%. This generally allows an accurate classification of clothing according to the Australian standard. This low-cost UV meter can also help in the creation of public awareness about the UV transmittance of clothing.

## Influencing Factors

Over the last 5 years knowledge about the UV-protective properties of clothing and the factors influencing them has increased considerably (Osterwalder et al. 2000). This has mainly been due to information campaigns by dermatologists and non-profit organizations such as the Swiss Cancer League or the Skin Cancer Foundation. Rules of thumb are summarized in Table 1.

A frequently asked question concerns the influence of colors. Figure 3 helps answer this question. UVR is the part of the total spectrum of electromagnetic waves adjacent to the visible range. Colors by definition absorb somewhere in this visible range from 400–700 nm. The colors yellow, red and turquoise are shown in the Fig. 3 (W. Schlenker 2001, personal communication). Although our eyes are unable to detect absorption of these molecules in the UV range, we know that dyestuff molecules particularly absorb somewhere in the UV range. Absorption does not stop at wavelengths below 400 nm. Although the UV spectrum of the three colors in Fig. 3 cannot be predicted from the visible spectrum, it becomes clear that combinations of

**Table 1.** Rules of thumb for UV protection via textiles

| Characteristic | Good protection | Poor protection |
| --- | --- | --- |
| Fabric construction | Tightly woven/knitted | Loosely woven/knitted |
| Fabric weight | Heavy | Light |
| Type of fiber | Wool, polyester | Cotton, silk, polyamide, polyacryl |
| Textile color | Dark, bold | White, light, pastels |
| Moisture | Dry | Wet |
| Fit | Loose | Tight |

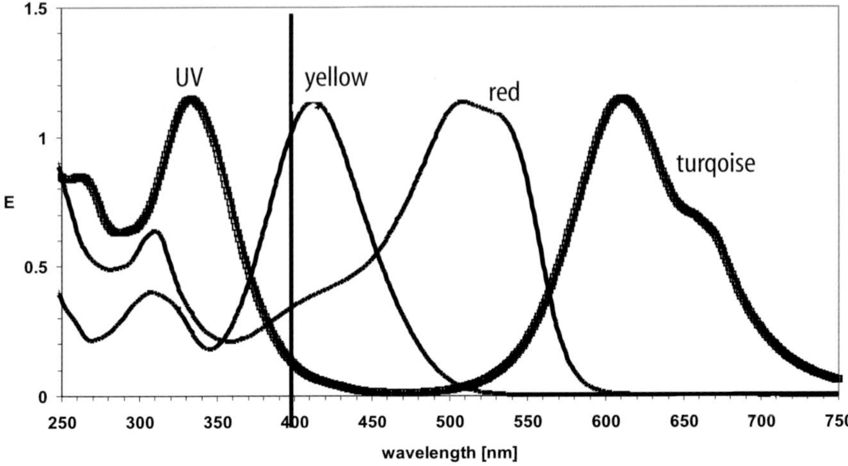


**Fig. 3.** Influence of colors on UV protection

colors, such as "black", are more likely to have a good UV absorption than "pure colors".

## How Can UV Transmittance be Reduced Along the Textile Chain

There are many ways to improve the UV protective properties of fabrics (Jöllenbeck et al. 2000). These may be discussed in terms of the textile chain (Table 2). Starting with the fiber, it is possible to incorporate UV absorbers or pigments such as titanium dioxide into man-made fibers. The construction of the fabric is crucial for its protective properties. The "cover factor" may be too low, i.e. the area of holes too large. If the area of the holes is say 2–5% or more, there is no chance that a fabric can qualify as protective clothing (Hilfiker et al. 1996). In the wet processing step, dyestuff molecules, as discussed above, improve UV protection. In this step, special colorless UV absorbers that are substantive such as textile dyes, can be added.

The last stage in the textile chain is fabric care. Laundering can improve garments by shrinking and pilling. Holes become smaller and the thickness increases. Optical brighteners (fluorescent whitening agents, FWA), present in most main laundry detergents, also contribute to better protection, mainly in the UVA range. FWA molecules transform UVA wavelengths into visible (bluish) wavelengths. The most recent approach to improving the UV-protective properties of fabrics is special UV absorbers that can be added to laundry products (Eckhardt and Osterwalder 1998).

## Application of UV Absorbers During Laundering

The application of UV absorbers during laundering to improve the UV protective property of fabrics is particularly attractive, because it can be carried out individually in every household (Kaskel et al. 2001). The principle of laundry application is similar to that of dyeing in the household washing machine. The only difference being that the "dye" is colorless and integrated into the laundry product.

**Table 2.** Improvement in UV protection along the textile chain

| | | |
|---|---|---|
| Fiber substrate | Fiber | |
| Fiber additives | | |
| Fabric construction | Fabric | |
| Dyes | Wet processing | Textile chain |
| Special UV absorbers | | |
| Shrinking and pilling | Fabric care | |
| Fluorescent whitening agents | | |
| UV absorbers for laundering | | |

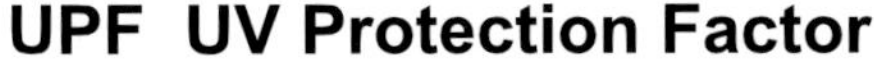

## UPF  UV Protection Factor

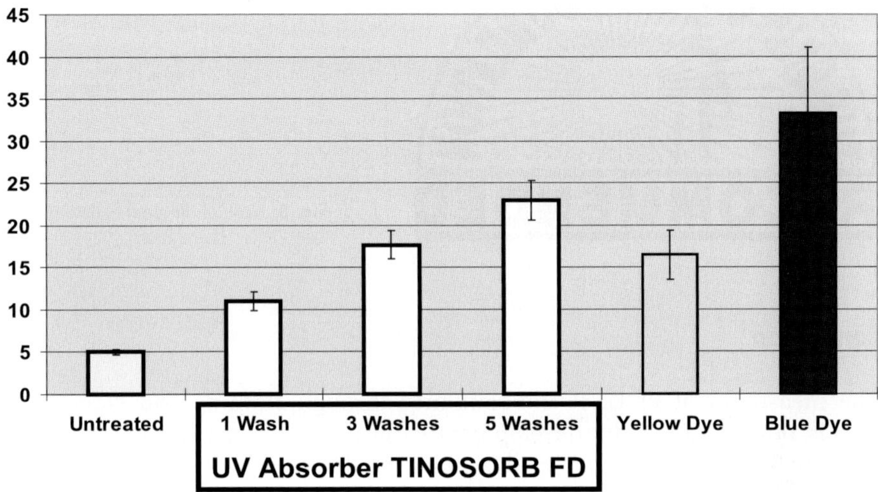


**Fig. 4.** Improvement in UV protection by the use of a UV absorber added to a laundry product in comparison with household textile dyeing

The UV absorber developed by Ciba Specialty Chemicals consists of a backbone that is substantive mainly to cotton fiber and provides some UVA absorption. Attachments to this backbone are responsible for the UVB absorption. Wang et al. (2001) studied this new laundry additive and compared it with household dyeing with a yellow and blue dye. The UV protection factor doubled even after the first wash (Fig. 4). After three washes UPF 15 was exceeded and so was the value provided by the yellow dye.

A UV absorber can be brought into contact with a fabric during the wash or rinse cycle of a laundry operation. The effect that can be achieved is enormous. The high UV transmittance of 30% of a thin, bleached cotton swatch in the dry state (UPF 3) can be reduced tenfold to about 3% (UPF >30) in ten wash cycles. The detergent should contain about 0.1–0.3% of the special UV absorber. The same effect can be achieved with only one wash cycle with a higher concentration provided by a special laundry additive. Yet another method of application is via a rinse cycle fabric conditioner (Rohwer and Kvita 1999). All three application methods have already been commercialized.

Improving UV-protective properties during laundering is a quite revolutionary concept for consumers as well as detergent manufacturers. The fact that the protective effect is invisible is recognized as a difficulty in promoting awareness of the concept, but a label on the laundry product provides a visual means of achieving this. The Skin Cancer Foundation does recognize this new approach to improving UV protection. The Seal of Recommendation (Fig. 5) is given to laundry products that meet a standard protocol. The objective is to achieve UPF 30 after ten washes starting at UPF < 5 on a standard cotton swatch.

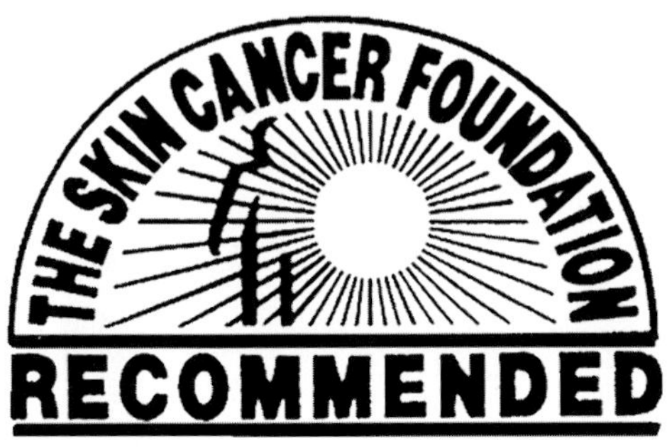

**Fig. 5.** Seal of Recommendation of the Skin Cancer Foundation

## Conclusion

The measurement of UVR transmittance through clothing and standardization is important for the development of protective clothing and also its popularity. Besides laboratory analyzers, a smaller, more cost-effective UV meter is available. The measurement and the knowledge about the factors that influence UVR transmittance is already quite widespread. This helps individuals and organizations engaged in the primary prevention of skin cancer.

There are various methods for improving UV protection by clothing in use today. Besides treatment of the textile during manufacture, there are now also household products available. To promote awareness of this new possibility of improving the UVR transmittance properties of fabrics, the Skin Cancer Foundation provides the opportunity for laundry products to qualify for their "Seal of Recommendation" as sun-protection products.

## References


BSI (1998) BS 7914. Method of test for penetration of erythemally weighted solar ultraviolet radiation through clothing fabrics. British Standards Institution, London

Dummer R, Osterwalder U (2000) UV protection factor of summer clothing in Switzerland and Germany. Dermatology 200:81–82

Eckhardt C, Osterwalder U (1998) Laundering clothes to be sun-protective. Proceedings of the Fourth World Conference on Detergents: Strategies for the 21st Century, Montreux. ISBN 1-893997-01-4

Hilfiker R, Kaufmann W, Reinert G, Schmidt E (1996) Improving sun protection factors of fabrics by applying UV-absorbers. Tex Res J 66:61–70

Hoffmann K, Laperre J, Avermaete A, Altmeyer P, Gambichler T (2001) Defined UV protection by apparel textiles. Arch Dermatol 137:1089–1094

Jollenbeck M, Härri HP, Schlenker W, Osterwalder U (2000) UV protective fabrics, functional finishes and high performance. American Association of Textile Chemists and Colorists Textiles Symposium, Charlotte, 27–28 January 2000

Kaskel P, Rohwer H, Osterwalder U, Peter RU (2001) Sonnenschutz aus der Waschmaschine. MMW Fortschr Med 143:40

Osterwalder U, Schlenker W, Rohwer H, Martin E, Schuh S (2000) Facts and fiction on ultraviolet protection by clothing. Radiat Protect Dosimetry 91:255–260

Quelle (1997) Fun in the sun, Katalog Frühjahr/Sommer 102:1–12

Rohwer H, Kvita P (1999) Sun protection of the skin with a novel UV absorber for rinse cycle application. Jorn Com Esp Deterg 29:115–125
Skin Cancer Foundation (2000) Sun and Skin News 17:1
Standards Australia/Standards New Zealand (1996) AS/MZS 4399. Sun protective clothing – evaluation and classification. Standards Australia/Standards New Zealand, Sydney/Wellington
Wang SQ, Kopf AW, Marx JM, Bogdan A, Polsky D, Bart RS (2001) Reduction of ultraviolet transmission through cotton T-shirt fabrics with low ultraviolet protection by various laundering methods and dyeing: clinical implications. J Am Acad Dermatol 44:767–774

# Dress Up for Sun Protection/Creation of Public Awareness

Pierre Césarini

## Abstract

A clear or white skin was a sign of distinction for millennia. However, white people, during the last century, sought a tan, which was thought a sign of good health and upper social class. Sun-seekers are now better aware of the risks to their health of UV exposure, but their behaviour has not improved significantly at a global level. The only country deviating from this observation is Australia where aggressive prevention campaigns, such as the "Slip, Slop, Slap" and "Sun Smart" campaigns, have been conducted with success over more than 30 years. However, the financial cost of such campaigns is high, and may be considered too high in countries where skin cancers are fortunately less frequent and/or the culture of public health is unfortunately less developed. The global solar UV index (UVI) program is a response to the increasing skin cancer rate in all white populations. Lead by WHO, the UVI program aims to help people to evaluate the maximum intensity of UV radiation on a given day and at a given location. Since the beginning of the 1990s, UVI forecasts have increasingly been broadcast with weather bulletins. In the matter of protection of the skin, the entire scientific community has agreed that avoiding sun exposure during the 3 to 5 h around noon and to be fully clothed should be recommended. However, for a lot of people to protect the skin means only to apply sunscreen, and these individuals need convincing that it is preferable to use clothes. It may be necessary to involve public health actors in the increasing efforts to educate people and persuade them to adapt their protection strategy to their skin type, to the UV intensity and to their daily activities.

A clear or white skin was a sign of distinction for millennia. Only agricultural workers and sailors including slaves whatever their country of origin were tanned. However, this situation was totally reversed over a few decades. When people started to have holidays with pay, tanning became fashionable.

Recent Results in Cancer Research, Vol. 160
© Springer-Verlag Berlin Heidelberg 2002

White people, since the middle of the last century have sought a tan, which is now often considered a sign of good health and upper social class.

However, sun-seekers are becoming more and more aware of the health risks of UV exposure, but their behaviour has not improved significantly at a global level. The only country deviating from this observation is Australia where aggressive prevention campaigns, such as "Slip, Slop, Slap" and "Sun Smart", have been conducted with success over more than 30 years. Australians have modified their behaviour and, as a consequence, the slope of increasing skin cancers is levelling. As a result of the epidemiological finding that one out of every two Australians will develop a skin cancer by the age of 50 years, governmental and non-governmental organizations have spent a lot of money, e.g. Aus.$ 0.14 per person in Victoria, on population information campaigns. This is too much for countries where skin cancers are fortunately less frequent and/or the culture of public health is unfortunately less developed.

The global solar UV index (UVI) program [1] is a response to the increasing skin cancer rate in all white populations. Lead by WHO, [2] the World Meteorological Organization (WMO) and the United Nation Environmental Program (UNEP) in collaboration with international organizations such as the International Commission on Non-Ionising Radiation Protection (ICNIRP) and the International Agency for Research Against Cancer (IARC) and national organizations, the UVI program aims to help people evaluate the maximum intensity of UV radiation on a given day and at a given location.

Since the beginning of the 1990s, UVI forecasts have increasingly been disseminated as part of weather bulletins [3]. Numerous studies conducted in Canada, the USA and France have shown that people are aware of this new meteorological data and understand its meaning. In January 2000 l'IFOP-Gallup conducted a telephone survey of a sample of 1004 individuals representative of the French population aged 15 years or older. The general degree of knowledge and awareness had significantly improved. This was particularly clear concerning the risk of sunburn in children, which was understood by three out of four French people (compared to one-half in 1995) as a risk factor for skin cancer, and the period between 3 and 4 p.m. was considered dangerous by more than one-half the population (compared with only one-third in 1997). Knowledge of the UVI was associated with recognition of, and a more in-depth knowledge of, the dangers of the sun. This improvement in awareness of the dangers of UV exposure are probably a result of the wide dissemination in the broadcast and print news media of messages such as "tomorrow between 12 and 4 p.m. the UV index will reach…"; "…be particularly vigilant with children" and "UV rays are invisible and produce no heat", which often accompany UVI reports. People who have not been reached by the campaign are largely uninformed on this topic.

Some sharp disparities between different sections of the population were observed. The young (less than 35 years old), parents, and therefore young parents (with children under 2 years of age) were clearly the best informed. Knowledge of risk decreased slightly among parents with children older than

2 years. The middle classes, and to a lesser degree the upper classes, were the best informed. The least informed by far were the elderly and the unemployed. Men and women had the same level of awareness.

The main thrusts of the Worldwide UVI program are:

- The weather forecast is of major interest to people and this guarantees a large and regular audience. For example, UVI dissemination in France reaches more than 85% of the population.
- The UVI reports clearly aim to increase awareness of the nature of UV rays and that their intensity varies.
- Dissemination of the UVI is also an opportunity to disseminate advice and recommendations which vary according to UV intensity and skin type.
- Since there is no necessity to buy time or space in the media, the campaign is very cost-efficient.

In the matter of protection of the skin, the entire scientific community has agreed to recommend first avoidance of sun exposure during the 3 to 5 h around the solar noon, second the wearing of a wide-brimmed hat and clothes and last the generous application of sunscreen. However, for a lot of people to protect the skin means only to apply sunscreen. The consumer perceives this as a double advantage: he or she can gain a tan and retain a clear conscience. Convincing people to use preferably clothes as the best protection would be possible either with a change in fashion (which would seem an unrealistic aim) or with the general use of self-tanning lotions. An intermediate path would be for increasingly educated consumers to use protection adapted to their skin type, to the UV intensity and to their activities.

## References


1. ICNIRP, WMO, WHO, UNEP (1995) Global Solar UV-Index, Oberschleissheim, Germany
2. OMS/WHO INTERSUN (1995) Protection against exposure to ultraviolet radiation. WHO/EHG/95.17, Geneva, Switzerland
3. Césarini P (1998) UV index and communicating UV information to the public. In: Mathes R, Sliney D (Eds) Measurements of Optical Radiation Hazards. ICNIRP – CIE 6/98, Munich, Germany – Vienna, Austria, pp 437–442

# Melanoma 3

## Pathogenesis
Epidemiology
Diagnostic
Therapy
Follow-up

# The Precursors of Malignant Melanoma

A. Neil Crowson, Cynthia M. Magro, Ignacio Sanchez-Carpintero, and Martin C. Mihm Jr

## Abstract

The precursors to melanoma are generally considered to be related to nevi of different types. Here we emphasize the dysplastic nevus, the congenital nevus, and lentigo maligna as specific lesions. The dysplastic nevus is discussed not only as a formal precursor but also as a marker of cutaneous melanoma. The clinical and histologic characteristics are outlined, as well as evidence of progression in dysplastic nevi. The congenital nevus is briefly reviewed and emphasis is placed upon clues to malignant degeneration. The concept of lentigo maligna as a precursor as distinct from an in situ phase is detailed.

## Introduction

In recent decades the systematic study of patients with malignant melanoma has revealed the presence in a significant number of patients of precursor lesions which appear to place patients at an increased risk for the development of malignant melanoma. We intend to elucidate recent advances in our understanding of those precursor lesions from the standpoint of the biologic events and the histologic clues which help to predict malignant transformation. These precursor lesions include, but are not restricted to: the dysplastic nevus, lentigo maligna, the congenital nevus, mucosal melanocytoses of conjunctival, nasopharyngeal, penile, vulvar and gastrointestinal tract mucosa, and the atypical Spitz tumor [1]. Only the first three of these lesional categories are considered here.

Recent Results in Cancer Research, Vol. 160
© Springer-Verlag Berlin Heidelberg 2002

## The Dysplastic Melanocytic Nevus and the Dysplastic Nevus Syndrome

In 1978, Lynch et al. [2] coined the term "familial multiple atypical mole melanoma syndrome" for a symptom complex of multiple atypical nevi which placed family members at increased risk for developing melanoma. Clark et al. [3] characterized the dysplastic nevus as a defining element of this syndrome. In 1992 the National Institutes of Health (NIH) Consensus Conference recommended supplanting the term dysplastic nevus with the appellation "nevus with architectural disorder and cytologic atypia" [4]. We use the original term "dysplastic nevus" with which clinicians are familiar, as subgroups of congenital and acquired nevi (such as those in acral and genital sites) manifest architectural disorder and cytologic atypia but have no association with subsequent malignant melanoma. The confusing NIH terminology, which also does not encompass grading that we believe is integral to assessment of any dysplastic nevus, has largely been abandoned.

The incidence of dysplastic nevi is likely in the 5–10% range in Caucasians [5]. The concern raised by the dysplastic nevus relates to the inherent risk of transformation to malignant melanoma and to its being a marker for the development of melanoma at other sites. Melanoma patients with two or more dysplastic nevi may also be at increased risk for a second primary. The risk of progression of a dysplastic nevus to melanoma is unknown. Up to 92% of melanomas occurring in patients with dysplastic nevus syndrome have evidence of a dysplastic nevus precursor, while dysplastic nevi are precursors for up to 18% of all nonfamilial melanomas [6]. Roughly 95% of malignant melanomas arising in dysplastic nevi are of superficial spreading type.

Patients with two or more dysplastic nevi greater than 8 mm in size are said to suffer from the dysplastic nevus syndrome, which may occur sporadically or in a familial complex with an autosomal dominant pattern of inheritance, the latter most commonly encoded by a gene found on chromosome 9 at 9p21 [7]. Dysplastic nevus patients with a family history of dysplastic nevi and melanoma are held to have a cumulative lifetime risk for the development of melanoma of 100% [8]. The features of sporadic dysplastic nevus syndrome may resemble those of familial dysplastic nevus syndrome by virtue of numerous large, atypical nevi that may appear at puberty and continue to appear throughout life. Such patients appear either to have expressed a spontaneous genetic event or to have family members with the syndrome who were never identified. Most patients with sporadic dysplastic nevus syndrome present in the fourth to fifth decades of life with only a few atypical moles on sun-exposed areas; UV radiation may play a role in the development of sporadic dysplastic nevi.

Mutations and loss of heterozygosity of p16 and p53 genes have been detected in blood lymphocytes from members of kindreds with hereditary cutaneous malignant melanoma, most of the mutations being of the $C \rightarrow T$ transitional type known to be a signature for UV light-induced point mutation. One study has shown areas of chromosomal loss at regions encoding for p16 (9p21–22) and p53 (17p13) in 78% of dysplastic nevi, with no loss of heterozygosity in benign intradermal nevi [9]. Loss of heterozygosity at 9p21 appears to be restricted to melanoma and to dysplastic, as opposed to banal nevi [10]. The *CDKN2A* gene responsible for melanoma susceptibility in most families with melanoma linked to 9p encodes a cyclin-dependent kinase inhibitor, the dysfunction of which is also implicated in several sporadic cancers. The second most frequent cancer in such kindreds linked to *CDKN2A* gene mutations is pancreatic carcinoma, which occurs in up to 17% of patients [11].

## Clinical Features

Patients with familial dysplastic nevi develop multiple large atypical moles distributed everywhere on the body surface including the scalp, doubly covered areas (breasts of women and the bathing trunk area of men and women), and lower legs. Banal acquired nevi usually spare the scalp, the doubly covered areas, and the legs. Dysplastic nevi have characteristic features: unlike common acquired nevi, they are more than 6 mm in diameter, have irregular borders and a variegated pattern of pigmentation with shades of tan, dark-brown, and black and even, rarely, hypopigmented macules. The great heterogeneity among lesions in a given patient contrasts with the less-numerous and more-homogeneous common acquired nevi, the latter having smooth borders, uniform pigmentation, and a diameter less than 6 mm. The presence of erythema often correlates with a brisk inflammatory host response, sometimes associated with the clinical halo phenomenon. Although this pattern of inflammation may herald progression to malignant melanoma, it is also seen as part of the host response to a dysplastic nevus. When regression occurs, a lesion may acquire zones of depigmentation.

Although dysplastic nevi may be flat or slightly raised, in our experience, most have a pebbled surface best appreciated with oblique or side illumination. Nevi only a few millimeters in diameter removed from patients with familial dysplastic nevus syndrome may manifest the classic dysplastic nevus histology. Patients with multiple primary melanomas with or without familial dysplastic nevus syndrome may show a diffuse pattern of irregular pigmentation resembling freckling, but with a histology comprising intraepidermal lentiginous melanocytic dysplasia.

Epiluminescence microscopy of dysplastic nevi reveals a pattern of patchy interruptions in the pigment network (the "broken network"), which is distinctive from common banal nevi and melanoma. We have established that the use of near-infrared spectroscopy to probe molecular vibration of chemical bonds and so to assay tissue biochemistry nondestructively can be applied in vivo to distinguish dysplastic nevi from banal nevi and from lentigines with a high degree of accuracy [12]. There is no doubt that dysplastic nevi differ from banal nevi from all of clinical, histologic, biochemical and molecular standpoints.

## Histology

The histology of the dysplastic nevus is so reproducible that a diagnosis can usually be rendered on scanning magnification. Interobserver variability lies in the area of grading of atypia, which should not be done at scanning magnification as it requires assessment of cytology which can only be assessed at 400× or higher magnification. The constellation of histologic findings in the dysplastic nevus encompasses two broad components: architecture and cytology [13].

## Major Criteria for Diagnosis of a Dysplastic Nevus

1. Asymmetric basilar proliferation of nevomelanocytes along the dermoepidermal junction extending laterally beyond the confines of a preexisting dermal component if present.
2. Cells have one or both of two characteristic cytologic and architectural intraepidermal patterns:
   a) Lentiginous dysplasia: randomly disposed single cells are located along and between elongate rete ridges with nests of varying sizes; nuclei are hyperchromatic, angulated and are similar in size to or larger than adjacent keratinocytes.
   b) Epithelioid dysplasia: epithelioid melanocytes are disposed in variably sized junctional nests as well as in a single-cell array along the dermoepidermal junction of an often normal or hyperplastic epidermis. The cells have round to oval nuclei with delicate chromatin, nucleoli, thick membranes, and diameters greater than those of adjacent keratinocytes. Rounded cytoplasmic contours encompass cytosols ranging from amelanotic to coarsely melanized with giant melanosomes.

## Minor Criteria for Diagnosis of a Dysplastic Nevus

1. Papillary dermal collagen shows concentric eosinophilic fibrosis in which a dense zone of hypocellular collagen envelops rete ridges and/or lamellar fibroplasia in which delicate layers of collagen are interspersed with presumptive neural crest-derived facultative fibroblasts laying collagen along the tips of hyperplastic retia in parallel arrays.
2. Lymphocytic infiltrates in the papillary dermis.
3. Telangiectasia and/or vascular proliferation.
4. Fusion of retia by confluent growth between adjacent melanocytic nests.

A diagnosis of dysplastic nevus is made when both major and at least two minor criteria are met. If a lesion exhibits cytologic without architectural atypia, or if all architectural features are present without cytologic atypia, the diagnosis rendered is junctional or compound nevus and a note is appended to the report to state that, in the absence of an adequate constellation of criteria, a diagnosis of dysplastic nevus cannot be rendered. Such lesions need not be reexcised.

Histologic features of dysplasia may be seen in other subtypes of nevi including congenital nevi, Spitz nevi, and neurotized nevi [14]. A variant of dysplastic nevus characterized by an exclusively lentiginous proliferation of atypical nevomelanocytes in concert with periretal stromal fibrosis is termed "de novo melanocytic dysplasia". A similar form of "lentiginous" dysplasia characterizes lentigo maligna and atypical mucosal melanocytic hyperplasias but, unlike these forms of preinvasive melanocytic proliferations, there is no upward migration of melanocytes or conspicuous nest formation in de novo dysplasia. Further, there is no retiform effacement, the retia appearing elongated with an irregular shape and fusion. There is increased vascularity, a sparse lymphocytic infiltrate and scattered dermal melanophages. Broad laminated superficial dermal fibroplasia as seen in the classic dysplastic nevus and lichenoid inflammation are absent.

We grade atypia as mild, moderate and severe for all forms of melanocytic dysplasia. Studies have shown that criteria can be learned and reproducibly applied by pathologists with a consistency that is maintained in both the three-tier grading system which we employ, namely mild, moderate and severe, or a two-tier system, namely low- and high-grade dysplasia [4, 13, 15]. Some observers have found reasonable concordance in grading of architectural, but not cytologic, features implying that the interpretation of cytology is more challenging [16]. We grade atypia on the basis of both architecture and cytology, which are assessed separately, although architectural and cytologic grades of atypia tend to correlate. A recent study has found a significant correlation, but by no means perfect concordance, between the degree of architectural and nuclear atypia [4]. For a comprehensive treatment of our grading criteria we refer the reader elsewhere [1].

## Management

At the first patient visit, we recommend that a clinically atypical nevus be excised to confirm the impression of dysplastic nevus. Any changing or suspicious lesion should be removed. It is our practice that excisional biopsy with a margin of a few millimeters is appropriate. If a partial biopsy has been performed, we advise removal of any clinically apparent residuum with a margin of a few millimeters. If slight atypia is present at a histologic margin without a clinically evident residuum, we do not advise reexcision. If moderate atypia is present at a margin, we advise conservative reexcision with a margin of a few millimeters. If severe dysplasia is present at a margin, or if a margin is only clear by a millimeter or two, we advise reexcision to obtain a 5-mm margin of normal skin. Follow-up of any patient is dependent on the number of lesions and the degree of clinical or histologic atypia. Photographic documentation is desirable.

# Lentigo Maligna

## Clinical Features

Lentigo maligna (LM) occurs on sun-exposed skin of Caucasians and predominantly affects the face, the head and neck and, less often, other sun-exposed areas of the body [17]. Extrafacial lentigo maligna melanoma (LMM) constitutes 18% of all cases and preferentially involves the trunk in men and lower legs in women, and presents at a thinner depth relative to LMM of the head and neck. LM has been designated a form of malignant melanoma in situ, although distinction between LM as a melanoma precursor and an in situ form of the disease has been proposed [18]. The term "lentigo maligna melanoma" is used when the tumor assumes invasive properties. The lifetime risk for developing LMM in a lesion of LM is estimated to be 5% [19]. Long-term exposure to UV irradiation is the greatest risk factor, and, in fact, the diagnosis of LM or LMM is not made if the lesion occurs on sun-protected skin or in the absence of solar elastosis. Other risk factors include rearrangement of chromosome 10 at the 10q24–26 region [20], use of estrogen, progesterone, and hair dyes [1]. Of all melanomas, 4–15% are LMM, and of all head and neck melanomas, 10–26% are LMM [1, 21].

The LM presents as a pigmented macule with a variegated tan to brown color and irregular borders. The initial presentation may be in the fourth decade of life or, rarely, earlier. There is a slight female predominance. From its initial small size it gradually evolves, sometimes to a size of 15–20 cm. One aspect of its evolution is partial regression evidenced by areas of light gray or blue-gray discoloration. The in situ lesion is nonpalpable, with areas of invasion evidenced by palpable nodularity. The fully evolved lesion is strikingly variegated, exhibiting colors of tan, brown, dark brown, and sometimes black admixed with gray or blue-black. As the lesion progresses, it may extend into the conjunctiva, oral mucosa, or external auditory canal. The characteristic evolution of this lesion takes anywhere from 10 to 50 years before invasion supervenes, at which time the average size is 6.0 cm. Controlled for level of invasion and thickness, there is no difference in survival in comparison with other subtypes of melanoma [21].

## Histology

The histology of LM is one of polygonal melanocytes with hyperchromatic, angulated nuclei dispersed as individual units, initially confined to the basal layer of the epidermis in a discontiguous fashion and extending along the eccrine ducts and the outer root sheath epithelium of hair follicles. Also characteristic is the multinucleated giant melanocyte set along the basal layer of the epidermis; termed "star-burst giant cells", these may contain more than 30 fully malignant nuclei and have been identified in up to 85% of cases [22]. Sun-damaged skin of the head and neck of the elderly may show multinucleation of melanocytes as a sequel of photoactivation, in which case nuclei of the multinucleated giant cells show only mild hyperchromasia with regular nuclear contours. The epidermis in LM is characteristically atrophic, manifesting thinning and loss of the retiform pattern overlying elastotic dermal collagen; telangiectasia and melanophages complete the picture [18]. As the lesion progresses, continuity of single-cell basilar melanocytic proliferation is observed, followed by variably sized dyshesive junctional theques along the dermoepidermal junction which assume a parallel disposition to the long axis of the epidermis and are referred to as "the swallow's nest sign". Foci of prominent pagetoid infiltration attend lesional progression. Nesting, confluence of melanocytes along the basal layer and pagetoid spread of neoplastic melanocytes, which we designate as melanoma in situ [18], are the harbingers of the next phase of lesional evolution, namely, dermal invasion.

Transition to microinvasive melanoma is accompanied by a lichenoid infiltrate with admixed melanophages in a sclerotic papillary dermis, findings which warrant careful scrutiny for singly disposed neoplastic melanocytes with a cytomorphology identical to those within the epidermis. These are typically epithelioid with abundant, variably pigmented cytoplasms. Their distinction from activated melanophages may be difficult. Under such circumstances we employ an HMB-45 or Melan-A preparation, preferably with a red as opposed to a brown chromagen. An S100 preparation is less desirable as many antigen-presenting dendritic cells stain positively in the dermis. Histologic features that define the progression of LMM to vertical growth phase include the formation of a nodule or fascicle within the dermis that exceeds the size of any theque within the epidermis. The cells in vertical growth phase melanoma often assume a spindled morphology with a variable stromal response. At times prominent desmoplasia may be observed, warranting the designation of desmoplastic melanoma; neurotropism is a frequent concomitant.

Assessment of level and depth of invasion in LMM can be difficult, as the dermis is usually thin and contains sparse collagen with abundant elastotic material complicating the distinction of papillary from reticular dermis. Invasion of the adventitial dermis of a follicle situated in the reticular dermis may be misinterpreted as level IV melanoma if the follicular epithelium is not apparent in the sections examined. The maximum depth should not be based on adventitial dermal involvement unless that is the only invasion discernible; then, the measurement should be to the point of infiltration of the adventitial dermis from the innermost layer of the outer root sheath epithelium.

Problematic is deciding whether a low-density proliferation of singly disposed atypical melanocytes in sun-damaged skin represents LM or photoactivation. Critical in this determination are the clinical circumstances. When in doubt, additional biopsies or complete removal of the lesion may be necessary. Novel application of topical biologic response modifiers such as Imiquimod may make this distinction less crucial in the near future.

## Congenital Nevi and the Risk of Malignant Transformation

Congenital nevi are identified in approximately 1% of newborn infants. This definition encompasses a broad category of lesions whose size varies from a few millimeters to many centimeters, sometimes extending over much or all of the body surface. The congenital nevus undergoes an evolutionary change with age. Some affect subcutaneous structures such as muscle, bone, lymph nodes and, in rare scalp lesions, the brain. Giant congenital nevi have been variously described as those covering a large area of the body, those resembling a garment covering a limb or the trunk, or those greater than 20 cm in diameter. Lesions located in the region of the head and neck may be associated with melanocytic proliferations of the meninges with rare extension into the cisterna magni causing secondary hydrocephalus. This phenomenon, termed neurocutaneous melanocytosis, may be associated with intracranial melanoma.

In one prospective series of 160 patients with large congenital nevi, all three patients who developed melanomas did so at extracutaneous sites: two in the central nervous system and one in the retroperitoneum [23]. The 5-year cumulative risk for developing melanoma was 2.3% and the relative risk was 101 [23]. The giant congenital nevus has a bimodal peak of incidence of melanoma, the first occurring in the first 5 years of life and the second occurring from puberty into adulthood. Small congenital nevi, on the other hand, are not reported to undergo malignant transformation during the first two decades of life, but the risk of malignancy appears during late adolescence, and the incidence then progressively rises in adult life. Epidemiologic studies impute an incidence of malignant transformation in small congenital nevi of approximately 1% and in giant congenital nevi of roughly 4–7%. Small- and intermediate-sized congenital nevi do not require excision, at least for the first two decades of life, because there appears to be no significant risk of developing malignant melanoma during this period. Congenital nevi covering 4% or less of the body surface may not be associated with a significant risk for malignant transformation [24].

The morphology of the congenital nevus changes with age, irrespective of the nevus size. There is darkening within the first 5–6 years of life and then again at puberty. The lesion is flat at birth and becomes progressively more palpable with age, gradually acquiring terminal hairs. As the patient ages, these lesions usually develop areas of hyperkeratosis, "doughy" alterations associated with mucinous degeneration, and the formation of neurofibromata. The appearance of firm nodules in congenital nevi is always of concern and any nodular proliferation should be excised for histologic evaluation to exclude malignant transformation. One diagnostic consideration in this setting is the development of proliferative nodules. Up to 5 mm in diameter with smooth or sometimes ulcerated surfaces, these are held to reflect self-limited, slowly growing and often spontaneously regressing proliferations [25].

## Treatment

We believe that no lesion should be prophylactically removed in its entirety. Each patient is carefully followed and evaluated with gross inspection and palpation for subcutaneous nodules, changes in lesional consistency, surface topography or coloration. Should any such change occur, an excision of this area with a margin of the nevus is recommended. We recommend complete excision or partial extensive excision of a giant congenital nevus in a patient in whom biopsy shows foci worrisome for evolution into melanoma or consistent with overt melanoma. Nevi up to 5 cm in size can be excised in a one-stage procedure, but larger lesions may mandate the use of a tissue expander, sometimes with staged therapy using full- or intermediate-thickness grafts following superficial partial removal of the nevus, with the proviso that no histologic evidence of atypia is identified.

## References


1. Crowson AN, Magro CM, Mihm MC Jr (2001) The melanocytic proliferations: a comprehensive textbook of pigmented lesions. Wiley-Liss, New York, pp 209–223, 225–280, 282–447, 162–175
2. Lynch HT, Frichot B, Lynch JF (1978) Familial atypical multi-mole melanoma syndrome. J Med Genet 15:352–356
3. Clark WH, Reimer RR, Greene M, Ainsworth AM, Mastrangelo MJ (1978) Origin of familial malignant melanomas from heritable melanocytic lesions. "The B-K mole syndrome". Arch Dermatol 114:732–738
4. Shea CR, Vollmer RT, Prieto VG (1999) Correlating architectural disorder and cytologic atypia in Clark (dysplastic) melanocytic nevi. Hum Pathol 30:500–505
5. Nordlund JJ, Kirkwood J, Forget BM, et al (1985) Demographic study of clinically atypical (dysplastic) nevi in patients with melanoma and comparison subjects. Cancer Res 45:1855–1861
6. Grob JJ, Andrac L, Romano MH, et al (1988) Dysplastic naevus in non-familial melanoma. A clinicopathological study of 101 cases. Br J Dermatol 118:745–752
7. Cannon-Albright LA, Meyer LJ, Lewis CM, et al (1994) Penetrance and expressivity of the chromosome 9p melanoma susceptibility locus (MLM). Cancer Res 54:6041–6044
8. Greene MH, Clark WH, Tucker MA, Kraemer KH, Elder DE, Fraser MC (1985) High risk of malignant melanoma in melanoma-prone families with dysplastic nevi. Ann Intern Med 102:458–465
9. Park WS, Vortmeyer AO, Pack S, et al (1998) Allelic deletion at chromosome 9p21(p16) and 17p13(p53) in microdissected sporadic dysplastic nevus. Hum Pathol 29:127–130
10. Birindelli S, Tragni G, Bartoli C, et al (2000) Detection of microsatellite alterations in the spectrum of melanocytic nevi in patients with or without individual or family history of melanoma. Int J Cancer 86:255–261
11. Vasen HF, Gruis NA, Frants RR, van der Velden PA, Hille ET, Bergman W (2000) Risk of developing pancreatic cancer in families associated with a specific 19 bp deletion of p16 (p16-Leiden). Int J Cancer 87:809–811
12. McIntosh LM, Summers R, Jackson M, et al (2001) Towards non-invasive screening of skin lesions by near-infrared spectroscopy. J Invest Dermatol 116:175–181
13. Clemente C, Cochran AJ, Elder DE, et al (1991) Histopathologic diagnosis of dysplastic nevi: concordance among pathologists convened by the World Health Organization Melanoma Programme. Hum Pathol 22:313–319

14. Toussaint S, Kamino H (1999) Dysplastic changes in different types of melanocytic nevi. A unifying concept. J Cutan Pathol 26:84–90
15. Murphy G, Mihm MC Jr (1999) Recognition and evaluation of cytological dysplasia in acquired melanocytic nevi. Hum Pathol 30:506–512
16. Hastrup N, Clemmensen OJ, Spaun E, Sondergaard K (1994) Dysplastic naevus: histopathologic criteria and their inter-observer reproducibility. Histopathology 24:503–509
17. Clark WH, Mihm MC (1969) Lentigo maligna and lentigo maligna melanoma. Am J Pathol 55:39–54
18. Tannous ZS, Lerner LH, Duncan LM, Mihm MC Jr, Flotte TJ (2000) Progression to invasive melanoma from malignant melanoma in situ, lentigo maligna type. Hum Pathol 31:705–708
19. Weinstock MA, Sober AJ (1987) The risk of progression of lentigo maligna to lentigo maligna melanoma. Br J Dermatol 116:303–310
20. Grammatico P, Modesti A, Steindl K, et al (1992) Lentigo maligna: cytogenetic, ultrastructural, and phenotypic characterization of a primary cell culture. Cancer Genet Cytogenet 60:141–146
21. Koh HK, Michalik E, Sober AJ, et al (1984) Lentigo maligna melanoma has no better prognosis than other types of melanoma. J Clin Oncol 2:994–1001
22. Cohen LM (1995) Lentigo maligna and lentigo maligna melanoma. J Am Acad Dermatol 33:923–936
23. Bittencourt FV, Marghoob AA, Kopf AW, Koenig KL, Bart RS (2000) Large congenital melanocytic nevi and the risk for development of malignant melanoma and neurocutaneous melanocytosis. Pediatrics 106:736–741
24. Swerdlow AJ, English JS, Qiao Z (1995) The risk of melanoma in patients with congenital nevi: a cohort study. J Am Acad Dermatol 32:595–599
25. Lowes MA, Norris D, Whiteld M (2000) Benign melanocytic proliferative nodule within a congenital naevus. Austr J Dermatol 41:109–111

# Interferon-$\alpha$ Sensitivity in Melanoma Cells: Detection of Potential Response Marker Genes

Ulrich Certa, Monika Seiler, Elisabetta Padovan, and Giulio C. Spagnoli

## Abstract

Interferon alpha (IFN-$\alpha$) represents an adjuvant therapy of proven effectiveness in increasing disease-free interval and survival in subgroups of melanoma patients. Since high doses of cytokine are required, the treatment is often accompanied by toxic side effects. In addition, naturally occurring insensitivity to IFN-$\alpha$ may hamper its therapeutic efficacy. Clinical, molecular or immunological markers enabling the selection of potential responders have not so far been identified. To explore the molecular basis of IFN-$\alpha$ responsiveness, we analyzed the expression pattern of about 7000 genes in IFN-$\alpha$-sensitive and IFN-$\alpha$-resistant cell lines using high-density oligonucleotide arrays. Melanoma cell lines were screened for their sensitivity to proliferation inhibition and HLA class I induction by IFN-$\alpha$ by standard $^3$H-thymidine incorporation and flow cytometry. Total cellular RNA from four sensitive and two resistant cell lines was extracted, reverse-transcribed and hybridized to high-density oligonucleotide arrays. The comparative analysis of gene expression in either set of cell lines allowed the identification of four genes (RCC1, IFI16, hox2 and h19) preferentially transcribed in sensitive cells and two (SHB and PKC-$\zeta$) preferentially expressed in resistant cells.

These data may provide a useful basis for the development of diagnostic tools to select potential IFN-$\alpha$ responders as eligible for treatment, while avoiding unnecessary toxicity to nonresponders.

This work was partially funded by a research grant from the Swiss National Fund for Scientific Research (no. 31-57'473.99 to G.C.S.)

Recent Results in Cancer Research, Vol. 160
© Springer-Verlag Berlin Heidelberg 2002

## Introduction

Interferon alpha (IFN-$\alpha$) is widely used in the therapy of melanoma (Agarwala and Kirkwood 1996; Kirkwood et al. 1997; Grob et al. 1998). In spite of its relative toxicity (Vial and Descotes 1994), in some subgroups of patients this treatment has clear clinical efficacy, but no clinical, immunological or molecular features allowing predictions of treatment outcomes have been identified as yet (Kirkwood 1998).

A central element of modern pharmacogenomics is the identification of surrogate markers for drug efficacy using multiparallel approaches. The availability of tumor cell lines that are sensitive or resistant to well-defined effects of IFN-$\alpha$ provides tools that can be used to search for genes whose expression is restricted to either cell type in the absence of cytokine exposure. These can lead to the development of diagnostic reagents, such as antibodies or enzyme assays.

In this work we used high-density oligonucleotide arrays (Schena et al. 1995, 1996; DeRisi et al. 1996; Heller et al. 1997) to analyze the expression of about 7000 genes in RNA samples from melanoma cell lines sensitive or resistant to IFN-$\alpha$ induced inhibition of proliferation and HLA class I induction.

We report here on the identification of gene patterns of potential diagnostic relevance that are preferentially expressed in either IFN-$\alpha$ sensitive or IFN-$\alpha$-resistant melanoma cell lines.


## Materials and Methods

### Cell Lines and Culture Conditions

ME15, ME51, ME59, and ME67 cell lines were generated in our laboratory on culture of cell suspensions derived from surgically excised melanoma metastases (Lüscher et al. 1994). The A375 cell line was a gift from Dr. Eberle (Basel, Switzerland), while the D10 cell line was provided by Dr. Rimoldi (Lausanne, Switzerland). All cell lines were cultured in RPMI medium supplemented with 10% FCS, glutamine (2 mM), sodium pyruvate (1 mM), nonessential amino acids, and HEPES buffer (10 mM) (all from Gibco Life Sciences, Paisley, UK).


### Proliferation Assays and HLA Class I Expression Analysis

Cell proliferation was evaluated on culture of 5000 cells per well in flat-bottom 96-well plates (Becton Dickinson Labware, Franklin Lakes, N.J., USA) in the presence or absence of the indicated concentrations of IFN-$\alpha$ over a 5-day period. De novo DNA synthesis was measured by $^3$H-thymidine incorporation following overnight incubation in the presence of the tracer.

Surface expression of HLA class I was quantitatively monitored (mean fluorescence intensity: MFI) by flow cytometry, using a FITC-labeled mAb specific for a monomorphic determinant of HLA-A-B-C heavy chain or control, isotype-matched reagents (Pharmingen, San Diego, Calif.), in cells cultured for 48 h in the presence or absence of IFN-$\alpha$.

## Oligonucleotide Array Hybridization and Data Analysis

Cultured melanoma cells were harvested by scraping, and total cellular RNA was extracted (Mahadevappa and Warrington 1999; Certa et al. 2001). Ten micrograms from each sample was used directly as a template for cDNA synthesis using a commercial kit (Roche Molecular Biochemicals, Rotkreuz, Switzerland). The T7 promoter sequence incorporated into the cDNA synthesis primer allowed template amplification and biotin labeling by in vitro transcription using a commercial kit (Affymetrix, Santa Clara, Calif.). After alkaline heat fragmentation, cDNA was hybridized to the array and all subsequent steps were performed following standard procedures as supplied with the arrays (Affymetrix, Santa Clara, Calif.). Raw data were collected with a confocal laser scanner (Hewlett Packard, Palo Alto, Calif.) using GeneChip software v3.1 (Affymetrix, Santa Clara, Calif.) and normalized on the basis of the total signal of chips hybridized with ME15-derived cDNA. The normalized average difference (nAD) between the signals of the perfect and of the mismatch probe sets for each gene was used as the expression level of a given gene. Array-to-array variations did not exceed 2% according to the hybridization of one sample to five arrays from the same batch in a pilot study.

## Results

### Identification of IFN-$\alpha$-sensitive and -insensitive Melanoma Cell Lines

Established melanoma cell lines were assayed for their sensitivity to IFN-$\alpha$ by testing the capacity of the cytokine to inhibit their proliferation and to increase their surface expression of HLA class I determinants. Two cell lines (D10 and ME67) were found to be insensitive to the antiproliferative effects of IFN-$\alpha$, which inhibits the proliferation of ME51 and ME59 by at least 50% even in concentrations as low as 10 U/ml, whereas A375 and ME15 required 10 times the dose to elicit similar effects (data not shown). The up-regulation of HLA class I expression by IFN-$\alpha$ closely matched its antiproliferative effects, and in no case was a dissociation of the two activities observed.

## Detection of Potential Marker Genes for IFN-$\alpha$ Responsiveness

Following hybridization to high-density oligonucleotide arrays, the availability of large mRNA expression data sets from six human melanoma cell lines well characterized for their responsiveness to IFN-$\alpha$ raised the possibility of identifying genes preferentially expressed in sensitive or resistant lines in the absence of cytokine treatment. Microarray data of all genes from the responder (ME15, ME51, ME59 and A375) cells and all from the nonresponder (D10, ME67) cells were combined, resulting in two averaged data sets. These data were then screened for genes that were up-regulated more than three-fold in either group.

This analysis resulted in the identification of a group of four genes preferentially expressed in IFN-$\alpha$-sensitive cell lines (Fig. 1, panel A). Two of them, *IFI16* and *RCC1*, encode nuclear proteins endowed with mitotic regulation and transcriptional activation capacities, respectively (Bischoff and Ponstingl 1991; Trapani et al. 1994). A third is the *hox2* homeobox gene (Acampora et al. 1989), whereas the fourth, *h19* gene, encodes an untranslated RNA involved in the DNA methylation and genetic imprinting processes (Brannan et al. 1990). Notably, however, RCC1 gene was not expressed in one IFN-$\alpha$-sensitive cell line (ME51).

On the other hand, two genes encoding likely components of signal transduction pathways, *SHB* and *PKC-$\zeta$* (Barbee et al. 1993; Welsh et al. 1994) appeared to be preferentially expressed in IFN-$\alpha$-resistant D10 and ME67 cell lines (Fig. 1, panel B).


## Discussion

IFN-$\alpha$ treatment is an adjuvant therapy that has proven effective in increasing disease-free interval and overall survival following potentially curative surgery in patients with malignant melanoma, (Agarwala and Kirkwood 1996; Kirkwood et al. 1997; Grob et al. 1998). However, relatively high doses are required, frequently resulting in severe toxicity (Vial and Descotes 1994), while so far no clinical, immunological, or molecular features that would allow targeted selection of patients likely to benefit from the treatment have been identified (Kirkwood 1998). The identification of criteria predicting the potential effectiveness of IFN-$\alpha$ therapy would be high desirable insofar as nonresponders would be spared unnecessary toxicity and it would be possible to select specific subgroups of patients who could be expected to be responders.

In this work we addressed the genetic profile of melanoma cell lines classified according to their sensitivity or insensitivity to critical direct effects of IFN-$\alpha$, namely the inhibition of proliferation and the up-regulation of HLA class I expression.

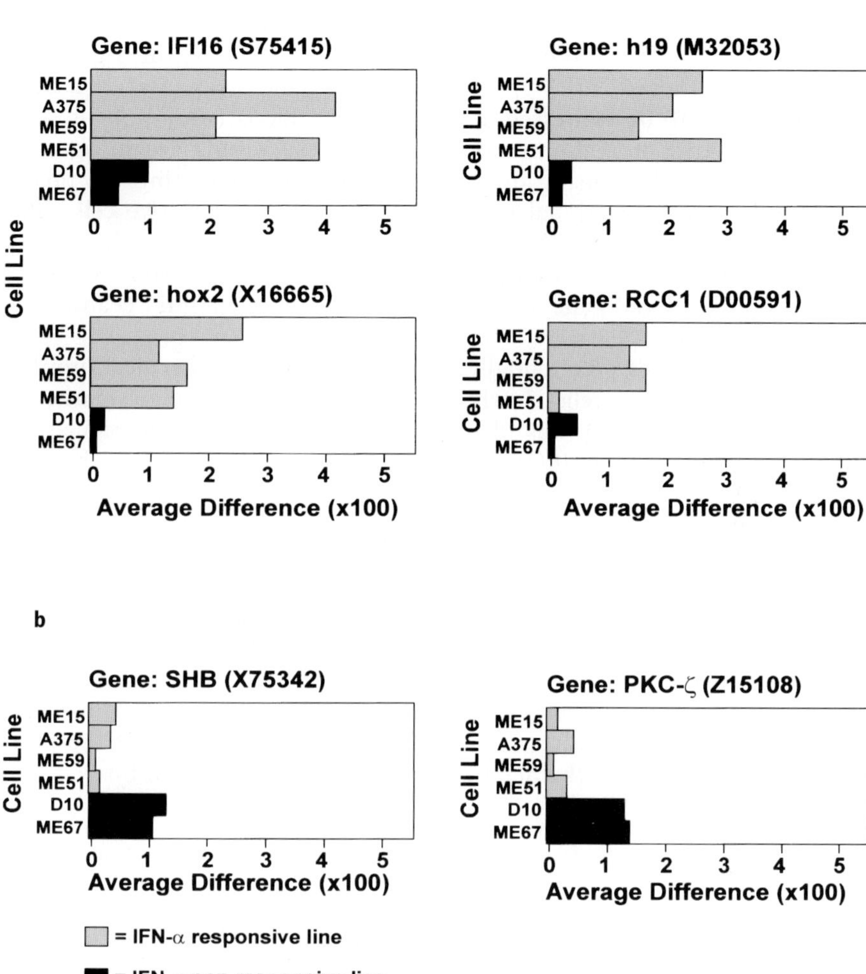



**Fig. 1 a, b.** Genes preferentially expressed in IFN-α-sensitive (**a**) and IFN-α-resistant (**b**) melanoma cell lines. Oligonucleotide array expression data were collected from untreated melanoma cells. Data from the sensitive (ME15, A375, ME59, ME51) or resistant (D10, ME67) lines were combined into two data sets. Average values for individual genes were then filtered to identify genes that were up-regulated at least threefold in either group. Data are presented as average differences in signal intensity between match and mismatch probe sets. Expression patterns of potential interferon-α response marker genes. *Bars* representing sensitive lines are filled in *gray* and those representing resistant lines, in *black*

The use of the oligonucleotide microarray technology makes it possible to investigate the expression of large panels of genes and appears to be ideally suited to the analysis of relatively simple cellular systems (Marton et al. 1998; Iyer et al. 1999; Pollack et al. 1999).

Resistance to the antiproliferative and HLA class I-inducing effects of IFN-$\alpha$ does not appear to be related to major differences in the expression of genes encoding IFN-$\alpha$ receptors or key players in the specific signal transduction chain. Indeed, *STAT* genes detectable by the array (Stat 2, 4, 5a and 5b) were found to be expressed at relatively low levels (nAD $\leq$50) in all cell lines, irrespective of IFN-$\alpha$ responsiveness. These results are in agreement with data obtained by using different technologies, suggesting the presence of relatively functional signal transduction in IFN-$\alpha$-insensitive cells (Ralph et al. 1995; Wong et al. 1997). Interestingly, similar results were also obtained when some of the cell lines under investigation in the current work were tested by conventional gene and protein expression techniques (Pansky et al. 2000).

A pattern of genes preferentially expressed according to typical profiles in sensitive and resistant cells clearly emerges, although no single marker specific for IFN-$\alpha$ sensitivity was identified. Genes involved in the regulation of cell proliferation, such as *IFI16*, *h19* and *RCC1*, but also *hox2*, which was not widely thought to have a role in this context, were found to be preferentially expressed in sensitive cell lines. Intriguingly, genes encoding SHB and PKC-$\zeta$ proteins, which are known components of defined signal transduction pathways, appear to be preferentially expressed in IFN-$\alpha$-resistant cells. These puzzling data suggest that IFN-$\alpha$ resistance could result from a series of active events, as opposed to a merely defective activation.

Taken together our data provide a database of potential relevance in the investigation of the molecular background of IFN-$\alpha$ sensitivity of melanoma cells. Ongoing studies addressing the validation of these data at the protein level might result in the characterization of reagents of clinical interest.

**Acknowledgements.** Thanks are due to Prof. A. Eberle (Basel, Switzerland) and Dr. D. Rimoldi (Lausanne, Switzerland) for providing cellular reagents and to Prof. P. Ruinart (Reims, France) for supplying liquid media.

## References

Acampora D, D'Esposito M, Faiella A, Pannese M, Migliaccio E, Morelli F, Stornaiuolo A, Nigro V, Simeone A, Boncinelli E (1989) The human HOX gene family. Nucleic Acids Res 17:10385–10402

Agarwala SS, Kirkwood JM (1996) Interferons in melanoma. Curr Opin Oncol 8:167–174

Barbee JL, Loomis CR, Deutscher SL, Burns DJ (1993) The cDNA sequence encoding human protein kinase C-zeta. Gene 132:305–306

Bischoff FR, Ponstingl H (1991) Catalysis of guanine nucleotide exchange on Ran by the mitotic regulator RCC1. Nature 354:80–82

Brannan CI, Dees EC, Ingram RS, Tilghman SM (1990) The product of the H19 gene may function as an RNA. Mol Cell Biol 19:28–36

Certa U, de Saizieu A, Mous J (2001) Hybridization analysis of labeled RNA by oligonucleotide arrays. Methods Mol Biol 170:141–156

DeRisi J, Penland L, Brown PO, Bittner ML, Meltzer PS, Ray M, Chen Y, Su YA, Trent JM (1996) Use of a cDNA microarray to analyse gene expression patterns in human cancer. Nat Genet 14:457–460

Grob JJ, Dreno B, de la Salmonière P, Delaunay M, Cupissol D, Guillot B, Souteyrand P, Sassolas B, Cesarini J-P, Lionnet S, Lok C, Chastang C, Bonerandi JJ (1998) Randomised trial of interferon $\alpha$-2a as adjuvant therapy in resected primary melanoma thicker than 1.5 mm without clinically detectable node metastases. Lancet 351:1905–1910

Heller RA, Schena M, Chai A, Shalon D, Bedilion T, Gilmore J, Woolley DE, Davis RW (1997) Discovery and analysis of inflammatory disease-related genes using cDNA microarrays. Proc Natl Acad Sci USA 94:2150–2155

Iyer VR, Eisen MB, Ross DT, Schuler G, Moore T, Lee JCF, Trent JM, Staudt LM, Hudson J, Boguski MS, Lashkari D, Shalon D, Botstein D, Brown PO (1999) The transcriptional program in the response of human fibroblasts to serum. Science 283:83–87

Kirkwood JM (1998) Adjuvant IFN alpha$_2$ therapy of melanoma. Lancet 351:1901–1903

Kirkwood JM, Resnick GD, Cole BF (1997) Efficacy, safety, and risk-benefit analysis of adjuvant interferon alfa-2b in melanoma. Semin Oncol 24:16–23

Lüscher U, Filgueira L, Juretic A, Zuber M, Lüscher NJ, Heberer M, Spagnoli GC (1994) The pattern of cytokine gene expression in freshly excised human metastatic melanoma suggests a state of reversible anergy of tumor-infiltrating lymphocytes. Int J Cancer 57:612–619

Mahadevappa M, Warrington JA (1999) A high-density probe array sample preparation method using 10- to 100-fold fewer cells. Nat Biotechnol 17:1134–1136

Marton MJ, DeRisi JL, Bennett HA, Iyer VR, Meyer MR, Roberts CJ, Stoughton R, Burchard J, Slade D, Dai H, Bassett DE, Hartwell LH, Brown PO, Friend SH (1998) Drug target validation and identification of secondary drug target effects using DNA microarrays. Nat Med 4:1293–1301

Pansky A, Hildebrand P, Fasler-Kann E, Baselgia L, Ketterer S, Beglinger C, Heim MH (2000) Defective Jak-STAT signal transduction pathway in melanoma cells resistant to growth inhibition by interferon-$\alpha$. Int J Cancer 85:720–725

Pollack JR, Perou CM, Alizadeh AA, Eisen MB, Pergamenschikov A, Williams CF, Jeffrey SS, Botstein D, Brown PO (1999) Genome-wide analysis of DNA copy-number changes using cDNA microarrays. Nat Gen 23:41–46

Ralph SJ, Wines BD, Payne MJ, Grubb D, Hatzinisiriou I, Linnane AW, Devenish RJ (1995) Resistance of melanoma cell lines to interferons correlates with reduction of IFN-induced tyrosine phosphorylation. Induction of the anti-viral state by IFN is prevented by tyrosine kinase inhibitors. J Immunol 154:2248–2256

Schena M, Shalon D, Davis RW, Brown PO (1995) Quantitative monitoring of gene expression patterns with a complementary DNA microarray. Science 270:467–470

Schena M, Shalon D, Heller R, Chai A, Brown PO, Davis RW (1996) Parallel human genome analysis, microarray-based expression monitoring of 1000 genes. Proc Natl Acad Sci USA 93:10614–10619

Trapani JA, Dawson M, Apostolidis VA, Browne KA (1994) Genomic organization of IFI16, an interferon-inducible gene whose expression is associated with human myeloid cell differentiation: correlation of predicted protein domains with exon organization. Immunogenetics 40:415–424

Vial T, Descotes J (1994) Clinical toxicity of Interferons. Drug Safety 10:115–150

Welsh M, Mares J, Karlsson T, Lavergne C, Breant B, Claesson-Welsh L (1994) Shb is a ubiquitously expressed Src homology 2 protein. Oncogene 9:19–27

Wong LH, Krauer KG, Hatzinisiriou I, Estcourt MJ, Hersey P, Tam ND, Edmonson S, Devenish RJ, Ralph SJ (1997) Interferon-resistant human melanoma cells are deficient in ISGF3 components, STAT1, STAT2, and p48-ISGF3gamma. J Biol Chem 272:28779–28785

# Molecular Cytogenetics as a Diagnostic Tool for Typing Melanocytic Tumors

Boris C. Bastian


## Abstract

The melanocyte can give rise to a variety of both benign and malignant lesions that differ in their clinical and histopathological appearance. It is likely that genetic changes underlie this phenotypic diversity. Comparative genomic hybridization (CGH) is a genome-wide scanning technique that permits the measurement of copy number aberrations in archival tumors. Using CGH, we have demonstrated significant differences in the frequency of chromosomal aberrations in primary cutaneous melanomas and Spitz nevi. Whereas the majority of melanomas have aberrations frequently involving chromosomes 9, 10, 7, and 6, most Spitz nevi do not show aberrations. However, a small subset of Spitz nevi show an isolated gain of the short arm of chromosome 11p. As this aberration has not been observed in melanomas, the measurement of chromosomal aberrations should be further evaluated as a diagnostic tool for ambiguous melanocytic tumors.


## Current Problems in the Histopathological Classification of Melanocytic Tumors

The melanocyte can give rise to a multiplicity of tumors that differ substantially in clinical and histological appearance and in prognosis. The benign tumors are generally termed melanocytic nevi, and the malignant ones are termed melanoma. Melanoma is an important clinical problem, as it is the seventh most common malignancy in the United States. In 2000, it is estimated that 47 700 cases of invasive malignant melanoma and 20 000–40 000 cases of melanoma in situ were newly diagnosed in the U.S. (Rigel and Carucci 2000). Melanoma has been increasing in incidence and mortality more rapidly than any other malignancy except lung cancer in women. Rising awareness in the public and medical arenas has led to a dramatic increase in


Recent Results in Cancer Research, Vol. 160
© Springer-Verlag Berlin Heidelberg 2002

excision of suspicious lesions in recent decades. The vast majority of tumors excised are benign (Del Mar et al. 1994).

Histopathology is the gold standard for diagnosis of pigmented lesions of the skin. In spite of very wide morphologic variability, the majority of cases can be classified reliably with current pathological criteria. However, there is a significant subset of cases that are so ambiguous that no consensus can be reached even among expert pathologists (Cook 1997; Corona et al. 1996; Farmer et al. 1996; Jackson 1997; Kempf et al. 1998; Piepkorn and Odland 1997; Wakely et al. 1998). The effect of the ambiguity on standard clinical practice is illustrated in a recent study from The Netherlands. An expert panel reviewed 1069 consecutive melanocytic lesions that had been submitted for review by clinical pathologists to identify the most common diagnostic problems. In 14% (22/158) of the cases that had initially been classified as invasive melanoma the panel considered the lesions were benign, and in 16.6% (85/513) the panel considered malignant what had been diagnosed as benign (Veenhuizen et al. 1997). Together with lymphoma, melanoma heads the list of tumors concerned in pathology malpractice claims (Troxel and Sabella 1994).

Diagnostic uncertainty of these dimensions has significant adverse consequences for patients (Goldes et al. 1984). Misclassifying a melanoma as benign may be fatal, and diagnosing a benign lesion as malignant can result in significant morbidity. Current medical practice with equivocal cases is to proceed as if they were definitely malignant. However, the morbidity of the therapeutic options – wide re-excision, sentinel lymph node biopsy, and adjuvant alpha interferon – coupled with the diagnostic uncertainty frequently leads to a less aggressive treatment regimen. This typically includes a limited re-excision and close clinical follow-up. Thus, patients with benign lesions still suffer the side effects of significant surgery and the emotional strain of the diagnosis, while patients who in fact do have a melanoma may not receive the optimal treatment.

Currently there is no method of definitively resolving these ambiguities. A clinical test that could enhance established diagnostic procedures would be of significant clinical benefit.

Such a test would need to be applicable to routinely fixed tissue, because diagnostic problems typically arise after the specimen has already been processed. There are several routes that it seems could conceivably lead to the identification of markers detectable by such a test. Screening approaches permitting an analysis of thousands of markers are the most powerful of these. However, most of these approaches rely on RNA as a source, which cannot currently be extracted from formalin-fixed tissue in sufficient amounts and quality. By contrast, DNA can be readily extracted from formalin-fixed tissue in quantities and quality that are adequate for a variety of analyses. We have relied on genomic analyses to identify potential diagnostic markers for melanocytic tumors.

## Comparative Genomic Hybridization

As originally described (Kallioniemi et al. 1992), comparative genomic hybridization (CGH) detects and maps DNA sequence copy number variation throughout the entire genome onto a cytogenetic map supplied by metaphase chromosomes (Fig. 1, left). Recently, an implementation of CGH has been described in which the metaphase chromosomes are replaced by arrays of genomic bacterial artificial chromosomes (BAC) clones (Fig. 1, right) (Pinkel et al. 1998). The relative copy number can then be measured at loci specified by the BAC clones by hybridization of fluorescently labeled test and reference DNAs, as in conventional CGH. The use of metaphase chromosomes as the hybridization target has previously limited the resolution of CGH to 10–20 Mb, made the resolution of closely spaced aberrations impossible, and only allowed linkage of CGH results to genomic information and resources with cytogenetic accuracy. In array CGH, the resolution is determined by the genomic spacing and/or length of the target clones, and the positions of the clones are accurately known on the human DNA sequences, because each clone contains a sequence tag. Array CGH allows accurate quantification of DNA copy number variations over a wide dynamic range, including reliable detection of single copy deletions and duplications (Albertson et al. 2000). Array CGH provides substantially better resolution and sensitivity than does conventional CGH in the analysis of tumor genomes.

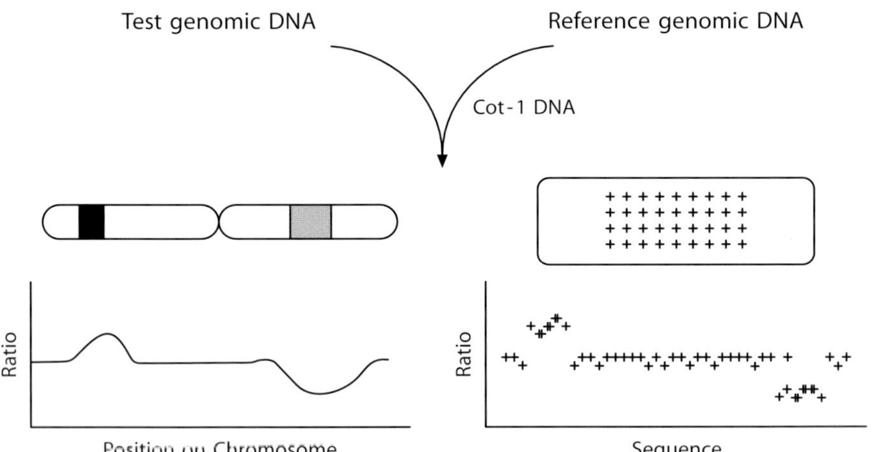


**Fig. 1.** Comparative genomic hybridization. *Left*: Total genomic DNAs are isolated from a "test" and a "reference" cell population, labeled with different fluorochromes, and hybridized to normal metaphase chromosomes. Cot-1 DNA is used to suppress hybridization of repetitive sequences. The resulting ratio of the fluorescence intensities of the two fluorochromes at a location on a chromosome is approximately proportional to the ratio of the copy numbers of the corresponding DNA sequences in the test and reference genomes. *Right*. A similar hybridization to an array of mapped clones permits measurement of copy number with resolution determined by the length of the clones and/or their map spacing

## DNA Copy Number Changes in Primary Cutaneous Melanoma

We have performed conventional CGH on several hundred formalin-fixed, paraffin-embedded primary melanocytic lesions, mostly melanomas. In an initial survey we screened 32 randomly selected primary cutaneous melanomas for chromosomal alterations using CGH (Bastian et al. 1998) (Fig. 2). Most of these were superficial spreading melanomas (SSM), the most common type in a light-skinned population. This was the first comprehensive analysis of chromosomal gains and losses in primary melanoma. The most frequent aberrations were losses of chromosome 9 (81% of the tumors), most commonly affecting the p-arm. Further common losses occurred on chromosomes 10 (63%), 6q (28%), and 8p (22%). Gains in copy number involved chromosomes 7 (50%), 8q (34%), 6p (28%), 1q (25%), 20 (13%), 17 (13%), and 2 (13%) (Bastian et al. 1998). Most of these aberrations involved large chromosomal regions. One acral lentiginous melanoma (ALM) was included in this group, and it had high-level amplifications of several small chromosomal regions. This prompted a larger investigation of the genomic aberrations in 15 ALM. All the ALMs had at least one (mean 2.0) gene amplification, significantly more than in a control set of 15 SSMs of comparable tumor thickness, in which only 2 of the 15 (13%) had one amplification each ($P < 0.0001$). At least 15 different genomic regions were amplified in ALM. These involved small portions of chromosomal arms, sometimes including oncogenes specifically implicated in melanoma. The most frequently amplified regions in ALMs were 11q13 (47%), 22q11–13 (40%), and 5p15 (20%).

ALM exhibits several clinical and epidemiological features that distinguish it from the SSMs. For example, the incidence of ALM is approximately equal across all racial groups, and it develops on palmar, plantar, and subungual skin, sites that have little exposure to sunlight and are protected from ultraviolet radiation by a thick stratum corneum. However, its classification as a distinct type of melanoma has been controversial. Our findings of the different characters of the genetic events that are involved in ALM and SSM, coupled with its clinical features, support the classification of ALM as a distinct melanoma subtype.


## DNA Copy Number Changes in Spitz Nevi

Problems of diagnostic ambiguity most commonly arise with Spitz nevus. Sophie Spitz initially described this condition as "juvenile melanoma" and regarded it as a subset of childhood melanoma that followed a benign course (Spitz 1948). It is now regarded as benign. Spitz nevi account for about 1% of surgically removed melanocytic nevi (Casso et al. 1992) and occur most frequently, but not exclusively, in children. Spitz nevi, like melanoma, can display a composition of melanocytes with abundant cytoplasm and large nuclei that contain macronucleoli. Mitotic figures can be numerous in either condition (Piepkorn 1995; Weedon 1997). This overlap can make it impossi-

# Loss of Heterozygosity and Microsatellite Instability in Acquired Melanocytic Nevi: Towards a Molecular Definition of the Dysplastic Nevus

Albert Rübben, Inja Bogdan, Elke-Ingrid Grußendorf-Conen, Günter Burg, and Roland Böni

## Abstract

Acquired melanocytic nevi may show signs of histological dysplasia, and epidemiological studies have demonstrated that dysplastic melanocytic nevi (DMN) are associated with an elevated melanoma risk. Nevertheless, the concept of DMN as precursors of melanoma has remained a concept, in view of the difficulty of establishing unambiguous cytological and histological criteria for DMN. Recent molecular data suggest that genetic instability is more frequent in DMN than in benign acquired melanocytic nevi. We have analyzed 54 benign melanocytic nevi and 6 DMN for loss of heterozygosity (LOH) at microsatellite markers D9S171, IFNA, D9S270, D9S265. LOH at one or more loci was detected in 17 out of 54 benign nevi and in 4 out of 6 DMN. LOH was demonstrated at 26 out of 103 amplified and informative microsatellites in benign nevi and at 6 out of 11 microsatellites in DMN. In addition, 6 benign nevi and 6 DMN were microdissected in 4–15 regions per lesion and analyzed for LOH and microsatellite instability (MSI) at D9S162 and D14S53. Both LOH and MSI were detected more frequently in dysplastic nevi (LOH frequency 0.61 vs 0.18; MSI frequency 0.27 vs 0.05). These results confirm that genetic instability is more prevalent in DMN than in benign acquired melanocytic nevi. Therefore, DMN might be defined as a monoclonal and genetically unstable, but limited, melanocytic proliferation that distinguishes this entity from the benign nevus and from malignant melanoma.

## Introduction

The concept of the dysplastic melanocytic nevus as a precursor of malignant melanoma has been the subject of an ongoing debate since the initial description of the B-K mole syndrome in 1978 (Clark et al. 1978; Clark and Ackerman 1989). The histological criteria established by Clark and coworkers, and especially the definition and nature of the dysplastic or atypical nevus cell, have

Recent Results in Cancer Research, Vol. 160
© Springer-Verlag Berlin Heidelberg 2002

been criticized as subjective (Ackerman 1988). On the other hand, as long ago as in 1988, Hecht and Hecht presented data indicating that the dysplastic nevus syndrome (DNS) is characterized by genetic instability, and they concluded: "The DNS road to malignancy may logically proceed by genomic alterations including translocations, duplications, and deletions." In this view, the dysplastic nevus cell is characterized by a mutator phenotype (Loeb 2001). This conclusion was derived from laborious cell culture experiments and only focused on dysplastic nevi of members of melanoma prone families, and it therefore did not find its way into the fierce controversy on the nature of the dysplastic nevus, which was fought basically with histological and cytological arguments.

The elucidation of the molecular mechanisms responsible for hereditary nonpolyposis colorectal cancer (HNPCC) did not only support the notion that genetic instability might be critical for tumorigenesis, but also provided the technical basis for a molecular test (Ionov et al. 1993; Aquilina et al. 1994). Colon tumors of HNPCC patients harbor germ-line mutations in genes responsible for repair of DNA mismatches. As a result, these tumors acquire abundant mutations in short repetitive DNA sequences named microsatellites, which can easily be analyzed by polymerase chain reaction (Weber and May 1989). This form of genetic instability is named microsatellite instability (MSI) and has been demonstrated in various other malignant tumors (Atkin 2001).

Defects in the repair of double-strand DNA breaks (Lopes et al. 1999) and anomalies of centrosome function (Ghadimi et al. 2000) and spindle assembly in tumor cells may lead to chromosomal instability characterized by losses or duplications of long stretches of chromosomal DNA. DNA deletions induced by chromosomal instability can be identified by LOH of microsatellite DNA.

MSI seems to be more prevalent in diploid cancers, while LOH is more common in aneuploid cancers (Sugai et al. 2000). The analysis of microsatellite DNA enables the detection of both mechanisms of genetic instability and is thus a powerful tool for the diagnosis and characterization of malignant tumors.

LOH and MSI have also been detected in malignant melanoma (Dracopoli et al. 1985; Peris et al. 1995; Boni et al. 1998a; Rübben et al. 2000) as well as in dysplastic nevi (Healy et al. 1996; Lee et al. 1997; Boni et al. 1998b). The predominant form of genetic instability in malignant melanoma seems to be the occurrence of structural mutations and especially of large deletions, rather than mismatch repair deficiency (Ohta et al. 1996; Wagner et al. 1998).

Recent studies using microsatellite analysis have evaluated the occurrence of LOH and MSI in both benign (common) and dysplastic melanocytic nevi. Park et al. detected LOH only in dysplastic nevi and not in benign nevi. Birindelli and coworkers (2000) found a higher incidence of MSI in dysplastic nevi than in benign nevi (31% vs. 23%), and they also noted that LOH was restricted exclusively to dysplastic nevi and melanomas and was not detected within benign lesions. Hussein et al. (2001b) analyzed a larger number of melanocytic lesions and detected MSI in 28% of dysplastic nevi but not in any benign melanocytic nevi. The discrepancies between the studies may reflect differences in technique and in the definitions used for LOH and MSI (Hussein et al. 2001 a). Nevertheless, these data suggest that genetic instability is associated with the dysplastic nevus and thus support the initial findings of Hecht and Hecht (1988).

Our own results from microsatellite analysis of benign and dysplastic melanocytic nevi confirm this conclusion. The methodology used in our laboratory is based on the molecular analysis of multiple microdissected regions of a mole, and thus enables detection of LOH or MSI with a high sensitivity. Furthermore, our data delineates critical parameters for a future standardization of LOH/MSI analysis of melanocytic nevi. On the basis of our results and of findings from previous studies we would like to propose a molecular definition of the dysplastic nevus.

## Materials and Methods

### Biopsy Specimens

A total of 60 benign and 12 dysplastic melanocytic nevi were analyzed. Dysplastic nevi were diagnosed by experienced dermatopathologists (G.B., E.-I. G.-C.) according to the criteria defined by the WHO panel 1985 (Clemente et al. 1991).

### Microdissection and DNA extraction

Microdissection was performed on 5- to 10-µm-thick deparaffinized tissue sections under a light microscope (magnification 200×). Nevus cells were removed either with a disposable 30-G needle or with adhesive to pick them up, as described elsewhere (Turbett et al. 1996). With this technique we isolated nevus cell clusters containing approx. 50–1000 cells. Cells of the unaffected dermis were used for the extraction of control DNA. The microdissected cells were digested with proteinase K (2.5 mg/ml) in a total volume of 20 µl overnight at 37 °C. Proteinase K was inactivated by boiling for 10 min at 94 °C. When the microdissected area contained fewer than 100 cells, 1.5 µl of the solution was used directly as template DNA. Otherwise, the DNA was eluted into 50 µl $H_2O$ using the Qiagamp Tissue Kit (Qiagen, Hilden, Germany) according to the manufacturer's recommendations, and 10 µl of this solution was used for each PCR.

### Microsatellite PCR

54 benign nevi and 6 dysplastic nevi were analyzed for LOH at microsatellite markers D9S171, IFNA, D9S270 and D9S265. PCR was performed in 10 µl volume with Taq-polymerase AmpliTaq Gold (Perkin Elmer, Roche Diagnostics, Basel, Switzerland) according to the manufacturer's recommendations.

Amplification consisted of 35 cycles with 1 min at 55 °C, 1 min at 72 °C and 1 min at 94 °C. Labeling of PCR products was accomplished by incorporation of $^{32}$PdCTP (6000 Ci/mmol). Separation of PCR-products was done in an 8% acrylamide gel (Gel-Mix8, Gibco BRL). Autoradiography was performed with Typon X-Ray DX-41 film (Typon, Burgdorf, Switzerland).

In addition, 6 benign nevi and 6 dysplastic lesions were analyzed at 4–15 microdissected regions per lesion for LOH as well as for MSI at markers D9S162 and D14S53. Oligonucleotides were labeled 5' with fluorescent dyes (HEX, 6-FAM) (Microsynth, Balgach, Switzerland). Separation of PCR products was performed in a 6% acrylamide gel (Gel-Mix6, Gibco BRL) using an automated sequencer (Applied Biosystems ABI-PRISM 373).

Complete loss of a single band (peak) or greater than 80% reduction of the band (peak) of higher molecular weight or greater than 50% reduction of the band (peak) of lower molecular weight was scored as LOH.

## Results

LOH at one or more markers on the short arm of chromosome 9 (D9S171, IFNA, D9S270, D9S265) was detected in 17 out of 54 benign nevi and in 4 out of 6 dysplastic nevi. On average, 2 microsatellite markers were informative for each lesion. LOH was demonstrated at 26 out of 103 amplified and informative microsatellites (25%) in benign nevi and at 6 out of 11 amplified and informative microsatellites (54%) in dysplastic nevi. Figure 1 displays

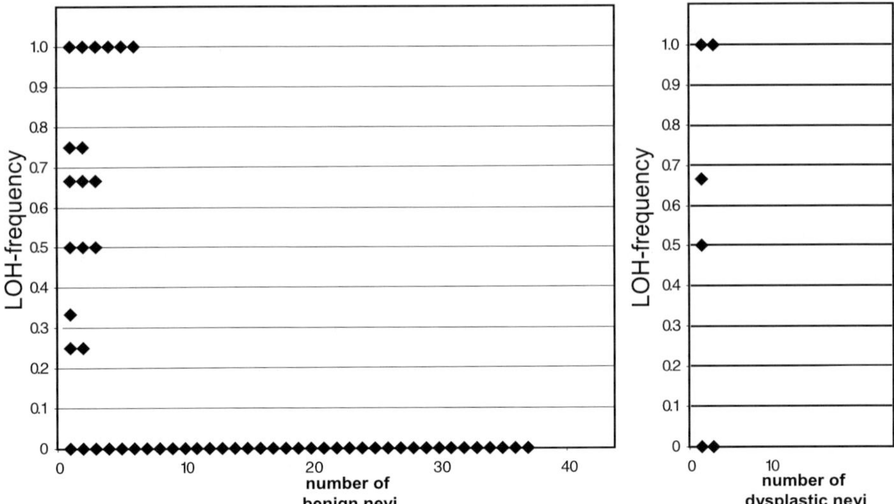


**Fig. 1.** Loss of heterozygosity (LOH) mutation frequencies at D9S171, IFNA, D9S270, D9S265 in benign and dysplastic melanocytic nevi (mutation frequency = number of LOH detected at informative microsatellite markers/total number of amplified informative microsatellite markers)

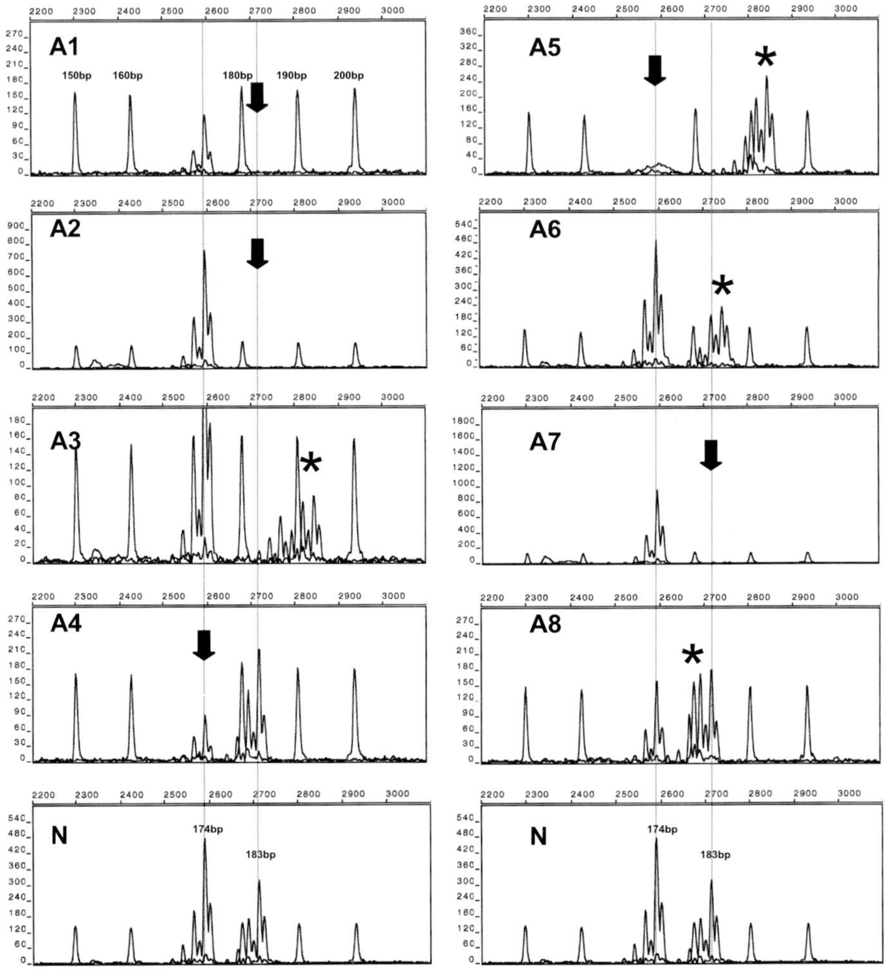

**Fig. 2.** Electropherogram analysis of LOH (*arrows*) and microsatellite instability (MSI; *stars*) at marker D9S162 in 8 microdissected areas (*A1–A8*) of a dysplastic melanocytic nevus (case 11). Electropherogram *N* shows the two alleles of 174 bp and 183 bp present in the normal tissue of the patient. The *dotted lines* indicate the positions of the normal alleles in all electropherograms. The molecular size marker GENESCAN 400HD shows peaks of 150, 160, 180, 190 and 200 bp

the frequency of LOH (LOH at informative markers/total number of informative markers analyzed per lesion) for all benign and dysplastic lesions. Most benign nevi demonstrated zero or low LOH frequency, while dysplastic nevi showed a more heterogeneous pattern. In order to determine LOH and MSI frequencies more accurately we analyzed 6 additional benign nevi and 6 dysplastic nevi at multiple (4–15) microdissected regions (on average 9 areas per lesion) for LOH or MSI at markers D9S162 and D14S53, two regions that have previously been shown to be lost frequently in melanoma (Rübben et

**Table 1.** Analysis of benign and dysplastic melanocytic nevi at multiple microdissected regions for loss of heterozygosity (LOH)[a] and microsatellite instability (MSI)[a]

| Case no. | Diagnosis | D9S162 | | | D14S53 | | | Frequency | |
|---|---|---|---|---|---|---|---|---|---|
| | | LOH (n) | MSI (n) | Regions analyzed (n) | LOH (n) | MSI (n) | Regions analyzed (n) | LOH (n) | MSI (n) |
| 1 | Compound nevus | 0 | 0 | 10 | 1 | 0 | 7 | 0.06 | 0.00 |
| 2 | Compound nevus | 5 | 0 | 8 | 3 | 1 | 8 | 0.50 | 0.06 |
| 3 | Compound nevus | 0 | 1 | 15 | 5 | 2 | 15 | 0.17 | 0.10 |
| 4 | Compound nevus | 0 | 1 | 14 | 3 | 2 | 14 | 0.11 | 0.11 |
| 5 | Compound nevus | 1 | 1 | 8 | 1 | 0 | 11 | 0.11 | 0.05 |
| 6 | Compound nevus | 3 | 0 | 11 | 0 | 0 | 5 | 0.14 | 0.00 |
| 7 | Dysplastic compound nevus | 8 | 1 | 8 | 1 | 0 | 10 | 0.55 | 0.06 |
| 8 | Dysplastic compound nevus | 5 | 2 | 7 | 4 | 0 | 9 | 0.58 | 0.13 |
| 9 | Dysplastic compound nevus | 2 | 1 | 4 | 6 | 3 | 8 | 0.63 | 0.33 |
| 10 | Dysplastic compound nevus | 6 | 0 | 6 | 9 | 9 | 11 | 0.91 | 0.53 |
| 11 | Dysplastic compound nevus | 5 | 4 | 8 | 2 | 1 | 4 | 0.56 | 0.42 |
| 12 | Dysplastic compound nevus | 2 | 2 | 10 | 5 | 1 | 8 | 0.41 | 0.17 |

[a] Frequency of LOH and MSI were calculated as: (number of microdissected regions showing LOH or MSI at D9S162 + number of microdissected regions showing LOH or MSI at D14S53)/(total number of regions analyzed for LOH or MSI at D9S162 + total number of regions analyzed for LOH or MSI at D14S53)

al. 2000). Figure 2 shows the electropherogram result obtained in a dysplastic nevus (case 11) analyzed at 8 regions with marker D9S162. LOH could be shown in areas 1, 2, 4, 5, and 7, while MSI was found in areas 3, 5, 6, and 8. It is interesting to note that areas 1, 2, and 7 have lost the allele with the higher molecular weight, while areas 4 and 5 show loss of the lower allele. The data are summarized in Table 1 and displayed graphically in Fig. 3. The mean frequency of LOH was 0.18 for benign nevi and 0.61 for dysplastic nevi. MSI was also more frequent in dysplastic lesions than in benign nevi

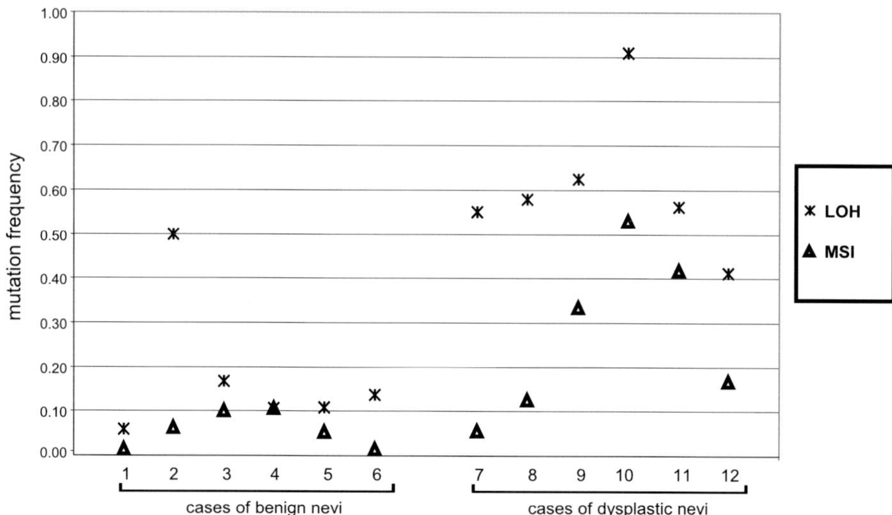


**Fig. 3.** LOH- and MSI-mutation frequencies at D9S162 and D14S53 in microdissected benign and dysplastic melanocytic nevi (cases 1–12)

(0.27 vs 0.05). Nevi with higher LOH frequency also tended to have higher MSI frequency.

## Discussion

Our results confirm the observation of other groups (Park et al. 1998; Birindelli et al. 2000; Hussein et al. 2001 a) that genetic instability is more prevalent in dysplastic nevi than in benign nevi, and we found that both forms of genetic instability, i.e. chromosomal instability as detected by LOH and microsatellite instability, occurred at higher frequencies in dysplastic lesions.

Analysis of multiple microdissected areas of a lesion showed that both LOH and MSI occurred focally in the nevi. This observation has two important implications. First, it indicates that LOH and MSI evolve during the proliferation of nevus cells. As a melanocytic nevus is the result of monoclonal growth of nevus cells (Robinson et al. 1998), mutations such as LOH or MSI will accumulate during nevus maturation. The linkage between LOH and proliferation has already been demonstrated in malignant melanoma (Boni et al. 1998 a). Second, analysis of the lesion as a whole or only at a few areas might underscore the true genetic instability within the tumor. Thus, analyzing multiple microdissected regions at multiple microsatellite markers should provide a more accurate estimate of the genetic instability in the nevus.

Our data and earlier observations may be integrated into a molecular definition of the dysplastic nevus. Figure 4 exemplifies the basic concept. A benign nevus begins as a junctional nevus, then evolves into a compound ne-

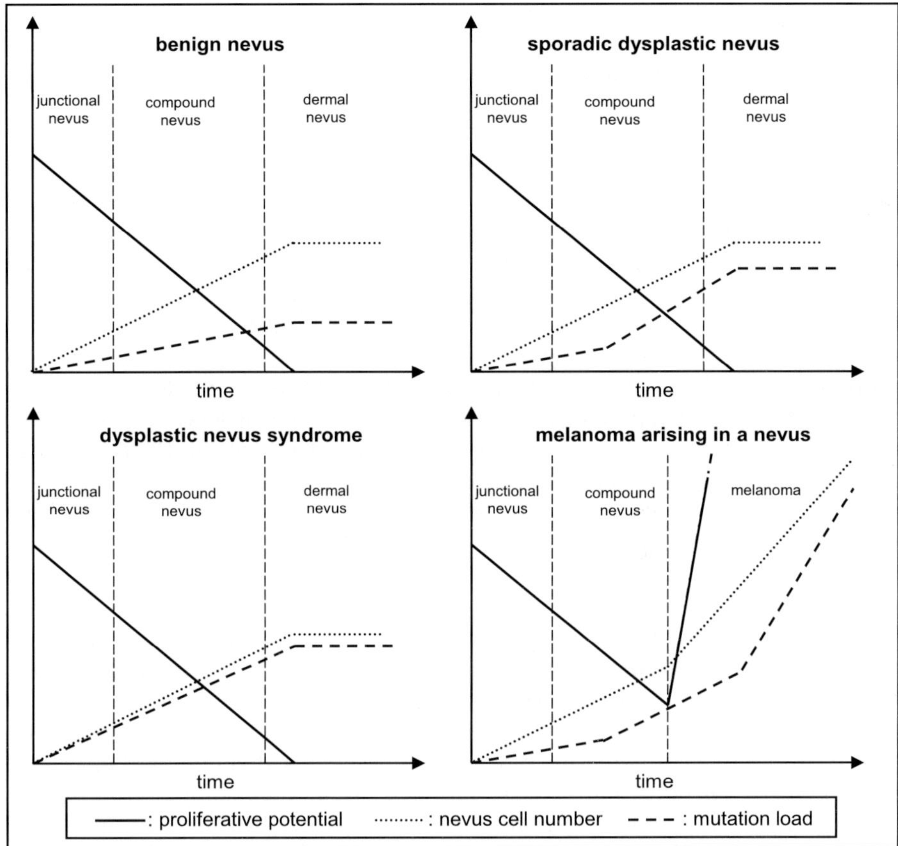



**Fig. 4.** A molecular concept of the dysplastic melanocytic nevus: DMN is a monoclonal and genetically unstable but limited melanocytic proliferation

vus and matures to a dermal nevus. During this process, the proliferative potential of the nevus cells diminishes, the number of cells in the nevus increases and the nevus cells accumulate some mutations. A dysplastic nevus will be characterized by an enhanced mutation rate, which might affect all nevus cells or only a subset of the nevus cell population. We might speculate that in the dysplastic nevus cell syndrome all nevi and all nevus cells within a single lesion yield an enhanced mutation rate, as proposed by Hecht and Hecht in 1988. On the other hand, in sporadic dysplastic nevi, mutations leading to genetic instability might reflect secondary events arising during nevus growth. In both cases, the nevus cells accumulate more mutations during the process of nevus maturation. Once the nevus is mature, the nevus cells do not accumulate further mutations as they cease to proliferate. Cytological signs of atypia may be more prominent in the case of chromosomal instability associated with aneuploidy than in dysplastic nevi harboring only microsatellite instability. Furthermore, signs of atypia may not be detected within mature nevus cells in dermal nevi, although the mutation load should reach its maximum at the end of the proliferative phase. Therefore, cytological signs of atypia may not be an accurate representation of the mutation load in the lesion, which can only be measured by molecular techniques, such as microsatellite analysis. In this model, a melanoma evolving from a nevus is characterized by the occurrence of a cell population that has both an unlimited proliferative potential and an enhanced mutation rate. Only if these assumptions are correct might the melanoma cells accumulate the further mutations necessary to gain the full malignant and metastatic phenotype. As dysplastic cells are thought to accumulate more mutations than benign nevi they will carry a higher risk of malignant transformation. Furthermore, once the dysplastic nevus has matured, the risk of malignant progression is greatly reduced. The model also supports the observation that large nevi are a risk factor for malignant melanoma (Grob et al. 1990), as large nevi are able to accumulate more mutations.

The proposed definition of the dysplastic nevus as a monoclonal and genetically unstable but limited melanocytic proliferation separates this entity from the benign nevus and from malignant melanoma. Genetic instability may not be detected unambiguously by cytological or histological features, which also explains the long-lasting controversy over the pathological criteria required to make the diagnosis. Microsatellite analysis of microdissected nevus cell nests might represent one approach to measuring genetic instability. The technique still lacks standardization. Therefore, consensus must be obtained on the most suitable microsatellite markers for this analysis, the method to be used for detection of LOH and MSI, the number of analyzed regions per lesion and the number of microdissected cells per PCR before microsatellite analysis might become a reference test for diagnosis and risk assessment of dysplastic nevi.

## References


Ackerman AB (1988) What naevus is dysplastic, a syndrome and the commonest precursor of malignant melanoma? A riddle and an answer. Histopathology 13:241–256

Aquilina G, Hess P, Branch P, MacGeoch C, Casciano I, Karran P, Bignami M (1994) A mismatch recognition defect in colon carcinoma confers DNA microsatellite instability and a mutator phenotype. Proc Natl Acad Sci USA 91:8905–8909

Atkin NB (2001) Microsatellite instability. Cytogenet Cell Genet 92:177–181

Birindelli S, Tragni G, Bartoli C, Ranzani GN, Rilke F, Pierotti MA, Pilotti S (2000) Detection of microsatellite alterations in the spectrum of melanocytic nevi in patients with or without individual or family history of melanoma. Int J Cancer 86:255–261

Boni R, Matt D, Voetmeyer A, Burg G, Zhuang Z (1998a) Chromosomal allele loss in primary cutaneous melanoma is heterogeneous and correlates with proliferation. J Invest Dermatol 110:215–217

Boni R, Zhuang Z, Albuquerque A, Vortmeyer A, Duray P (1998b) Loss of heterozygosity detected on 1p and 9q in microdissected atypical nevi. Arch Dermatol 134:882–883

Clark WH, Ackerman AB (1989) An exchange of views regarding the dysplastic nevus controversy. Semin Dermatol 8:229–250

# The Changing Incidence and Mortality of Melanoma in Australia

Robin Marks

## Abstract

For many years Australia has had the highest incidence and mortality rates in the world for melanoma. The incidence rate has been increasing at around 5% per year and the mortality rate, at a rate slightly lower than that. Epidemiology studies have shown clearly that there is both a constitutional and an environmental contribution to melanoma risk, with sunlight being the major risk factor in the environment. The data also clearly show that the thickness of a melanoma at the time it is removed is one of the major determinants of the likelihood of metastasis and thus of the long-term prognosis. Both of these components have been incorporated into major public health programmes aimed at melanoma control in Australia over the last 25 years. Primary prevention programmes have been aimed at reducing the desire for a tan and subsequent overexposure to sunlight. Secondary prevention (early detection) programmes have encouraged people in the community to seek early attention if they notice a new or changing pigmented lesion. Although the age-adjusted incidence and mortality rates for Australia continue to rise, cohort analysis of both incidence and mortality rates reveals that the overall rise is not reflected in all age groups. In the younger cohorts – groups that it has been possible to influence by our public health campaigns in recent decades – both incidence and mortality rates are dropping.

## Introduction

The incidence and mortality rates for melanoma rose during the last century in most developed countries throughout the world. In Australia, mortality attributable to melanoma, which was recorded throughout much of the twentieth century, rose by an increment of around 6% per year in men and 3% per year in women (Giles et al. 1996). The incidence rate for melanoma, which has only been recorded throughout the country in the last several decades,

Recent Results in Cancer Research, Vol. 160
© Springer-Verlag Berlin Heidelberg 2002

had been rising at an annual rate of around 6.5% in men and boys and 4.4% in women and girls (Giles et al. 1989). In 1990, the age-adjusted annual incidence rate for melanoma was 27.6 per 100 000 persons, whereas the age-adjusted mortality rate for that year was 4/100 000 persons (Jelfs et al. 1996). In 1990, the estimated number of person-years of life lost as a result of all melanoma in Australia was in the order of 10 500, being 6500 for men and just over 4000 for women. This was due to a higher mortality rate for males in 1990: 5/100 000 males compared with 2.6/100 000 females in that year.

A comparison with other developed countries whose populations are of mainly European origin shows similar increases in incidence and mortality rates to those in Australia, but at levels that are substantially lower than in Australia (Armstrong and Kricker 1994; Parkin et al. 1992). In other words, Australia has the highest incidence and mortality rates in the world for melanoma. In the age group 15–44, melanoma has become the most common cancer in men and is now second only to breast cancer in women. Overall, melanoma is now the fourth most common cancer occurring in men, being surpassed by cancer of the lung, bowel and prostate, and is the third most common in women, being surpassed by bowel and breast cancers only.

As a result of these figures, which clearly show that melanoma has become a major public health problem in Australia, there have been a variety of public health approaches to try to control both the incidence and the mortality attributable to this tumour.

## Data Underpinning the Public Health Approach to Melanoma Control

There have been many epidemiology studies looking at the causation of melanoma in populations that may be susceptible, such as that of Australia. The earliest paper suggesting the possibility that sunlight exposure might be contributing to melanoma was published in the 1950s from Australia (McGovern 1952). Since then a substantial body of literature has accumulated suggesting that there are both constitutional and environmental factors that determine the eventual expression of the disease in adults. Constitutional risk factors have included fair skin with a tendency to burn easily rather than tan when exposed unprotected to sunlight and a tendency to develop a large number of moles, both common acquired and dysplastic, with a risk gradient related to total number of naevi (Evans et al. 1988). The inherited condition xeroderma pigmentosum, which is characterised by a defect in DNA repair following exposure to ultraviolet radiation (UVR), is very strongly associated with the risk of development of melanoma, along with other sunlight-related skin cancers, at a very young age in the people affected (Harper 1998). Although extensive research has been undertaken in the search for the particular genotype at risk of melanoma, it appears at this stage that it is unlikely to be clearly related to a single gene.

There is no doubt that the major environmental factor coming out in all epidemiological studies as the single most important contributor to risk of melanoma is exposure to sunlight. Exposure to very large amounts of sunlight in early childhood, if sufficient to cause sunburn that will be remembered many years later, is a major determinant. It appears that intermittent overexposure to sunlight, whether in childhood or during leisure time in adulthood, is associated with a higher risk than is regular exposure to sunlight in a way that does not lead to sunburn (Elwood and Jopson 1997). Nevertheless, regular sunlight exposure in outdoor workers in a country such as Australia does increase the risk of melanoma over and above the rates seen in people with similar constitutions living in other countries, e.g. the United Kingdom, so that it is not merely intermittent overexposure that increases the risk (Green and O'Rourke 1985).

It is the UVR spectrum in sunlight that appears to be the most likely aetiological component of solar radiation. Initial work focused on the UVB range, but some more recent data have raised the question of whether UVA may contribute (Swerdlow and Weinstock 1998). As yet, there are no data showing a correlation with the visible or infrared spectrum of solar radiation. There is some interest in which particular wavelengths of the solar spectrum are likely to be most carcinogenic, but it must be remembered that for the vast majority of people who have developed melanoma in the last 100 years, it has been exposure to the whole of sunlight, not just particular wavelengths, that has resulted in their developing the tumours that have been recorded in epidemiological studies.

An important approach to cancer control is the so-called secondary prevention. This is an attempt to detect a cancer at an early stage while it may still be possible to remove it with a very high chance of cure. In other words, it is important to know what the characteristics, both clinical and histological, of early tumours are, which indicate that they are still in an early stage and on which public and professional education programmes can be based in an attempt to have people seen and treated while still at a curable stage. The most important feature to emerge from studies over the last several decades has been that the major histopathological determinant of risk of metastasis is the thickness of the tumour, measured in millimetres at the time of removal (Balch et al. 1985). This translates clinically into the fact that flat or macular pigmented tumours are the early tumours, regardless of their diameter, which is a feature to be promoted in a public education programme. The public perception of the word mole is of a lesion that is raised (Borland et al. 1992). Thus, the actual effect of an education programme explicitly promoting a search for moles may well in fact be that the public looks out for elevated pigmented lesions, i.e. late melanomas. Other correlations with prognosis include: site (lesions on the head, neck and trunk are more likely to metastasise early than lesions on the limbs), sex (tumours in male subjects are more likely to metastasise early than those in women or girls when all other prognostic indicators are the same), the presence of microscopic ulceration and, to a lesser degree, Clark's levels and the number of mitoses (Balch et al. 1985).

Before public and professional education programmes could be developed for primary and secondary prevention of melanoma, research was necessary to determine what was current practice amongst professionals in Australia and what attitudes, knowledge, beliefs and behaviours relating to sunlight and suntans were prevalent in the Australian population.

In Australia, general practitioners are the primary medical practitioners, to whom members of the public are recommended to turn in the first instance if they notice a new or changing pigmented lesion. Studies in Australia have shown that the ratio of benign to malignant pigmented lesions removed is substantially higher amongst general practitioners than the ratio amongst specialists, such as plastic surgeons or dermatologists (Marks et al. 1997). In other words, professional education is an important part of the approach to melanoma control that must precede measures to induce members of the public to seek attention if they are concerned about a particular lesion. Randomised controlled studies have shown that smaller excision margins for early melanomas are unlikely to alter the long-term prognosis, and it is also important to insert this type of information into professional education programmes.

Behavioural research data collected on members of the Australian public in the 1980s had shown that there was a substantial desire for a suntan, not only for its perceived ability to make people look more attractive, but also because it was believed to be healthy (Hill et al. 1992). The latter belief may have stemmed from the promotion of exposure to sunlight in the early twentieth century as good for health. Thus, a public education programme focusing on changing attitudes to suntans and changing behaviours in sunlight needed to focus not only on the fact that it is not necessary to change one's skin colour (develop a suntan) to be attractive, but also on the message that a suntan is not a sign of improved health.

## The Public Health Approach to Skin Cancer Control in Australia

### Early Detection

Early detection programmes were developed in Australia in the 1970s as the first approach to dealing with the increasing incidence and mortality rates for melanoma. These programmes dealt with persons who had a tumour at the time, rather than taking the long-term approach of trying to prevent tumours from developing in the future.

There have been extensive education programmes for professionals and for members of the public. The public education programmes have focused on the nature of melanoma: the fact that early tumours are flat, looking like unusual freckles, being stressed rather than the earlier concentration on moles; the fact that the lesions are generally asymptomatic; and that they look different from surrounding pigmented lesions. Booklets showing the signs of melanoma have been produced and displayed in medical practices, pharmacies, sports areas, hairdressers' salons, physiotherapists' and chiropractors' rooms and other areas throughout the community.

In 1985, a coalition of the Australian Cancer Society and the Australasian College of Dermatologists developed the National Skin Cancer Awareness Programme, which has continued ever since (Noy and Houston 1986). An early part of that programme involved developing professional education material, which was sent to every general practitioner in the country, giving details of the signs of early melanoma and the treatment that would be appropriate when any patient presented with one of these tumours.

A variety of public education activities using screening caravans, such as the "battle stations" in use in New South Wales and the "spot checks" offered in Queensland, Western Australia and Victoria, have been provided at beaches and other public open spaces during summer. These are not a long-term screening programme, but more of an educational exercise, to show members of the public that they should seek medical attention for a changing pigmented lesion. Australia does not have a formalised screening programme, despite the fact that it has the highest incidence of melanoma in the world. Opportunistic screening of patients by general practitioners, particularly of elderly patients if they present with other illnesses or to ask for repeat prescriptions for their medication, has been widely promoted.

A number of specialised melanoma units, such as the Queensland Melanoma Project, the Sydney Melanoma Unit and the Victorian Melanoma Service, have been established for specialist referral where necessary. Nevertheless, the majority of people with pigmented lesions are seen by general practitioners, whereupon their lesions are either excised locally or they are referred further to a specialist dermatologist or plastic surgeon for treatment in their rooms. The vast majority of people in Australia do not require the care of highly specialised melanoma units. In Australia, legislation requires the registration of all new melanomas in the State Cancer Registries, so that details not only of the incidence of these tumours, but also of the pathology (e.g. thickness, level and histological subtype) are recorded.

## Primary Prevention

Because of the very high incidence of melanoma in Australia, the long-term approach of trying to prevent these tumours has been widely promoted in the last two decades. In the early 1980s the Slip! Slop! Slap! programme developed by the Anti-Cancer Council of Victoria became the national primary prevention programme. There have been variations on this programme, including SunSmart, which was developed in 1987, Me No Fry, and others, throughout the country. These have been public education programmes with extensive material and activity throughout the whole of the community (Marks 1999).

There are professional education programmes as well, which are aimed at teachers, pharmacists, unions, sports organisations, and many other institutions responsible for the environment or for activities undertaken by members of the public whilst they are outdoors. One of the activities has been sponsorship of sporting events to which young people are attracted. Funding for the sponsorship has come through various state-based health promotion foundations, which receive income from the taxation on tobacco products. Accompanying the education programmes has been structural change (Marks 1996). Structural change includes legislation to remove sales tax from approved sunscreens and the development of standards by which sunscreens are tested and promoted; institution of sun protection policies in schools and sporting organisations; creation of shade in school yards and other public open spaces by means of constructed canopies or natural canopies from tree planting; and rescheduling so that work or sport activities are kept away from the middle of the day.

Sunscreens, although widely promoted for photoprotection, are also clearly stated to be a second-line approach to melanoma prevention, rather than the primary approach. Natural protection, including hats, clothing and avoidance of exposure to the sun around the middle of the day, are promoted as the first-line approach, and sunscreens are an adjunct to that approach, and not a substitute for it. Despite the continuing pressure from the commercial sunscreen manufacturers to promote high SPF numbers, a ceiling on the number that it was felt could be publicly promoted in Australia was set initially at 15, and more recently at 30. Anything above that was labelled either 15+ or 30+. The recommendation on which particular SPF number to select has continued to be 15 or higher, the selected product to have added broad-spectrum cover to provide protection from UVA as well.

Australia has been very active in campaigning to reduce the manufacture, distribution, use, and release of ozone-depleting substances. Even though ozone depletion is unlikely to have contributed substantially to the high incidence of melanoma in Australia, those countries with high insolation and high incidence rates, such as Australia, are affected more by minor changes in ozone levels than low-insolation countries.

In summary, the public and professional education programmes for melanoma control in Australia have been extremely widespread and comprehensive in the last two decades. Virtually every person in the country has been reached by one or more of these programmes over the years.

## Changes in the Incidence and Mortality Rates of Melanoma in Australia

### Mortality Rate

The major outcome variable of interest for early detection programmes is mortality rate. If tumours are detected at a sufficiently early stage and treated adequately, then the mortality rate should level off and eventually fall.

An earlier outcome measure of success in early detection programmes is assessment of the thickness of the tumours. A reduction in the thickness of tumours with which people are diagnosed should occur as a result of the education program. In the 1950s, the case fatality rate for melanoma was in the order of 50%. It is now less than 20%, and this reduction is associated with a substantial reduction in the average thickness of all melanomas now removed (Armstrong and Kricker 1994). The majority are less than 1 mm thick. It has now got to the stage where the question of whether or not a proportion of these early melanomas being removed may not have progressed on to metastasising tumours has been raised (Burton and Armstrong 1995). Although this is an interesting rhetorical question, we do not yet have biological markers that enable us to answer it.

An even earlier stage assessment of an early detection programme is a check on whether or not there has been an increase in public knowledge about melanoma and its signs. Over 90% of the Australian population now understand about melanoma (Borland et al. 1992). They recognise that this cancer can be dangerous, and many can give details of the signs of these tumours unprompted. However, there is still more work to be done, particularly on the misconception that all moles are raised and that most melanomas develop from moles.

However, the outcome of most interest is mortality, and the mortality data have shown a plateauing for both men and women since 1985. In the period 1990–1994 the rate rose by 3.7% in men to 5/100 000 men and fell by 5.2% to 2.38/100 000 women (Giles et al. 1996).

Cohort analysis of mortality data shows that the mortality rates in men rose steeply in the cohorts born before around 1930, were stable in cohorts born between 1930 and 1950, and began to fall in the more recent cohorts (Giles et al. 1996). The mortality rates in women showed similar changes, but occurring around 5 years earlier. It has been suggested that an overall reduction in the age-adjusted mortality rate for melanoma will be seen in Australia over the next decade or so.


## Incidence Rate

The earliest change likely to be recorded as the result of a primary prevention programme (whose long-term outcome of interest is a reduction in incidence rates) is a change in knowledge, beliefs and attitudes vis-à-vis protection from sunlight and the development of suntan. There have certainly been changes in all age groups throughout the Australian community in these areas (Hill et al. 1993). The desire for a suntan has decreased and been replaced by a desire for a lighter tan in a large proportion of the population, while a substantial number of people now desire no suntan at all. Along with these changes have been behaviour changes in photoprotection, including the use of hats, clothing and sunscreen and the avoidance of exposure to the sun around the middle of the day. Measures of sunburn frequency have shown a concurrent reduction over time (Hill et al. 1993). Although these are short-term measures, in the long term they are likely to be translated into an effect on incidence rates. Economic modelling of the cost-effectiveness of primary prevention based on these data has shown that a national programme would be excellent value for money in terms of deaths avoided and cost per life-year saved (Carter et al. 1999).

The incidence rate for melanoma has continued to rise. However, the rate of increase in both men and women peaked in 1988, and the incidence has risen more slowly since then, the rise being 5% per annum in men and 3% per annum in women from the years 1991–1993. Based on these rates of increase, the age-adjusted incidence rate for melanoma in Australia for 2001 is likely to be around 40/100 000 persons per year. However, as with mortality rates, age-adjusted rates are a simplification. Although they may be of value for national and international comparisons, they are a reduction of masses of data to a single figure. Use of this figure involves the risk of covering up changes by averaging out many different components. Breaking down the age-adjusted figure and undertaking cohort analysis by gender and date of birth reveals that the overall rise in incidence rate is not reflected in all age groups. The incidence rate continues to rise in the elderly cohorts in both men and women (Giles and Thursfield 1996). On the other hand, the rate in the younger cohorts has peaked and started to fall, particularly for those born since 1950 onwards. It is the younger cohorts who have been in a position to be influenced by our primary prevention programmes over the past two decades.

In summary, for many decades Australia has led the world with the highest incidence and mortality rates for melanoma for the periods in which they have been recorded. As a result of this, extensive public health programmes have been instituted, focusing on both early detection of melanoma occurring in people now and prevention of melanoma that might otherwise occur in the long term. These programmes have now been going for over three decades and have resulted in changes in both mortality and incidence rates in the age cohorts at which the public health programmes have been substantially directed. Although we have a long way to go, changes in mortality and incidence rates are finally becoming apparent after many years of extensive work by a large group of dedicated people working together with a unified aim, i.e. long-term melanoma control.

## References


Armstrong B, Kricker A (1994) Cutaneous melanoma. Cancer Surv Trends Cancer Incidence 19:219–239

Balch CM, Soong SJ, Shaw HM et al (1985) An analysis of prognostic factors in 4000 patients with cutaneous melanoma. In: Balch CM, Milton GW (eds) Cutaneous melanoma: clinical management and treatment results worldwide. Lippincott, Philadelphia, pp 321–352

Borland R, Marks R, Noy S (1992) Public knowledge about characteristics of moles and melanoma. Aust J Public Health 16:370–375

Burton RC, Armstrong BK (1995) Current melanoma epidemic: a non-metastasizing form of melanoma? World J Surg 19:330–333

Carter R, Marks R, Hill D (1999) Could a national skin cancer primary prevention campaign in Australia be worthwhile? An economic evaluation. Health Promotion Int 14:73–82

Elwood M, Jopson J (1997) Melanoma and sun exposure: an overview of published studies. Int J Cancer 73:198–203

Evans RD, Kopf AW, Lew RA et al (1988) Risk factors for the development of malignant melanoma. I. Reviews of case-control studies. J Dermatol Surg Oncol 14:393–406

Giles G, Thursfield V (1996) Trends in skin cancer in Australia. Cancer Forum 20:188–191

Giles G, Dwyer T, Coates M et al (1989) Trends in skin cancer in Australia: an overview of the available data. Trans Menzies Found 15:143–147

Giles GG, Armstrong BK, Burton RC, Staples MP, Thursfield VJ (1996) Has mortality from melanoma stopped rising in Australia? Analysis of trends between 1931 and 1994. BMJ 312:1121–1125

Green AC, O'Rourke MG (1985) Cutaneous malignant melanoma in association with other cancers. J Natl Cancer Inst 74:977–980

Harper J (1998) Genetics and genodermatoses. In: Champion H, Burton JL, Burns DA, Breathnach SM (eds) Textbook of dermatology, 6th edn. Blackwell Scientific Publications, Oxford, pp 407–412

Hill D, White V, Marks R et al (1992) Melanoma prevention: behavioural and non-behavioural factors in sunburn among an Australian population. Prev Med 21:654–669

Hill D, White V, Marks R, Borland R (1993) Changes in sun-related attitudes and reduced sunburn prevalence in a population at high risk of melanoma. Eur J Cancer Prev 2:447–456

Jelfs P, Coates M, Giles GG et al (1996) Cancer in Australia, 1989–1990 (with projections to 1995). Aust Institute Health Welfare, Canberra, p 147

Marks R (1996) Prevention and control of melanoma: the public health approach. CA Cancer J Clin 46:199–216

Marks R (1999) Two decades of the public health approach to skin cancer control in Australia: why, how and where are we now? Aust J Dermatol 40:1–5

Marks R, Jolley D, McCormack C, Dorevitch AP (1997) Who removes pigmented skin lesions? A study of the ratio of melanoma to other benign pigmented skin tumours removed by different category of physician in Australia, 1989 & 1994. J Am Acad Dermatol 36:721–726

McGovern VJ (1952) Melanoblastoma. Med J Aust I [Suppl 10]:139–143

Noy S, Houston J (1986) National Skin Cancer Awareness Week 1985: a new initiative in public education about skin cancer. Cancer Forum 10:88–91

Parkin DM, Muir CS, Whelan SL et al (1992) Cancer incidence in five continents, vol 6. (IARC scientific publications 120) IARC, Lyon

Swerdlow AJ, Weinstock MA (1998) Do tanning lamps cause melanoma? An epidemiologic assessment. J Am Acad Dermatol 38:89–90

# Why Is Epiluminescence Microscopy Important?

Klaus Wolff

## Abstract

The new morphological information provided by epiluminescence micro-scopy (ELM) requires a fresh approach to the analysis of pigmented lesions. It necessitates a learning process that pertains to the recognition of hitherto unknown morphological features and is based on the discrimination of these features and their combination into two different patterns. ELM has been shown to improve the sensitivity and specificity of the diagnosis of melano-ma and other pigmented lesions by 25–30%. Digitized ELM (DELM) pro-vides an unlimited capacity for data storage and retrieval. It is a computer-ized imaging method, objective and noninvasive; it provides objective evi-dence of lesional changes on follow-up; documents growth and any changes in the structure and shape of lesions; and thus helps in decisions on whether to excise them or not. It provides for quality control by means of the afore-mentioned documentation, which may also serve as back-up in the case of medico-legal problems. In addition, the spectrum is widened by the dimen-sion of teledermatology and cybernet computer-assisted diagnosis, which holds great promise for the future. ELM and DELM are thus the most impor-tant single development of the past three decades in the early diagnosis of melanoma.

## Introduction

During recent decades, the incidence of melanoma has been rising faster than that of most other human cancers (Armstrong 1996; Garbe 2000; Hall et al. 1999; Jemal et al. 2001). Because melanoma occurs at an earlier age than most cancers it is one of the leading cancers in terms of potential life-years lost per person and loss of productivity (Elwood and Koh 1994; Kittler et al. 2001; Lee 1992; MacKie 1994; Weinstock 1993, 1998). The most effective approach to the management of cutaneous melanoma is early recognition fol-

Recent Results in Cancer Research, Vol. 160
© Springer-Verlag Berlin Heidelberg 2002

lowed by surgical excision, and there is consensus that the current impressive 5-year survival rates of patients with melanoma are attributable solely to early diagnosis. While the majority of pigmented lesions can be diagnosed correctly on the basis of established clinical criteria, there remains a surprisingly high number of small melanocytic lesions in which a distinction between benign and malignant is difficult or even impossible to make on clinical grounds alone. Data indicating that even in specialized centers the diagnostic accuracy for early malignant melanoma is only slightly better than 60% (Grin et al. 1990) may be sobering, but they have to be accepted as fact.

## Epiluminescence Microscopy

Epiluminescence microscopy (ELM) is a noninvasive in vivo technique that has the potential to correct these diagnostic limitations, because it permits the recognition of malignant pigmented lesions much earlier than is possible by clinical inspection alone (Binder et al. 1995; Pehamberger et al. 1987; Soyer et al. 1989; Steiner et al. 1987; Wolff et al. 1994). ELM makes subsurface structures of the skin accessible to visual examination in vivo by using surface microscopy with oil immersion. In other words, ELM takes in vivo skin microscopy one step further than surface microscopy, because it allows the observer to look not only at, but also into, the superficial skin layers (Wolff et al. 1994). The subject has been expertly reviewed in two recent publications (Argenziano and Soyer 2001; Soyer et al. 2001).

Different terms have been used to describe this new technique, and they range from ELM and dermatoscopy to dermoscopy, skin surface microscopy and melanoscopy. They all describe the same approach and are synonymous. It must be understood that ELM is a diagnostic method, a technique, and thus a tool whose use has to be learned for it to be mastered. Looking into the surface layers of the skin by ELM reveals a new dimension of morphological features, colors and patterns, which cannot be understood without new learning criteria (Pehamberger et al. 1993; Wolff et al. 1994). Methods have been sought and found to make ELM analysis of lesions relatively reliable and reproducible: pattern analysis (Pehamberger et al. 1987; Wolff et al. 1994), the ABCD rule for dermoscopy (Nachbar et al. 1994; Stolz et al. 1994), the negative/positive features rule (Menzies et al. 1996), the seven-point checklist rule (Argenziano et al. 1998), and the ABCDE rule (Kittler et al. 1999). Interpreting an ELM image is like learning to read. The ELM criteria described can be compared to the letters of the alphabet, which have to be identified and assembled as letters are assembled into words which thus can be read and provide a meaning. The different approaches to the ELM analysis of pigmented lesions were compared at the Consensus Net Meeting on Dermoscopy 2000 (Argenziano and Soyer 2001), and all have been found to be useful, with pattern analysis having a slight edge over the others.

This new morphology provided by ELM requires a fresh approach to the analysis of pigmented lesions. It necessitates a learning process that pertains to the recognition of hitherto unknown morphological features and is based on discrimination of these features and their combination into different patterns. Based on the examination of many thousands of lesions and eventual verification of the diagnosis by histopathological examination, ELM has been shown to improve the sensitivity and specificity of the diagnosis of melanoma and other pigmented lesions by 25–30% (Mayer 1997; Steiner et al. 1987; Wolff et al. 1994). Nonetheless, even exact pattern analysis does not eliminate diagnostic errors completely, so that ELM cannot replace histopathological examinations at present.

What, then are the situations in which ELM can be most useful to the clinician? It does not add to the diagnostic armamentarium available for unequivocal classic lesions, but it has significant value in the case of those equivocal small pigmented skin lesions that pose major diagnostic problems even for experienced clinicians. ELM increases the diagnostic accuracy in pigmented skin lesions in that it helps to distinguish between melanocytic and nonmelanocytic lesions and between benign and malignant growth patterns. ELM has already proved to be of great practical value in many centers and offices worldwide, by increasing the probability that early melanoma will not be overlooked and by helping to prevent unnecessary major surgery in patients in whom nonmelanocytic or benign pigmentary lesions are suspected on visual inspection alone to be melanomas. It has proved practical in patients with dysplastic nevi, by helping to determine which lesions need to be removed.

Of course, ELM has its limitations. It does not provide 100% diagnostic accuracy and is of little help in the case of small lesions that are pigmented maximally and uniformly or of completely amelanotic lesions, because not all of these reveal the criteria necessary for ELM pattern analysis. Experience with a large number of lesions has also revealed a number of other limitations of the ELM technique. Because pattern analysis and the other approaches to analysis of ELM images are based on the detection and combination of certain criteria, the presence of such criteria is more important than their absence. Therefore, the absence or nonvisibility of defined criteria, for instance as a result of heavy overall pigmentation, may render diagnosis by ELM impossible. Because pattern analysis depends on the combination of criteria, a single criterion is usually insufficient for diagnosis, and years of experience with this technique have revealed that some criteria are more important than others (Steiner et al. 1993).

Like any other technique, ELM has to be learned. We have demonstrated that dermatologists not formally trained in the use of ELM surprisingly performed worse in terms of diagnosis when diagnosing images provided by ELM, in contrast to those who had been trained in this technique (Binder et al. 1995). On the other hand, we have also shown that even a short formal training in ELM will have a tremendous effect on novices in this field, improving their diagnostic performance by a significant 8.4% (Binder et al. 1997). This leads to the important conclusion that formal training is required for the useful application of ELM and that ELM should thus be restricted to dermatologists trained in its use.

## Digital Epiluminescence Microscopy

In essence, digital ELM (DELM) combines ELM with a computer requiring a CCD chip hand microscope, a light source, a frame grabber, and the appropriate computer software (Binder et al. 1994; Braun et al. 1998; Kittler et al. 2000a; Stolz et al. 1996). It is a noninvasive dermatological imaging method that provides objective evidence of lesional changes at follow-up; it documents growth and changes in the structure and shape of lesions, and is therefore very helpful when it is necessary to decide whether a lesion should be excised or not. Since the patient can follow the examination and analysis of his/her lesions on the computer screen, DELM does not exclude the patient. One of the main assets of this procedure is that it provides quality control by way of documentation, and since it has unlimited storage capacity and provides instant retrieval of all data stored, it is a wonderful device to fall back on for back-up in the event of medico-legal problems.

This method has so far been found most useful in follow-up of melanocytic skin lesions (Braun et al. 1998; Kittler et al. 2000a), and in particular atypical nevi (Kittler et al. 2000b). Atypical or dysplastic nevi share some ELM features with early melanoma, and a correct diagnosis cannot be established by ELM in all cases. Especially in the evaluation of patients with multiple atypical nevi, the choice between no therapeutic intervention and excision is always crucial. The clinical evaluation of and the decision on management of a single melanocytic lesion have to be viewed in the context of the number and the clinical appearance of all lesions of the patient concerned (Halpern et al. 1993). In patients with multiple dysplastic nevi, excision of all atypical lesions is impracticable and would be associated with significant morbidity, disfigurement, and cost. While there is no doubt that melanocytic skin lesions with ELM signs of malignancy or with a severely atypical appearance should be excised to rule out or confirm melanoma, the majority of lesions show only minimal or moderate clinical signs of atypia, which may not justify wholesale removal (Rhodes 1998). Follow-up with DELM is therefore particularly suitable for patients with multiple atypical nevi. In one study we demonstrated that follow-up DELM helps to identify patterns or modifications over time that are typical for early melanoma (Kittler et al. 2000b). These modifications over time then provided the decisive information allowing differentiation between early melanoma and benign melanocytic skin lesions, and sequential DELM thus serves to improve the follow-up of patients with multiple atypical nevi.

DELM is also suited to cybernet computer-assisted diagnosis. Artificial neural networks (ANN) are computational models based on the principles of neural propagation and processing, which are being used increasingly for better recognition in various investigative and clinical fields. Studies have attempted to determine whether ELM criteria can be used in an observer-independent objective computerized system and whether the clinical diagnosis of pigmented skin lesions, particularly the discrimination between benign nevi and malignant melanomas, can be done with the help of ANN (Binder et al.

1994). The basic element of this system is the simulated neuron. A defined number of input patterns (ELM criteria) are processed by this neuron, and through a learning process it produces an output pattern. Upon completion of learning the ANN was able to classify a total of 86% of the ELM patterns presented in a test database of 100 pigmented skin lesions correctly. Malignant melanomas were diagnosed correctly in 95%, of cases common nevi in 87%, and dysplastic nevi in 73% of cases (Binder et al. 1994). In contrast, investigators experienced in the use of ELM correctly recognized 88% of all pigmented lesions, 95% of melanomas, 97% of common nevi, and 70% of dysplastic nevi. Thus, the results achieved by the computer using ANN were comparable to those obtained by trained investigators using ELM pattern analysis in clinical diagnosis. In a dichotomized model comparing compound and dysplastic nevi versus malignant melanomas, the sensitivity and specificity of human diagnosis were 95% and 91%, respectively, and the sensitivity and specificity of ANN diagnoses were 95% and 90%, respectively (Binder et al. 1998). Similar results have been obtained by other groups (Andreassi et al. 1999; Menzies et al. 1997; Seidenari et al. 1998, 1999; Menzies 1999; Schindewolf et al. 1993; Stolz et al. 1996) and by us (Ganster et al. 2001). Thus, the criteria used for ELM are consistent enough to allow a computerized system to make classifications and yield diagnoses with a high degree of accuracy. This system is presently being evaluated in depth by testing several classifiers, including standard statistical procedures and classifiers from the field of artificial intelligence, such as ANNs, k-nearest neighbor, decision trees, and support vector machines (Dreiseitl et al. 2001); by incorporating clinical information the impact of this information on the classification process has also been evaluated (Binder et al. 2000), as has the performance of an automated trichotomous classification (Dreiseitl et al. 2000). While it is still too early to incorporate automated diagnosis into routine clinical practice, the research results obtained so far suggest that this will become a reality in the future (Binder et al. 2000). Finally, DELM is extremely well suited to transmission via telecommunication, in that it permits instant transmission of computerized ELM images between offices (Kittler et al 1998), institutions, and research centers and also across continents, and is therefore a wonderful tool for the exchange of information for the purposes of consultation and teaching.

Why then are ELM and DELM important? ELM is a noninvasive technique that provides a significant improvement in the accuracy of diagnosis of pigmented lesions, and thus of melanoma. It helps to verify the diagnosis of nonmelanocytic pigmented lesions and is thus a decisive help in reducing the number of unnecessary surgical procedures performed. DELM, a classic example of dermatological imaging, carries all this one step further by providing objective evidence of lesional changes on follow-up and documenting growth and changes in structure and shape of lesions; and it is indispensable in decision-making processes on whether to excise or not; it allows quality control by providing documentation, unlimited storage capacity, and instant retrieval of data. The spectrum is widened by the new dimension of teledermatology and cybernet computer-assisted diagnosis, which holds great promise for the future. ELM is thus the most important single development of the past three decades in the early diagnosis of melanoma.


# References


Andreassi L, Perotti R, Rubegni P, Burroni M, Cevenini G, Biagioli M et al (1999) Digital dermoscopy analysis for the differentiation of atypical nevi and early melanoma: a new quantitative semiology. Arch Dermatol 135:1459–1465

Argenziano G, Soyer P (2001) Dermoscopy of pigmented skin lesions: a valuable tool for early diagnosis of melanoma. Lancet Oncol 2:443

Argenziano G, Fabbrocini G, Carli P, De Giorgi V, Sammarco E, Delfino M (1998) Epiluminescence microscopy for the diagnosis of doubtful melanocytic skin lesions. Comparison of the ABCD rule of dermatoscopy and a new 7-point checklist based on pattern analysis. Arch Dermatol 134:1563–1570

Armstrong B (1996) Melanoma incidence in Europe. Cancer Causes Control 7:195–196

Binder M, Steiner A, Schwarz M, Knollmayer S, Wolff K, Pehamberger H (1994) Application of an artificial neural network in epiluminescence microscopy pattern analysis of pigmented skin lesions: a pilot study. Br J Dermatol 130:460–465

Binder M, Schwarz M, Winkler A et al (1995) Epiluminescence microscopy: a useful tool for the diagnosis of pigmented skin lesions for formally trained dermatologists. Arch Dermatol 131:286–291

Binder M, Puespoeck SM, Steiner A, Kittler H, Muellner M, Wolff K et al (1997) Epiluminescence microscopy of small pigmented skin lesions: short-term formal training improves the diagnostic performance of dermatologists. J Am Acad Dermatol 36:197–202

Binder M, Kittler H, Seeber A, Steiner A, Pehamberger H, Wolff K (1998) Epiluminescence microscopy-based classification of pigmented skin lesions using computerized image analysis and an artificial neural network. Melanoma Res 8:261–266

Binder M, Kittler H, Dreiseitl S, Ganster H, Wolff K, Pehamberger H (2000) Computer-aided epiluminescence microscopy of pigmented skin lesions: the value of clinical data for the classification process. Melanoma Res 10:556–561

Braun BP, Lemonnier E, Guillod J, Skaria A, Salomon D, Saurat JH (1998) Two types of pattern modification detected on the follow-up of benign melanocytic skin lesions by digitized epiluminescence microscopy. Melanoma Res 8:431–437

Dreiseitl S, Ohno-Machado L, Binder M (2000) Comparing three-class diagnostic tests by three way ROC analysis. Med Decis Making 20:323–331

Dreiseitl S, Ohno-Machado L, Kittler H, Vinterbo S, Billhardt H, Binder M (2001) A comparison of machine learning methods for the diagnosis of pigmented skin lesions. J Biomed Inform 34:28–36

Elwood JM, Koh HK (1994) Etiology, epidemiology, risk factors, and public health issues of melanoma. Curr Opin Oncol 6:179–187

Ganster H, Prinz A, Rohrer R, Wildling E, Binder M, Kittler H (2001) Automated melanoma recognition. IEEE Trans Med Imaging 20:233–239

Garbe C (2000) Increasing incidence of malignant melanoma. Hautarzt 51:518

Grin CM, Kopf AW, Welkovich B, Bart RS, Levenstein MJ (1990) Accuracy in the clinical diagnosis of malignant melanoma. Arch Dermatol 126:763–766

Hall HI, Miller Dr, Rogers JD, Bewerse B (1999) Update on the incidence and mortality from melanoma in the United States. J Am Acad Dermatol 40:35–42

Halpern AC, Guerry D, Elder DE, Trock B, Synnestvedt M, Humphreys T (1993) Natural history of dysplastic nevi. J Am Acad Dermatol 29:51–57

Jemal A, Devesa SS, Hartge P, Tucker MA (2001) Recent trends in cutaneous melanoma incidence among whites in the United States. J Natl Cancer Inst 93:678–683

Kittler H, Seltenheim M, Pehamberger H, Wolff K, Binder M (1998) Diagnostic informativeness of compared digital epiluminescence microscopy images of pigmented skin lesions compared with photographs. Melanoma Res 8:255–260

Kittler H, Seltenheim M, Dawid M, Pehamberger H, Wolff K (1999) Morphologic changes of pigmented skin lesions: a useful extension of the ABCD rule for dermatoscopy. J Am Acad Dermatol 40:558–562

Kittler H, Seltenheim M, Dawid M, Pehamberger H, Wolff K, Binder M (2000a) Frequency and characteristics of enlarging common melanocytic nevi. Arch Dermatol 136:316–320

Kittler H, Pehamberger H, Wolff K, Binder M (2000b) Follow-up of melanocytic skin lesions with digital epiluminescence microscopy: patterns of modifications observed in early melanoma, atypical nevi, and common nevi. J Am Acad Dermatol 43:467–476

Kittler H, Binder M, Wolff K, Pehamberger H (2001) A ten-year analysis of demographic trends for cutaneous melanoma: analysis of 2501 cases treated at the University Department of Dermatology in Vienna (1990–1999). Wien Klin Wochenschr 113:321–327

Lee JA (1992) Trends in melanoma incidence and mortality. Clin Dermatol 10:9–13

MacKie RM (1994) Strategies to reduce mortality from cutaneous malignant melanoma. Arch Dermatol Res 287:13–15

Mayer J (1997) Systematic review of the diagnostic accuracy of dermatoscopy in detecting malignant melanoma. Med J Aust 167:206–210

Menzies SW (1999) Automated epiluminescence microscopy: human vs machine in the diagnosis of melanoma. Arch Dermatol 135:1538–1540

Menzies SW, Ingvar C, Crotty KA, McCarthy WH (1996) Frequency and morphologic characteristics of invasive melanomas lacking specific surface microscopic features. Arch Dermatol 132:1178–1182

Menzies SW, Bischof L, Peden G (1997) Automated instrumentation for the diagnosis of invasive melanoma: image analysis of oil epiluminescence microscopy. In: Altmeyer P, Hoffman K, Stucker M (eds) Skin cancer and UV radiation. Springer, Berlin Heidelberg New York

Nachbar F, Stolz W, Merkle T et al (1994) The ABCD rule of dermatoscopy. High prospective value in the diagnosis of doubtful melanocytic skin lesions. J Am Acad Dermatol 30:551–559

Pehamberger H, Steiner A, Wolff K (1987) In vivo epiluminescence microscopy of pigmented skin lesions. I. Pattern analysis of pigmented skin lesions. J Am Acad Dermatol 17:571–583

Pehamberger H, Binder M, Steiner A, Wolff K (1993) In vivo epiluminescence microscopy – improvement early diagnosis of melanoma. J Invest Dermatol 100:S356–S362

Rhodes AR (1998) Intervention strategy to prevent lethal cutaneous melanoma: use of dermatologic photography to aid surveillance of high-risk persons. J Am Acad Dermatol 39:262–267

Schindewolf T, Stolz W, Albert R, Abmayr W, Harms H (1993) Comparison of classification rates for conventional and dermatoscopic images of malignant and benign melanocytic lesions using computerized colour image analysis. Eur J Dermatol 3:299–303

Seidenari S, Pellacini G, Pepe P (1998) Digital videomicroscopy improves diagnostic accuracy for melanoma. J Am Acad Dermatol 39:175–181

Seidenari S, Pellacani G, Giannetti A (1999) Digital videomicroscopy and image analysis with automatic classification for detection of thin melanomas. Melanoma Res 9:163–171

Soyer HP, Smolle J, Hoedl S, Pachernegg H, Kerl H (1989) A new approach to the diagnosis of cutaneous pigmented tumors. Am J Dermatopathol 11:1–10

Soyer HP, Argenziano G, Chimenti S et al (2001) Dermoscopy of pigmented skin lesions. An atlas based on the consensus net meeting on dermoscopy 2000. EDRA Medical Publishing and New Media, Milan

Steiner A, Pehamberger H, Wolff K (1987) In vivo epiluminescence microscopy of pigmented skin lesions. II. Diagnosis of small pigmented skin lesions and early detection of malignant melanoma. J Am Acad Dermatol 17:584–591

Steiner A, Binder M, Schemper M, Wolff K, Pehamberger H (1993) Statistical evaluation of epiluminescence microscopy criteria for melanocytic pigmented skin lesions. J Am Acad Dermatol 29:581–588

Stolz W, Riemann A, Cognetta AB, Pillet L, Abmayr W, Hoelzel D et al (1994) ABCD rule of dermatoscopy: a new practical method for early recognition of malignant melanoma. Eur J Dermatol 4:521–527

Stolz W, Schiffner R, Pillet L, Vogt T, Harms H, Schindewolf T et al (1996) Improvement of monitoring of melanocytic skin lesions with the use of a computerized acquisition and surveillance unit with a skin surface microscopic television camera. J Am Acad Dermatol 35:202–207

Weinstock MA (1993) Epidemiology of melanoma. Cancer Treat Res 65:29–56

Weinstock MA (1998) Issues in the epidemiology of melanoma. Hematol Oncol Clin North Am 12:681–698

Wolff K, Binder M, Pehamberger H (1994) Epiluminescence microscopy: a new approach to the early detection of melanoma. Adv Dermatol 9:45–56

# Sentinel Node Biopsy: Not Only a Staging Tool?

Richard Essner and Alistair J. Cochran

## Abstract

The management of clinically negative regional lymph nodes in early-stage melanoma has been controversial for at least a century. While some surgeons offer elective lymph node dissection (ELND), others recommend treatment of the primary alone and only perform a therapeutic dissection (TLND) for cases of recurrence in the nodal basin. The rationale for ELND is based on the concept that metastases occur via the sequential passage of tumor from the primary site to the regional lymph nodes and then to more distant sites. If this theory is correct then early dissection of the regional lymph nodes will disrupt the metastatic cascade and prevent further spread of disease. On the other hand, advocates of the "wait and watch" approach suggest that metastases to the regional lymph node basin are only a marker of disease progression and that distant disease can occur in the absence of lymph node metastases. Four randomized prospective studies have examined the efficacy of ELND versus TLND. While all four studies have failed to demonstrate a survival advantage of ELND, there is some suggestion that patients with metastases in the regional basin may benefit from ELND.

As an alternative approach to this controversy, Morton and associates at the John Wayne Cancer Institute devised the technique of intraoperative lymphatic mapping and sentinel lymphadenectomy (LM/SL). This minimally invasive operative procedure allows the surgeon to identify the first or sentinel lymph (SN) in the regional basin. The technique is predicated on accurate mapping of the cutaneous lymphatics by lymphoscintigraphy and the intraoperative use of a vital blue dye to lead the surgeon to the SN and allow the pathologists to identify metastases in the lymph nodes. Patients with tumor-positive dissections would undergo complete lymph node dissection (CLND), and for those without metastases the complications and costs associated with

This work was supported by National Cancer Institute (USA) grant CA 29605 and funding from the Wrather Family Foundation and the Saban Family Foundation (Los Angeles, Calif.)

CLND could be avoided. The success of the procedure depends on the completion of a learning phase and on the cooperation of nuclear medicine physicians, surgeons, and pathologists. While this technique has become almost standard practice in the United States and around the world, we await the results of several important clinical trials to determine whether LM/SL will replace ELND or the wait and watch approach in the management of early-stage melanoma.

## Introduction

The controversy regarding the surgical management of the regional lymph nodes in early-stage melanoma began over 100 years ago. In 1892, Herbert L. Snow, in his lecture "Melanotic Cancerous Disease," advocated wide excision and elective lymph node dissection (ELND) as a method of controlling lymphatic permeation of metastases (Snow 1892). His studies suggested a direct connection of the primary site with the regional lymph nodes, indicating that treatment of melanoma should routinely include excision of the draining lymph nodes. ELND for patients with early-stage melanoma has remained controversial since Dr. Snow first proposed this management approach. Arguments in favor of it include the substantially better survival of patients with clinically negative, histologically positive lymph nodes than of patients with clinically apparent metastases to the regional lymph nodes (Balch et al. 1981, 1992; McCarthy et al. 1985; Morton et al. 1991; Reintgen et al. 1983; Roses et al. 1985). A major argument against ELND is that, if all individuals with high-risk melanoma are subjected to ELND, 70–80% will undergo an unnecessary surgical procedure that carries significant morbidity and a small possibility of operation-associated death. Multiple retrospective studies suggest a survival benefit for patients treated with ELND, and yet the therapeutic benefit of removing clinically normal lymph nodes has never been proven by randomized prospective studies (Balch et al. 1996; Cascinelli et al. 1998; Sim et al. 1986; Veronesi et al. 1977, 1982). Although ELND is considered a valuable staging procedure, its cost, morbidity, and overall low yield of tumor-containing nodes have led most surgeons to abandon this procedure as a routine part of patient care. The tumor status of the regional lymph nodes has become exceedingly important for determining patient prognosis and directing the use of adjuvant therapy (Kirkwood et al. 1996; Morton and Barth 1996).

In recent years, detection of occult regional lymph node metastases has been improved by intraoperative lymphatic mapping and sentinel lymphadenectomy (LM/SL). This technique, devised by Morton and associates at the John Wayne Cancer Institute, enables the surgeon to map the direct route of lymphatic spread from the primary lesion to the regional drainage basin and then selectively excise the first ("sentinel") lymph node(s) (SN) (Cochran et al. 1992; Morton et al. 1992 a). Because the SN has been shown to be the most likely site of tumor cells in the regional drainage basin, focused pathological examination of the SN specimen is a useful method of ultrastaging the regional nodes. LM/SL can be performed with minimal morbidity and expense, and has proven to be highly accurate and sensitive in detecting occult regional metastases in patients with early-stage melanoma.

## Methods

LM/SL is preceded by preoperative cutaneous lymphoscintigraphy. The technique was first devised from the work of Morton and his associates in 1977, when they reported on the use of intradermal injections of colloidal gold to document the lymphatic pathways from truncal melanoma (Robinson et al. 1977). Until that time, the lymphatic drainage patterns from these lesions were only predicted on the basis of the anatomical site of the primary. This study confirmed the belief held by many investigators that both dual and unexpected lymphatic patterns are common (Norman et al. 1991; Wanebo et al. 1985). With the development of LM/SL, cutaneous lymphoscintigraphy has been refined so that nuclear medicine physicians need to identify both the pattern of lymphatic drainage and the site of each SN. Cutaneous lymphoscintigraphy is performed in the United States primarily with technetium-99m ($^{99m}$Tc)-labeled sulfur colloid (SC), while other colloids are used in Europe and Australia. In brief, the procedure is performed with an intradermal injection of up to 18 MBq (0.5 mCi) radiopharmaceutical at the primary melanoma site or around the biopsy wound. Injections are given in four surrounding quadrants, and the skin is gently palpated to allow passage of the radiopharmaceutical into the lymphatics. A scintillation camera is used to document the drainage pattern from the primary to the dermal lymphatics and to the regional lymph nodes. The skin overlying the SN is marked. Because there is some variation in transit time of the radiopharmaceuticals to the regional lymph nodes, the nuclear medicine physician must perform dynamic images and be careful to differentiate SN from non-SN. We have found it quite useful for the nuclear medicine physicians to mark the body outline on the images. The outline provides a reference to the location and orientation of the SN. It is imperative that the surgeon is provided with these films while in the operating room.

In our experience the SN can be identified as early as 1 min and usually no later than 30 min after injection (depending on the agent and the distance between the primary and the regional nodes). By 4 h the SN can no longer be differentiated from the adjacent non-SN (Glass et al. 1998). We typically perform lymphoscintigraphy on the day of surgery, to allow the radiopharmaceutical to be used for intraoperative SN identification (Essner 1997). Lymphoscintigraphy is used to determine the regional lymph node basin at risk for metastases and is particularly helpful in sites on the head and neck or torso, which may have ambiguous lymph drainage (Shah et al. 1991).

Common problems encountered by the novice are: (1) excessive dose of radiopharmaceutical (dose should be ≤18 MBq, to avert unnecessary local radiation to the patient), (2) waiting too long to image after injection of the agent, (3) improper positioning of patient (e.g., not using oblique views of the axilla with the arm elevated), (4) not outlining the body on the images, and (5) not accurately and precisely marking the location of the SN on the skin (Glass et al. 1999). Attention to detail will result in accurate localization of the SN and provide the surgeon with a valid roadmap. It is also important that the surgeons understand the utility of cutaneous lymphoscintigraphy and the limitations of the images created (Bennett and Lagos 1983; Lock-Andersen et al. 1989; Sullivan et al. 1981).

## Intraoperative Mapping and Sentinel Lymphadenectomy

We prefer to perform the operative procedure on the same day as the lymphoscintigraphy. After induction of local or general anesthesia, 0.5–1.0 ml of isosulfan blue dye (Lymphazurin, Tyco International, Exeter, N.H., USA) is injected i.d. using a 25-G needle at the site of the primary melanoma. If the primary lesion has already been excised, the injection is given on either side of the scar. An incision is made over the regional lymph node basin and oriented so that a complete lymphadenectomy can be performed if needed. The skin flap closest to the primary is dissected free of the underlying tissue, and the subdermal lymphatics are observed as they and the SN turn blue. The blue dye typically takes 5–20 min to reach the regional nodes, and the transit time can usually be predicted from the distance between the primary and the dissected basin. The further apart the primary and regional lymph node basin, the greater the transit time. Injections are repeated every 20 min during the procedure if this is necessary to locate the SN. The SN is excised and evaluated for the presence of metastases (usually by permanent section analysis). If metastases are demonstrated CLND is performed at a later date.

In 1992 Morton and associates published their initial experience with LM/SL (Morton et al. 1992a; Cochran et al. 1992). They were able to identify a blue-stained SN in 194 (82%) of 237 regional lymphatic drainage basins. All 223 patients concerned underwent CLND regardless of the pathology of the SN. Of these specimens, 40 (21%) contained metastases in at least one lymph node. In only 2 of 194 CLND specimens were non-SN the exclusive site of regional metastases, a false-negative rate of 1%. These results are quite remarkable considering that in most cases preoperative lymphoscintigraphy was not used and the kinetics of the blue dye had not been well defined (Wong et al. 1991). Yet this early report demonstrates the strength of LM/SL as a staging procedure (Table 1).

LM/SL is a relatively difficult procedure, but its learning curve is steep. During their initial 58 cases, Morton identified only 81% of blue-stained SN; however, during the next 58 cases, his rate of SN identification increased to 96%, and it is now approaching 100%. The surgeon with the most experience with the procedure achieved an early success rate of 96%, while the surgeon with the least experience had the lowest level of success, 72% ($P < 0.01$). The gradual improvement in the rate of SN detection is partially based on the in-

**Table 1.** Results of blue-dye-directed sentinel lymphadenectomy for early-stage melanoma. Individual series demonstrate accuracy rates for sentinel node identification. In most studies, complete lymph node dissection (SCLND) was performed to verify the accuracy of the procedure

| Reference | N | Basins | SCLND all cases | Accuracy rate (%) |
|---|---|---|---|---|
| Morton et al. (1992a) | 223 | All | + | 82 |
| Morton et al. (1993) | 72 | Neck | + | 90 |
| Essner et al. (1993) | 128 | Groin | + | 97 |
| Reintgen et al. (1994) | 42 | All | + | 100 |
| Thompson et al. (1995) | 118 | All | + | 96 |
| Karakousis et al. (1996) | 55 | All | + | 93 |
| Belli et al. (1998) | 74 | All | – | 90 |

creased experience with the technique. We have found that the blue-stained afferent lymphatics and nodes can be difficult to identify. Most surgeons have little experience in dissecting the lymphatic channels prior to ever performing LM/SL. We have found that patients who have undergone wide excision of the primary with $\geq$1.5 cm margins or have had any procedure that disrupts the lymphatic drainage are not candidates for LM/SL (Kelemen et al. 1999).

In order to improve on the accuracy rate and diminish the learning curve for LM/SL, we devised the technique of radiopharmaceutical-directed LM/SL (Essner et al. 1994). Radiolymphoscintigraphy was first performed with a combination of blue dye injected intraoperatively and 18 MBq of $^{99m}$Tc HSA (approximately 0.5 cc) at the primary site. A hand-held gamma counter (Neoprobe 1000, Neoprobe, Dublin, Ohio) was used to follow the radioactive dye into the regional basin. Morton's group originally tested radiolymphoscintigraphy in 30 melanoma patients. Thirty-four lymph node basins were identified by preoperative lymphoscintigraphy. At least one SN was identified in each basin; the blue dye identified 36 SN, and the gamma probe detected all 36 nodes plus an additional six nodes. Overall, blue-stained SN had radioactive counts roughly 2-fold those of adjacent nonblue nodes, and up to an 8-fold the level of radioactivity in the lymph basin or background. Although none of the additional nodes contained metastatic disease, this study demonstrates the utility of the hand-held gamma counter to help identify blue-stained SN and the close concordance between the findings yielded by blue dye and by a radiopharmaceutical.

However, one of the difficulties with the combined technique is the logistics of injecting the radiopharmaceuticals in the operating room. Glass and associates at the John Wayne Cancer Institute examined the use of the three radiopharmaceuticals commonly used for lymphoscintigraphy, in the hope that this would provide some guidance as to which agents would best be suited for radiolymphoscintigraphy (Glass et al. 1998). They compared the three agents ($^{99m}$Tc AC, $^{99m}$Tc SC, and $^{99m}$Tc HSA) for their utility to identify the afferent lymphatics and SN. Using early (up to 30-min) images the three agents were equally effective for identifying the SN. On average two lymph nodes were identified in each basin. When they delayed their images up to 4 h after the injection of radiopharmaceutical the average number of nodes visualized did not change significantly. However, there appeared to be a wide variation from patient to patient in the number of lymph nodes seen by lymphoscintigraphy: [99m]Tc AC (range 1–7), [99m]Tc SC (range 1–14), and [99m]Tc HSA (range 0–9). The results from these experiences led the authors to examine the utility of all the three radiopharmaceuticals for radiolymphoscintigraphy.

Bostick and associates recently reviewed the John Wayne Cancer Institute experience with radiolymphoscintigraphy and LM/SL in 100 lymph node basins from 87 patients (Bostick et al. 1999a). All patients underwent lymphoscintigraphy with one of the three commonly used radiopharmaceuticals. LM/SL was performed with either concurrent injection of blue dye and [99m]Tc HSA or [99m]Tc SC injected up to 4 h before the operative procedure. One hundred thirty-six blue-stained and radioactive lymph nodes and eight additional non-blue-stained but hot nodes were removed in 98 lymph node basins (success rate 98%). A hand-held gamma probe (Neoprobe 1500) was used to determine the radioactive counts over the blue nodes, adjacent non-blue nodes, and an irrelevant background site. In 92% of the blue stained lymph nodes there was an in vivo count-to-background ratio of $\geq 2$, and 87% had in vivo count ratios $\geq 3$. There were metastases in 17 SN from 15 basins: 16 were located with blue dye and gamma probe, and 1 was found with blue dye alone. None of the tumor-positive lymph nodes were identified with gamma probe alone. Using the definition of a radioactive SN as having an in vivo count ratio $\geq 2$, a success rate of 85% would be achieved. When the in vivo count ratio was increased to $\geq 3$ to improve the specificity of the technique the success rate decreased to 78%. The concordance between the two techniques was not 100%. Not all blue-stained lymph nodes will have an elevated count ratio, and conversely not all nodes with an elevated count ratio will be blue. In fact when the in vivo count ratios were examined for all the blue-stained lymph nodes this revealed a wide variation between $<1$ and $100:1$. Similar results were observed when the ex vivo count ratio of the nodes was examined, suggesting that the radiopharmaceuticals alone can be misleading in LM/SL. Both of the radiopharmaceuticals were found to give similar count ratios for radiolymphoscintigraphy and lead to surgical excision of similar numbers of lymph nodes. At our center we have little difficulty with performing lymphoscintigraphy and LM/SL on the same day, but logistically this approach can be difficult. We believe concurrent use of the blue dye and [99m]Tc SC (filtered) injected on the same day lead to the highest level of concordance between the techniques and less doubt about the true SN (Table 2) (Essner et al. 2000).

**Table 2.** Accuracy rates for probe-assisted sentinel lymph node dissection. Multiple series demonstrate high accuracy rates for sentinel node dissection based on localizing a "hot" node. In many series, blue dye (+) was also employed

| Reference | N | Accuracy rate (%) | Blue dye |
|---|---|---|---|
| Krag et al. (1995) | 121 | 98 | +/- |
| Pijpers et al. (1995) | 41 | 100 | + |
| Mudun et al. (1996) | 13 | 100 | - |
| Albertini et al. (1996) | 106 | 96 | + |
| Thompson et al. (1997) | 21 | 100 | + |
| Bostick et al. (1997) | 23 | 98 | + |
| Leong et al. (1997) | 163 | 98 | + |
| Essner et al. (2000) | 247 | 98 | + |
| Murray et al. (2000) | 360 | 99 | – |
| Jansen et al. (2000) | 200 | 99 | + |

## Pathological Aspects

The pathological evaluation of the SN may be the most important component of the technique. Detection of micrometastatic disease in the lymph nodes has been made possible by the development of specific antibodies to melanoma-associated proteins, such as S-100 (Cochran et al. 1982, 1983; Gaynor et al. 1980, 1981; Moore 1965; Wen et al. 1983), HMB-45 (Gown et al. 1986), Melan-A (Chen et al. 1996; Fetsch et al. 1997), and NKI/C3 (Cochran et al. 1988), and our improved knowledge has led to more accurate expectations concerning the location of metastases in the nodes, which has reduced the number of pathology specimens that need to be evaluated. Prior to the development of LM/SL we demonstrated that conventional histology underestimated the number of patients with occult metastases in the regional nodes by 14%. Conventional histology also underestimated tumor positivity in ostensibly tumor-free nodes of patients with node-spread melanoma, by 30% (Cochran et al. 1988). In patients with nodal tumor identifiable only by immunohistology, the number of nodes containing occult tumor cells was small (usually only one or two) and the number of tumor cells present in an individual node was also small.

We developed the LM/SL technique by using intraoperative interpretation of frozen sections. Assessment of tumor status was based on evaluation of sections stained with hematoxylin and eosin (H&E) or with S-100 protein and HMB-45, using a rapid immunoperoxidase technique. If the SN was judged to be positive, CLND was undertaken. As the technique has evolved we have moved away from using frozen sections, believing that the "facing up" required to obtain a full-face frozen section preparation is wasteful of the tissue in which there is the greatest likelihood that occult tumor cells will be present (Cochran et al. 1988). Additionally, interpretation of H&E-stained frozen sections and sections stained by the rapid immunohistology approach is always more difficult, and thus more subject to error, than interpretation of well-fixed "permanent" material. We recommend that interpretation of SN be based on well-fixed full-face sections cut as close to the midline of the lymph node as possible.

There is a theoretical argument to be made that each SN should be serially sectioned to extinction, but such an approach would be impossibly expensive and is clearly impractical. Any practical approach to the SN must thus be a compromise between the ideal and the possible. Our present recommendation is that the lymph node is cut into two exactly equal halves through the longest circumference of the node. These two portions of the lymph node are placed cut face down in cassettes and fixed for at least 24 h. The technician is instructed to keep "facing-up" to a minimum. As soon as a full-faced section can be obtained, 10 serial sections are removed. Sections 1, 3, 5 (and possibly 10) are stained with H&E, section 2 for S-100 protein, and section 4 for HMB-45. Sections 6 and 7 are used for negative controls for the immunoperoxidase studies, and sections 8 and 9 are available to repeat any of the studies that are technically unsatisfactory or for additional immunohistochemistry. If suspicious or anomalous appearances are seen within the first 10 sections, additional groups of 10 sections can be examined (Fig. 1).

All SN must be examined by immunohistology using antibodies to S-100 protein and HMB-45 or Melan-A, unless the node contains overt tumor on gross inspection or review of H&E-stained slides. Immunohistology will always increase the frequency of SN found to contain tumor. The proportion of SN that requires immunohistology to identify occult tumor is decreasing sharply as pathologists gain experience in evaluating SN. This is the pathologists' equivalent of the surgeons' "learning curve."

Although we have found immunostaining essential for SN pathology, the technique has its pitfalls. S-100 protein is a highly robust marker for melanoma cells, staining virtually 100% of melanomas (Cochran et al. 1982; Wen et al. 1983). We look for epithelioid, oval, or spindle-shaped cells (usually located in the subcapsular sinus) which show S-100 protein positivity in both the cytoplasm and the nucleus. Other cells within the lymph nodes contain S-100 protein. The dendritic leukocytes of the paracortex are the most prominent of these confounding cells. Identification of these cells is not difficult in reactive paracortices where they are polydendritic. Difficulty may be encountered in inactive lymph nodes where the dendritic leukocytes show either minimal dendrite formation or none at all. S-100 protein positivity may also be found in capsular nevi (Carson et al. 1996) and in the Schwann cells of node-associated nerves (Cochran et al. 1997).

HMB-45 is a more specific marker for melanoma cells, but 10% and 15% of melanoma biopsies (especially metastatic melanoma) do not express this epitope. In contrast to S-100 protein, HMB-45-positive epitopes are confined to the cytoplasm. Antibodies to HMB-45 have the distinct advantage that they do not stain dendritic leukocytes and either do not stain capsular nevocytes or stain them at relatively low intensity. The antibody Melan-A may be used in a similar way to HMB-45, but suffers from the same defect that a proportion of melanomas do not stain positively with this reagent. We have

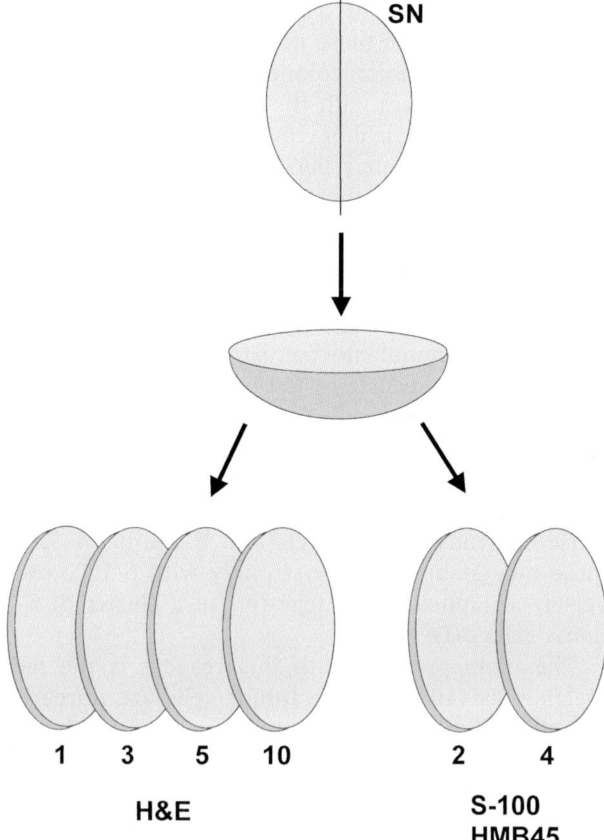


**Fig. 1.** Proposed scheme for evaluation of sentinel lymph nodes

utilized HMB-45 as our second antibody throughout the development of this technique and have found no compelling reason to change to Melan-A. One potential source of error with HMB-45 is that in lymph nodes with trabecular calcification (mainly in the groin or iliac area) extracellular HMB-45 reactivity may be seen.

In the initial series of LM/SL, SN identification was followed by CLND regardless of the tumor status of the SN. We evaluated 259 SN from 223 patients, an average of 1.2 SN per case. Tumor was identified in 47 of these 259 SN (18%). Tumor cells were identified by H&E alone in 83.2% of patients and in the remaining 16.7% by immunohistology alone. The tumor cells occurred as single cells, small clumps of tumor cells, and as larger colonies. We have found tumor in a non-SN in the absence of tumor in the SN in only 2 patients (1%), who were encountered very early in our experience with the technique.

Regardless of the tumor status of the SN, patients underwent CLND. We identified tumor-containing non-SN in 33% of patients with positive SN. We usually saw tumor in a single non-SN, less often in two or three. The amount of tumor in these non-SN is generally small and is distributed as single cells or small microcolonies, almost always in the subcapsular sinus.

A major problem with the immunostaining is the interpretation of S-100-positive dendritic leukocytes in the paracortex or sinuses. Dendritic leukocyte identification may be especially difficult if the dendritic leukocytes are nondendritic, as is often the case in immune-suppressed inactive SN. With good-quality immunohistochemical preparations, sinus macrophages do not stain for S-100 protein; however, if there is background staining these cells may present interpretative difficulties. Capsular nevocytes occur in more than 20% of patients undergoing LM/SL and are made more visible by means of immunohistochemistry. Capsular nevocytes are confined to the capsule and trabeculae of the lymph node. They are smaller and more cohesive than melanoma cells (with the possible exception of nevocytoid melanoma) and, while strongly S-100 protein-positive, express HMB-45 at a relatively weak level or not at all. Nevocytes often cluster around capsular vessels. The presence of neural tissue within the lymph node may occasionally cause difficulty in interpretation. If the nerve has associated Schwann cells, these may stain relatively strongly with S-100, and if the nerve is cut transversely an appearance suggestive of a cluster of S-100 protein-positive melanoma cells may result.

The main problem with this reagent is the fact that in a proportion of melanomas (10–15%) the tumor cells are unreactive with HMB-45. In hyalinized and calcified connective tissue within lymph nodes, especially lymph nodes from the groin and internal iliac areas, extracellular HMB-45 positivity may be seen and care is necessary to avoid overcalling this appearance.


## Discussion

LM/SL was devised as an alternative to either ELND or delayed therapeutic dissection for the management of the clinically negative lymph nodes in early-stage melanoma. The initial series from Morton and associates from the John Wayne Cancer Institute demonstrated the feasibility of this technique (Cochran et al. 1992; Morton et al. 1992 a, b).

A number of other investigators have also now reported their experience with LM/SL using blue dye alone (Reintgen et al. 1994; Thompson et al. 1995; Karakousis et al. 1996; Lingam et al. 1997). Most investigators with no prior experience of LM/SL achieved an accuracy rate of at least 90%. This relatively high rate of success is based on the more rapid learning of the technique through the experience gained by Morton and the other early pioneers of this procedure. The blue dye remains the gold standard for LM/SL.

In order to improve on the accuracy of LM/SL and diminish the learning curve of this procedure, a number of investigators have attempted to use radiopharmaceuticals for probe-directed LM/SL. Krag and associates were the first group to demonstrate a high success rate of SN identification with the use of a radiopharmaceutical alone (Krag et al. 1995). One hundred twenty-one patients underwent LM/SL, the majority with radiopharmaceutical alone. A SN was defined a node with at least 15 counts in 10 s and a count ratio three times background. Ninety-eight percent of patients had successful LM/SL. Yet the interval between injection of the radiopharmaceutical and surgery ranged from 15 min to 24 h. With this variation in technique we suspect that the true SN may have not always been properly identified. Other investigators have used an assortment of methods to define a radioactive SN (Table 2) (Albertini et al. 1996; Bostick et al. 1999a; Mudun et al. 1996; Pijpers et al. 1995). Our own data suggest that the in vivo count ratios for blue-stained lymph nodes can vary almost 100-fold even when surgery has been uniformly performed within 4 h after injection of the radiopharmaceutical (Bostick et al. 1999a). Although the use of radiopharmaceutical and probe alone for LM/SL would simplify the technique, our results with $^{99m}$Tc SC (filtered) suggest it is not ideal for this procedure. While larger particles, such as $^{99m}$Tc SC or AC, would be expected to be trapped in the afferent lymphatics of the SN, some of the particles are shunted through to adjacent lymph nodes. Similarly, our experience with $^{99m}$Tc HSA demonstrated that this agent passes quickly from the primary to the SN and to adjacent non-SN. The ideal radiopharmaceutical for this procedure would be one that travels quickly from the primary site to the SN and concentrates without leakage to adjacent lymph nodes. Until the kinetics of the radiopharmaceuticals are better defined for LM/SL, or better agents are developed, we recommend that these agents not be employed alone for LM/SL (Nathanson et al. 1997; Wong et al. 1997).

Most investigators now use blue dye and radiopharmaceuticals for LM/SL. Preoperative lymphoscintigraphy is performed using one of the colloid agents on the same day as surgery. At the time of surgery the hand-held gamma probe directs the surgeon to the site of the blue-stained SN. Occasionally the probe will lead the surgeon to an unexpected blue-stained lymph node (Joseph et al. 1997; Leong et al. 1997; Loggie et al. 1997; Miliotes et al. 1996; Reintgen et al. 1997; Nieweg et al. 1997; Van Der Veen et al. 1994). We have found the concordance between the two techniques to be at least 80%. While there are a variety of methods for defining a radioactive SN, a blue-stained lymph node remains the gold standard for this procedure.

The technique of LM/SL has been shown by a number of investigators to be a reliable indicator of the tumor status of the regional lymph nodes. Based on these studies LM/SL has become a popular alternative to conventional ELND and has become almost standard procedure for staging the regional lymph nodes. Yet, the successful performance of LM/SL is dependent on the experience of the multidisciplinary team of surgeon, pathologist and nuclear medicine physicians. We recommend that each team complete a learning phase of at least 15 cases (and perhaps up to 50) before LM/SL becomes routine procedure at any center (Morton 1997). Our studies clearly indicate that successful mapping of the SN is directly related to the surgeon's experience. While progressing through the learning phase the surgeon must perform CLND to monitor his or her own false-negative rate. Although the reported rates of missed SN is are extremely low, we have observed dissected basin recurrences as late as 5 years after negative LM/SL. The true accuracy rate of this technique has yet to be determined for the casual user. While this procedure has become increasingly popular, the therapeutic value is unproven.

Two major studies examining the utility of LM/SL are under way. In 1994 Morton and colleagues at the John Wayne Cancer Institute initiated an international multicenter randomized prospective trial comparing wide excision and LM/SL to wide excision alone in patients with clinical stage I melanoma (localized disease). Patients with intermediate (1–4 mm) thickness melanoma who have not had a wide excision (>1.5 cm margins), skin graft or other procedures that would alter the lymphatic drainage are eligible. CLND is performed only in lymphatic drainage basins containing tumor-positive SN. The purpose of this study is to determine the therapeutic benefit of LM/SL and the true accuracy of the technique on a large scale. As of August 2001 already 1826 patients had been accrued to the trial. The trial's organizers hope that LM/SL will eventually replace conventional ELND or the wait-and-watch approach as the standard of management for patients with clinical stage I melanoma (Morton et al. 1999). A second randomized prospective trial examines the efficacy of LM/SL as treatment for tumor-positive regional lymph nodes. The Sunbelt Melanoma Trial compares patients with one tumor-positive lymph node (following CLND) determined by conventional H&E or immunohistochemical techniques (followed by CLND) against those who are just observed or receive treatment with adjuvant interferon alpha (Schering-Plough, Kenilworth, N.J.). A second group of patients who had a tumor-positive SN on RT-PCR to melanoma associated gene products alone are randomized to observation, CLND, or CLND and interferon alpha. The organizer's of this study anticipate that this trial should provide further insight to the therapeutic value of LM/SL and the natural history for patients with a single tumor positive lymph node identified by either routine techniques or RT-PCR (Shivers et al. 1998; Bostick et al. 1999b).

Sentinel lymph node technology has become very widely adopted in the relatively few years since we first described the technique for application to melanoma. There is as yet no evidence that this approach is therapeutic. The technique certainly represents a considerable improvement in our ability to evaluate the tumor status of the regional lymph nodes for prognostication and may be useful in selecting patients for adjuvant therapy. Information as to the therapeutic relevance of the approach must await the outcome of the multicenter trials. While the concept of the approach is appealing and the techniques seem simple from the surgical, pathological and nuclear medicine standpoints, there are clearly pitfalls. The technique is also being used in a variety of other cancers, including breast cancer, colon cancer and vulvar carcinoma. It was previously applied to penile carcinoma (Cabanas 1977). While the broad lessons learned from our extensive experience with melanoma are likely to be applicable to other tumor systems, we urge caution and care in developing the techniques for each individual cancer system (Bilchik et al. 1998).

# References


Albertini JJ, Cruse CW, Rapaport D, et al (1996) Intraoperative radiolymphoscintigraphy improves sentinel lymph node identification for patients with melanoma. Ann Surg 223:217–224

Balch CM, Soong S-J, Murad TM, et al (1981) A multifactorial analysis of melanoma. III. Prognostic factors in melanoma patients with lymph node metastases (stage III). Ann Surg 193:377–388

Balch CM, Milton GW, Cascinelli N, Sim FH (1992) Elective lymph node dissection: pros and cons. In: Balch CM, Houghton AN, Milton GW, Sober AJ, Soong S-J (eds) Cutaneous melanoma, 2nd edn. Lippincott, Philadelphia, pp 345–366

Balch CM, Soong SJ, Bartolucci AA, Urist MM, Karakousis CP, Smith TJ, et al (1996) Efficacy of an elective regional lymph node dissection of 1 to 4 mm thick melanomas for patients 60 years of age and younger. Ann Surg 224:255–266

Belli F, Lenisa L, Clemente C, Tragni G, Mascheroni L, Gallino G, Cascinelli N (1998) Sentinel node biopsy and selective dissection for melanoma nodal metastases. Tumori 84:24–28

Bennett LR, Lago G (1983) Cutaneous lymphoscintigraphy in malignant melanoma. Semin Nucl Med 13:61–69

Bilchik AJ, Giuliano AE, Essner R, et al (1998) Universal application of intraoperative mapping and sentinel lymphadenectomy in solid neoplasms. Cancer J Sci Am 4:351–358

Bostick P, Essner R, Santarou T, Kelley M, Glass E, Foshag L, Stern S, Morton DL (1997) Intraoperative lymphatic mapping for early-stage melanoma of the head and neck. Am J Surg 174:536–539

Bostick PJ, Essner R, Glass E, Kelley M, Sarantou T, Foshag L, et al (1999a) Comparison of blue dye and probe-assisted intraoperative lymphatic mapping in melanoma to identify sentinel nodes in 100 lymphatic basins. Arch Surg 134:43–49

Bostick PJ, Morton DL, Turner RR, et al (1999b) Prognostic significance of occult metastases detected by sentinel lymphadenectomy and reverse transcriptase-polymerase chain reaction in early-stage melanoma patients. J Clin Oncol 17:3238–3244

Cabanas RM (1977) An approach to the treatment of penile carcinoma. Cancer 39:456–466

Carson KF, Wen D-R, Li P-X, Lana AM, Bailly C, Morton DL, Cochran AJ (1996) Nodal nevi and cutaneous melanomas. Am J Surg Pathol 20:834–840

Cascinelli N, Morabito A, Santinami M, Mackie RM, Belli F (1998) Immediate or delayed dissection of regional nodes in patients with melanoma of the trunk: a randomised trial. Lancet 351:793–796

Chen Y-T, Stockert E, Jungblith A, et al (1996) Serological analysis of Melan-A (MART-1), a melanocyte-specific protein homogenously expressed in human melanomas. Proc Natl Acad Sci USA 93:5915–5919

Cochran AJ, Wen D-R, Herschman HR, Gaynor RB (1982) Detection of S-100 protein as an aid to the identification of melanocytic tumors. Int J Cancer 30:295–297

Cochran AJ, Holland G, Wen D-R, Herschman HR, Lee WR, Straatsma BR (1983) Detection of S-100 protein in the diagnosis of primary and metastatic intraocular tumors. Invest Ophthalmol Vis Sci 24:1153–1155

Cochran AJ, Wen D-R, Morton DL (1988) Occult tumor cells in the lymph nodes of patients with pathological stage I malignant melanoma: an immunohistological study. Am J Surg Pathol 12:612–618

Cochran AJ, Wen DR, Morton DL (1992) Management of the regional lymph nodes in patients with cutaneous malignant melanoma. World J Surg 16:214–221

Cochran AJ, Bailly C, Paul E, Remotti F (1997) Melanocytic tumors: a guide to diagnosis. Lippincott-Raven, Philadelphia

Essner R (1997) The role of lymphoscintigraphy and sentinel node mapping in assessing patient risk in melanoma. Semin Oncol 24:S4–S10

Essner R, Wen DR, Cochran A, Morton DL, Ramming KP (1993) Lymphatic mapping and selective lymph node biopsy: an alternative to elective lymphadenectomy for early-stage melanomas of the trunk and lower extremity. Proc Am Soc Clin Oncol 12:396

tients with lymph node-confined disease in whom surgery might have an impact. It is hoped that, in the future, gene expression profiles of primary melanoma will help to pick out these patients. Multivariate analysis has shown that the sentinel node status is the most powerful prognostic factor in primary melanoma.

Sentinel node biopsy is a valuable tool for selecting patients for adjuvant treatments within the frame of clinical trials, in which micrometastatic and clinically involved lymph nodes are entered separately. In-transit metastases can be eradicated in 50% of cases by isolated limb perfusion with melphalan under mild hyperthermia. When in-transit metastases are recurrent, deep seated, or bulky, the combination of tumour necrosis factor (TNF) with melphalan and interferon gamma yields a complete response rate of around 80%. This is the first antiangiogenic treatment of cancer that is effective in clinical practice, but it has no effect on survival. Current better knowledge of melanoma biology indicates that local, limited surgery has an impact on local or regional spread only.

## Resection of Primary: Skin Margins

For many decades, standard practice was to perform a wide resection when removing a primary melanoma, because of its tendency to recur locally or regionally. Resection margins as wide as 5 cm from the melanoma border were applied. Surgical oncologists and dermatological surgeons believed, "It is better to have a large skin graft for ever than a small gravestone"! Thanks to a study of large databases, we have learned that a primary melanoma with a Breslow's thickness of 1.5 mm or more carries the risk that, within 5 years, regional lymph node metastases will develop in 20%, in-transit metastases in 5% and distant metastases in 20%, as the primary site of metastases. Therefore, it seemed better to remove the primary melanoma with minimal margins to keep the risk of local relapse as low as possible. The answer came from large-scale randomised studies.

The WHO Melanoma Group [14] undertook a comparison between margins of 3 cm and 1 cm for melanomas at any localisation and up to 2 mm thick. There were six recurrences in the small margins group and none in the wide margins group. However, there was no difference in survival between the two groups.

The American Melanoma Intergroup [2] studied limb melanomas between 2 and 4 mm thick. Randomization was between 2 and 4 cm margins. There were few recurrences, with similar recurrence rates in both groups and equivalent survival. On the basis of these trials, standard guidelines for melanoma resection margins can be summed up as follows: more than 3 cm is too much; 2 cm is enough for all primary melanomas 1 mm of more thick; 1 cm is enough for primary melanoma thinner than 1 mm.

## Regional Lymph Nodes

A frequent question is whether it is useful to remove impalpable lymph nodes. There is a speculative theory: if there are no palpable lymph nodes, there is still at least a 20% chance that, in patients with 1.5-mm-thick primary melanoma, regional lymph node metastases will develop within 5 years, and an "elective" regional lymph node dissection would eradicate microscopic lymph node metastases, preventing melanoma spread from extending beyond the first lymph node basin.

This theory needed to be evaluated in controlled studies. Four major randomised trials were published.

A WHO Melanoma Group worldwide randomised trial on limb melanoma of any thickness compared immediate elective lymph node dissection (ELND) and delayed lymph node dissection (DLND) – i.e. dissection when lymph node metastases appeared later [13]. There was no difference in survival. When this trial was designed, histological prognosis of melanoma was not yet established, and retrospective analyses were done after histological review of the slides. A trend for survival to be better was found in the intermediate-risk population with melanomas between 0.75 and 3 mm thick.

An American Intergroup study of patients with melanomas 2–4 mm thick showed no difference in overall survival, but retrospective subset analysis on nonulcerated melanoma showed some benefit [1].

A Mayo Clinic study [11] did not show any difference in survival, and the EORTC–WHO study on Isolated Limb Perfusion (ILP: see below), in which ELND was associated or not with ILP showed no influence of ELND on the survival curves [10].

It can be concluded that there is no evidence that ELND has any impact on survival. Subgroups retrospective analyses, although not methodologically orthodox, might suggest that some subpopulations of patients have regional micrometastases only and could hence benefit from lymph node dissection. Stringent criteria still need to be found.

The practice of ELND subjects patients to surgery that is unnecessary in up to 80% of cases and has significant side effects. One answer to this question emerged a decade ago: sentinel node biopsy. At present it appears to be the most powerful prognostic tool in melanoma [9].

If there are no palpable regional lymph nodes (N0), the histological status of the sentinel node is superior to Breslow's thickness as a prognostic indicator in multivariate analysis.

The clinical relevance of sentinel node biopsy has been covered in another paper during this congress (R. Essner, A. J. Cochran this volume). Briefly, our opinion is that this procedure is the most sensitive and accurate method allowing early detection of micrometastases. However, there is no evidence that sentinel node biopsy has any therapeutic value of its own. Currently, there is no evidence of improved survival after *selective* lymph node dissection. There are on-going studies [9] assessing the impact of sentinel node biopsy on survival, when it is followed by lymph node dissection in the case of a positive result, while observation alone is scheduled when it is negative. The value of the polymerase chain reaction is also being assessed in the "sunbelt" trial, in which patients are randomised to dissection or observation.

The main significance of sentinel node biopsy at present is as a selection criterion for controlled adjuvant treatment trials, where "true" stage II or III primary melanomas with negative sentinel nodes (N0) are separated off in a different stratification from those with positive sentinel node (N1).

## In-transit Melanoma Metastases of the Limbs

Approximately 5–10% of patients with high-risk limb melanoma develop in-transit metastases, i.e. lymph-borne metastases between the primary site and the lymph node drainage area. These metastases can increase in number and bulk, leading to haemorrhage, vascular compression and pain, sometimes to such an extent that amputation of the affected limb has to be considered. The method of mild hyperthermic isolated (ILP) perfusion with melphalan described by Stehlin [12] was in use by 1976 in most European centres. It was found to be safe and efficient, since toxicity was minimal and a substantial number of complete responses of unexcised metastases were observed. Complete responses were obtained in around 50% of the patients, a very high percentage compared with the few percent yielded by even the most effective systemic chemotherapy in melanoma [5].

Adding other chemotherapeutic drugs to melphalan does not seem to bring any benefit: it was reported that the addition of actinomycin-D to melphalan caused additional toxicity but no improvement of the therapeutic effect [5].

## Prophylaxis of In-transit Melanoma Metastases of the Limbs

Accepting the theory that melanoma progresses according to a stepwise order from the primary site to the regional lymph node basin, via the lymph channel, where satellite and in-transit metastases occur in about 5%, some authors designed isolated limb perfusion for in-transit metastases. It was used prophylactically against regional recurrences, both in primary melanoma and after resection of local recurrences or in-transit metastases. Uncontrolled studies were published, claiming a benefit, as survival curves were encouraging [5].

Therefore, adjuvant ILP with melphalan needed objective evaluation. A worldwide effort was devoted to the definitive assessment of the value of this sophisticated and expensive procedure. The EORTC Melanoma Group, the WHO Melanoma Programme and the North American Perfusion Group undertook a joint large-scale world multicentre phase III randomised study with 830 cases [10]. To be eligible, patients had to have a primary melanoma of a limb, which was required to be 1.5 mm thick or thicker. Patients were randomised to receive ILP with melphalan or not. All patients underwent wide excision of the primary site – i.e. with 3 cm margin – and the decision to perform or not perform an ELND was left to the local investigators' policy in all cases.

Patients were randomised to two groups: patients in arm 1 received ILP with melphalan under mild hyperthermia followed by resection of the primary site ± ELND; those in arm 2 underwent resection at the primary site only ± ELND.

The regional therapy was efficient in that ILP reduced the occurrence of in-transit metastases at the first recurrence site from 6% to 2.5%. There was a trend for disease-free survival to be longer after ILP, and there was no difference in overall survival.

It was concluded that prophylactic ILP with melphalan cannot be recommended as an adjunct to standard surgery in high-risk primary melanoma. Prophylactic ILP has now been abandoned by most centres in Europe.

## ILP with Tumour Necrosis Factor Is an Efficient Antiangiogenic Therapy of In-transit Melanoma Metastases of the Limbs

Cancer growth depends on angiogenesis which is promoted by angiogenic factors secreted by tumour cells. Old et al. discovered that tumour necrosis factor alpha (TNF) acted through a selective destruction of the tumour microvasculature. Most tumour models and human model xenografts on nude mice have shown that TNF has only a transient antitumour effect, because there is regrowth of the tumour after its necrosis. It was shown, however, that a definitive cure could be obtained in animals by combining TNF either with chemotherapeutic agents or with interferon (IFN) gamma. The effective dose of TNF in mice is around 50 µg/kg, and the maximal tolerated dose (MTD) is 350 µg/m$^2$ or 5 µg/kg. This one-tenth dose produced only anecdotal responses in humans. TNF causes a general vasoplegia leading to a decrease in vascular resistance. In 1988 we designed a protocol for the regional application of TNF by ILP with a dose of 10 times the MTD in humans and equivalent to the effective dose in animals: 3 mg for an upper limb and 4 mg for a lower limb, combined with 0.2 mg of IFN gamma and a high dose of melphalan (10 mg/l of limb volume for a lower limb and 13 mg/l of limb volume for an upper limb) [3, 6]. The first multicentre phase II study of this triple combination (TIM-ILP) yielded a 100% objective response rate, with 90% of complete responses [7].

The role of IFN gamma in this setting was evaluated by comparing TIM-ILP against TM (TIM minus IFN)-ILP in a randomised phase II trial. Results showed a 10% drop in the complete response rate when IFN gamma was omitted, but this difference was not statistically significant. A comparison with matched cases retrieved from a databank confirmed that melphalan only led to complete responses in 52% of cases [8]. Other European teams evaluated the double combination of TNF with melphalan, without IFN gamma (TM-ILP), and found a complete response rate ranging from 60% to 70% and an overall response (complete + partial) rate of 80–90% [4].

Despite the high response rates, TIM-ILP and TM-ILP are regional treatment modalities and have no impact on survival: survival curves of patients treated with melphalan alone and TNF-treated patients were similar, with a median survival of 2.5–5 years.

Further studies addressed the influence of tumour bulk on the complete response rate. The data from the Italian group and from the Boehringer Ingelheim databank (unpublished, 1999) showed a trend in favour of higher response rates after TNF and melphalan than after melphalan alone in bulky tumours, whilst small tumours seem to respond in a similar way to either of the two treatments. This is not surprising, since large tumours depend upon a more extensive and fragile angiogenesis. Current opinion is that ILP with TNF should be reserved for bulky melanoma metastases or for recurrences after ILP with melphalan alone.

## Future Prospects

With the new avenues that are opening up, such as molecular biology and immunology of melanoma, the role of surgery is changing: fresh tissue samples are essential for progress in these methods, and it is hoped that immunotherapy of melanoma will follow less aggressive but adequate surgery.

## References


1. Balch CM, Soong SJ, Bartolucci AA, Urist MM, Karakousis CP, Smith TJ, Temple WJ, Ross MI, Jewell WR, Mihm MC, Barnhill RL, Wanebo HJ (1996) Efficacy of an elective regional lymph node dissection of 1 to 4 mm thick melanomas for patients 60 years of age and younger. Ann Surg 224:255–263; discussion 263–256
2. Balch CM, Soong SJ, Smith, T, Ross MI, Urist MM, Karakousis CP, Temple WJ, Mihm MC, Barnhill RL, Jewell WR, Wanebo HJ, Desmond R (2001) Long-term results of a prospective surgical trial comparing 2 cm vs. 4 cm excision margins for 740 patients with 1–4 mm melanomas. Ann Surg Oncol 8:101–108
3. Lejeune FJ (1995) High dose recombinant tumour necrosis factor (rTNF alpha) administered by isolation perfusion for advanced tumours of the limbs: a model for biochemotherapy of cancer. Eur J Cancer 31:1009–1016
4. Lejeune FJ, Ruegg, C, Liénard D (1998) Clinical applications of TNF-alpha in cancer. Curr Opin Immunol 10:573–580
5. Lejeune FJ, Kroon B, Di Filippo F, Hoekstra HJ, Santinami M, Liénard D, Eggermont AMM (2001) Isolated limb perfusion: the European experience. Surg Clin North Am 10:821–832
6. Liénard D, Ewalenko P, Delmotte JJ, Renard N, Lejeune FJ (1992) High-dose recombinant tumor necrosis factor alpha in combination with interferon gamma and melphalan in isolation perfusion of the limbs for melanoma and sarcoma. J Clin Oncol 10:52–60
7. Liénard D, Eggermont AM, Schraffordt Koops H, Kroon BB, Rosenkaimer F, Autier P, Lejeune FJ (1994) Isolated perfusion of the limb with high-dose tumour necrosis factor-alpha (TNF-alpha), interferon-gamma (IFN-gamma) and melphalan for melanoma stage III. Results of a multi-centre pilot study. Melanoma Res 4 [Suppl 1]:21–26

8.  Liénard D, Eggermont AM, Koops HS, Kroon B, Towse G, Hiemstra S, Schmitz P, Clarke J, Steinmann G, Rosenkaimer F, Lejeune FJ (1999) Isolated limb perfusion with tumour necrosis factor-alpha and melphalan with or without interferon-gamma for the treatment of in-transit melanoma metastases: a multicentre randomized phase II study. Melanoma Res 9:491–502

9.  Morton DL, Ollila DW (1999) Critical review of the sentinel node hypothesis. Surgery 126:815–819

10. Schraffordt Koops HS, Vaglini M, Suciu S, Kroon BB, Thompson JF, Gohl J, Eggermont AM, Di Filippo F, Krementz ET, Ruiter D, Lejeune FJ (1998) Prophylactic isolated limb perfusion for localized, high-risk limb melanoma: results of a multicenter randomized phase III trial. (European Organization for Research and Treatment of Cancer Malignant Melanoma Cooperative Group Protocol 18832, the World Health Organization Melanoma Program Trial 15, and the North American Perfusion Group Southwest Oncology Group-8593) J Clin Oncol 16:2906–2912

11. Sim FH, Taylor WF, Pritchard DJ, Soule EH (1986) Lymphadenectomy in the management of stage I malignant melanoma: a prospective randomized study. Mayo Clin Proc 61:697–705

12. Stehlin JS, Giovanella BC, de Ipolyi PD, Muenz LR, Anderson RF (1975) Results of hyperthermic perfusion for melanoma of the extremities. Surg Gynecol Obstet 140:339–348

13. Veronesi U, Adamus J, Bandiera DC, Brennhovd O, Caceres E, Cascinelli N, Claudio F, Ikonopisov RL, Javorski VV, Kirov S, Kulakowski A, Lacour J, Lejeune F, Mechl Z, Morabito A, Rode I, Sergeev S, van Slooten E, Szczygiel K, Trapeznikov NN, Wagner RI (1982) Delayed regional lymph node dissection in stage I melanoma of the skin of the lower extremities. Cancer 49:2420–2430

14. Veronesi U, Cascinelli N, Adamus J, Balch C, Bandiera D, Barchuk A, Bufalino R, Craig P, De Marsillac J, Durand JC, et al (1988) Thin stage I primary cutaneous malignant melanoma. Comparison of excision with margins of 1 or 3 cm. N Engl J Med 318:1159–1162

# Perspectives of Pegylated Interferon Use in Dermatological Oncology

Hubert Pehamberger

## Abstract

The potent immunomodulatory, antiproliferative and antiviral properties of interferons (IFNs), together with their availability in large amounts thanks to the recombinant DNA technique, have resulted in their widespread clinical use in a variety of viral and nonviral proliferative disorders. In dermato-oncology, IFNs have been used primarily in melanoma, but also in nonmelanoma skin cancer, such as squamous and basal cell carcinomas, Kaposi sarcomas and lymphomas. Trials with IFNs have been performed in patients with melanoma in an adjuvant setting (stage II and III) and in metastatic disease (stage IV). While the response rates with IFNs as single agents in stage IV disease usually do not exceed 15%, the use of adjuvant IFNs has been claimed to increase disease-free survival (stage II), or even overall survival (stage III), in low- or high-dose regimens, respectively; the latter, however, involved numerous side-effects and were beset with lack of compliance and acceptance, as well as being very costly.

Pegylated IFN (PEG-IFN) is a form of recombinant human IFN that has been chemically modified by the covalent attachment of a branched metoxy-polyethylene glycol moiety. Pharmacogenetic and pharmacodynamic data obtained in animal and in phase I studies have indicated that PEG-IFN injected once a week has the potential to be superior in efficacy to human IFN injected three times a week. The safety profiles of PEG-IFN and IFN are comparable in healthy volunteers and in chronic hepatitis C (CHC) patients.

PEG-IFN is currently being evaluated for the treatment of CHC, renal cell carcinoma, chronic myelogenous leukaemia, and malignant melanoma, the last in both stage IV and stage III disease.

Recent Results in Cancer Research, Vol. 160
© Springer-Verlag Berlin Heidelberg 2002

## Interferons in Dermato-oncology

Interferons (IFNs) are a group of naturally occurring biological response modifiers that the recombinant DNA technique has now made available commercially for therapeutic purposes. After binding to specific cell surface receptors, IFNs activate cellular responses that have antiviral, antiproliferative, immunomodulatory and differentiating effects (Borden 1998; Edwards 2001).

The IFNs have been extensively studied in a variety of diseases and have been shown to exhibit therapeutic activity in dermato-oncological conditions, such as AIDS-associated Kaposi's sarcoma, basal cell carcinoma and cutaneous T-cell lymphoma (CTCL). In a phase I clinical study of 14 patients with stage II CTCL treated with combination therapy consisting of IFN-$\alpha$2a and extracorporeal photochemotherapy a total response rate of 56% was achieved (Wollina et al. 2001). Wennberg (2000) recently reviewed and reported on the efficacy of intralesional IFN-$\alpha$2b in patients with basal cell carcinoma. Four out of 15 patients were healed completely, and a 75% reduction was seen in 5 cases, with no serious side effects (Wennberg 2000). Dezube (2000) outlined the antineoplastic and antiretroviral efficacy of IFN-$\alpha$ in Kaposi's sarcoma. Of particular importance, however, is the emerging use of IFN-$\alpha$ in patients with high-risk melanoma.

Standard treatment for malignant melanoma is early detection and surgical excision, which cures 90% of cases, and the noninvasive technique of epiluminescence microscopy is one method that may improve diagnosis (Pehamberger et al. 1993). However, once the tumour has progressed, the chances of survival fall dramatically, with less than 3–5% of patients with stage IV disease surviving for longer than 5 years (Balch 2001).

Although it is generally agreed that the response rates to IFN in metastatic melanoma do not exceed 15%, accumulating clinical trial data support the use of adjuvant IFN-$\alpha$ treatment in patients with high-risk melanoma without evidence of metastases (Eggermont 2001; Grob et al. 1998; Kirkwood et al. 1996, 2000, 2001; Pehamberger et al. 1998; Wheatley et al. 2001). To date, two IFNs are approved for adjuvant use, IFN-$\alpha$2a (Roferon-A) and IFN-$\alpha$2b (Intron-A).

The first study, by Kirkwood et al. (1996), assessed relapse-free and overall survival in high-risk (stage IIb/III) resected melanoma patients treated with high-dose adjuvant IFN-$\alpha$ (induction dose of 20 MIU/m$^2$ daily for 1 month followed by 10 MIU/m$^2$ three times weekly for 48 weeks), compared with observation alone. Although in terms of relapse-free survival (RFS) (median increased from 1.0 to 1.7 years) and overall survival (OS) (median increased from 2.8 to 3.8 years) IFN-$\alpha$ had significant clinical benefit; the regimen was also associated with significant toxicity, indicating the need to investigate more tolerable IFN-$\alpha$-based regimens (Kirkwood et al. 1996).

In 1998 two studies appeared that demonstrated the effect of low-dose IFN-$\alpha$ in patients with no evidence of lymph node metastases (Grob et al. 1998; Pehamberger et al. 1998). Grob et al. studied IFN-$\alpha$2a as adjuvant therapy in patients with primary cutaneous melanoma. All patients in this phase

III trial ($n = 489$) had undergone surgical resection of a tumour thicker than 1.5 mm; 78% and 22% of the patients had AJCC clinical stage IIa and IIb, respectively. No patients had clinically detectable node metastases. Patients were randomised to receive either $3 \times 10^6$ IU (MIU) IFN-$\alpha$2a, s.c. three times weekly ($n = 244$) for 18 months or to observation alone ($n = 249$). Grob et al. confirmed that IFN-$\alpha$2a was significantly beneficial in terms of the disease-free interval ($P = 0.038$). A long-term analysis, after a median follow-up of 5 years, showed significantly longer RFS ($P = 0.035$) and a clear trend towards longer OS ($P = 0.059$) than in controls. Only 10% of patients experienced WHO grade 3 or 4 adverse events. Grob et al. concluded that adjuvant therapy of high-risk melanoma, with low doses of IFN-$\alpha$2a for 18 months, is safe and beneficial (Grob et al. 1998).

Pehamberger et al. (1998) studied the effects of adjuvant IFN-$\alpha$2a therapy compared with observation alone in a phase III prospective study. A total of 311 melanoma patients with a Breslow thickness $\geq 1.5$ mm and no clinically detectable lymph node involvement were randomised to receive either adjuvant IFN-$\alpha$2a treatment ($n = 154$) or observation ($n = 157$) following excision of the primary tumour. IFN-$\alpha$2a was given daily at a dose of 3 MIU s.c. for 3 weeks (induction phase), after which a dose of 3 MIU s.c. three times weekly was given over 1 year (maintenance phase). Significantly improved RFS was seen in the IFN-$\alpha$2a group ($P = 0.02$) compared with observation. Some 24% (37/154) of patients treated with IFN-$\alpha$2a relapsed, compared with 36% (57/157) in the control group. The mean observation period was 41 months, and every patient had at least 1 year of follow-up evaluation. Treatment-related side effects were limited primarily to WHO grades 1 and 2, a dose reduction being needed in 8 patients. Pehamberger et al. concluded that adjuvant IFN-$\alpha$2a treatment diminishes the occurrence of metastases, thus significantly prolonging disease-free survival (DFS) in stage II cutaneous melanoma patients (Pehamberger et al. 1998).

In the second paper Kirkwood et al. (2000) report on a phase III prospective, randomised, three-arm, intergroup trial evaluating the efficacy of high-dose IFN-$\alpha$2b (HDI) for 1 year and low-dose IFN-$\alpha$2b (LDI: 3 MIU three times weekly) for 2 years versus observation in high-risk (stage IIb and III) melanoma patients. A total of 642 patients were enrolled, and 608 proved eligible. At 52 months' median follow-up, HDI was superior to LDI in extending RFS. The 5-year estimated RFS rates for the HDI, LDI, and control arms were 44%, 40%, and 35%, respectively. The impact of HDI on RFS was significant ($P = 0.03$), and the benefit was equivalent for node-negative and node-positive patients. However, neither HDI nor LDI demonstrated an OS benefit (Kirkwood et al. 2000).

Evidence for a beneficial effect of HDI on OS came from a later study by this same group (Kirkwood et al. 2001). A large trial compared RFS and OS in patients receiving HDI versus antiganglioside GM2 melanoma vaccine. The patients enrolled in the trial had undergone resection of stage IIb/III melanoma and were stratified by sex and number of positive nodes. This trial demonstrated a significant benefit of HDI versus GM2 in terms of both RFS

(HR = 1.47, $P$ = 0.0015) and OS (HR = 1.52, $P$ = 0.009). The highly significant benefit of HDI compared with GMK forced the closure and unblinding of the trial after a median follow-up of 16 months. This large trial confirmed the benefit of HDI in terms of RFS that had already been observed in two earlier trials (Kirkwood et al. 1996, 2000), but in addition it provided evidence of an OS benefit.

Further efforts at refining the most tolerable and effective IFN-$\alpha$ regimen are being carried out by the European Organisation for Research and Treatment of Cancer (EORTC) Melanoma Group. Preliminary results of study EORTC 18952 have been reported (Eggermont 2001). This trial randomised 1418 patients with stage IIb/III melanoma to receive 10 MIU IFN-$\alpha$ daily for 4 weeks (induction) followed by either 10 MIU three times weekly for 1 year (group A) or 5 MIU three times weekly for 2 years (group B). These two active groups were compared with a third, in which observation alone was carried out (group C). The primary endpoint of distant-metastasis-free interval (DMFI) was not significantly affected in group A, but was significantly extended in group B ($P$ = 0.026, median follow-up of 1.6 years) compared with group C. Both regimens were relatively well tolerated. Dose-limiting adverse events were typical of IFN-$\alpha$ therapies, and grade-3 to grade-4 haematological, hepatic, cardiovascular and renal toxicities occurred in under 2% of patients. This study suggests that longer term maintenance therapy may significantly enhance clinical outcome and further emphasises the need for more tolerable regimens.

A recent meta-analysis of ten trials provides clear evidence for reduced risk of disease recurrence with adjuvant IFN-$\alpha$ treatment of melanoma (odds ratio 0.84, 95% CI = 0.77–0.92, $P$ = 0.0001) (Wheatley et al. 2001). Results for overall survival were less clear. There was no statistically significant evidence to show that high-dose IFN-$\alpha$ regimens were any more effective than lower dose regimens in these trials (Wheatley et al. 2001).

Despite clear therapeutic value, the clinical use of IFNs is impeded by their molecular size, which is correlated to their pharmacokinetic properties. IFN-$\alpha$ has a short plasma half-life owing to rapid clearance, enzymatic degradation, and innate immunogenic reactions (Wills 1990). This requires standard IFN-$\alpha$ to be administered frequently. Regimens usually require s.c. injections three times a week (low-dose interferon, LDI) or i.v. administration of high doses (high-dose IFN, HDI). However, even with daily administration, serum concentrations are not maintained over 24 hours; as well as limiting systemic exposure and therefore potential efficacy, the large peak-to-trough ratio caused by rapid clearance is associated with a number of acute side effects (Edwards 2001). Pioneering research has established the importance of pegylation to overcome these limitations and extend the clinical utility of IFNs.

## Pegylation: Enhancing the Clinical Utility of IFNs

Polyethylene glycol (PEG) is a chemically versatile yet biologically inert polymer, with both hydrophilic and hydrophobic features (Delgado et al. 1992). The attachment of PEG – pegylation – is an established method of altering the pharmacokinetic and pharmacodynamic properties of therapeutic proteins (Delgado et al. 1992; Francis et al. 1998). Chemical modification using PEG produces biologically active conjugates that can be used as unique pharmacological agents. These modified molecules exert enhanced therapeutic characteristics, whilst their main biological functions, such as enzymatic activity, are maintained (Veronese 2001).

PEG-IFNs have shown significant clinical value in hepatitis C (Zeuzem et al. 2000; Heathcote et al. 2000). Two PEG-IFNs, PEG-IFN-$\alpha$2a (PEGASYS), a large (40 kDa) branched structure, and PEG-IFN-$\alpha$2b (PEG-INTRON), a 12 kDa linear structure, are available. It has been shown down that once-weekly PEG-IFN-$\alpha$2a is more effective than three-times weekly IFN-$\alpha$2a (Zeuzem et al. 2000).

Data from Heathcote et al. (2000) substantiate this evidence of increased convenience and efficacy with PEG-IFN-$\alpha$2a in patients with hepatitis C and cirrhosis. In both of these trials the therapeutic level of PEG-IFN-$\alpha$2a was sustained at close-to-peak levels for a complete week (168 hours) after dose administration.

The efficacy, safety and tolerability – particularly the improvement in quality of life demonstrated with large, branched PEG-IFN-$\alpha$2a – shown in these trials demonstrates the benefit of PEG-IFNs in the clinical setting.

## Peg-IFNs: Extending Clinical Efficacy in Oncology

Enthusiasm for extending the benefits of pegylation to the oncology setting is emerging. Key features of this specific pegylation, such as a 100-fold increase in elimination half-life compared with IFN-$\alpha$ and sustained plasma absorption, will allow genuine once-weekly dosing and an improved tolerability profile (Motzer et al. 2001).

Indeed, PEG-IFN-$\alpha$2a has shown considerable potential in the treatment of advanced renal cell carcinoma (RCC) (Motzer et al. 2001). A phase I study by Motzer et al. was designed to determine the clinically effective dose of PEG-IFN in RCC and to establish the maximum tolerated dose (450 µg and 540 µg, respectively). It also suggests that PEG-IFN-$\alpha$2a has potential antitumour activity (Motzer et al. 2001). Therefore, although higher doses of PEG-IFN-$\alpha$2a are used, the benefits shown in CHC seem to remain. The pharmacokinetic and pharmacodynamic properties of PEG-IFN-$\alpha$2a shown in this trial suggest that it might be of potential use in the treatment of skin cancer, particularly melanoma.

There is an obvious need for more effective and more tolerable treatments for high-risk and metastatic melanoma. PEG-IFN-α2a has significant potential to advance the therapeutic treatment of this often refractory disease. This hypothesis is currently being tested in a phase II multicentre trial (Roche, protocol number NO16007). The trial aims to assess the tolerability, safety and efficacy of PEG-IFN-α2a as monotherapy in patients with stage IV melanoma. The EORTC Melanoma Cooperative Group performs a randomised trial (18991) comparing PEG-INTRON versus observation after regional lymph node dissection in ASCC stage III melanoma patients.

## Conclusion

Substantial evidence now confirms the benefits of adjuvant IFN a therapy in melanoma patients (Eggermont 2001; Grob et al. 1998; Kirkwood et al. 1996, 2000, 2001; Pehamberger et al. 1998; Wheatley et al. 2001). However, there is still much scope for improvement. Tolerability of long-term adjuvant immunotherapy is an important issue, as is the selection of patients most likely to benefit from such regimens. The recent refinements to the staging system (Balch 2001) will allow more accurate assessments of the benefits of immune therapy in subgroups of patients enrolled in clinical trials. This is where the therapeutic use of PEG-IFNs in melanoma could be beneficial. Pegylation is an efficient technique to enhance the pharmacokinetic and pharmacodynamic properties of therapeutic biological molecules. Significant evidence confirms that PEG modification extends the clinical benefits of interferons and allows more advantageous dosing schedules with fewer and less severe side effects and improved tolerability of therapeutic agents (Edwards 2001). PEG-IFN-α therapies offer the hope of overcoming the limitations of standard IFN treatment in melanoma and further improving its clinical management.

## References

Balch CM (2001) The revised melanoma staging system: its use in the design and interpretation of melanoma clinical trials. Paper presented at the 37th annual meeting of the American Society of Clinical Oncology, 12–15 May, San Francisco, Calif; 2001 Educational Book, pp 82–87

Borden EC (1998) Gene regulation and clinical roles for interferons in neoplastic diseases. Oncologist 3:198–203

Delgado C, Francis GE, Fisher D (1992) The uses and properties of PEG-linked proteins. Crit Rev Ther Drug Carrier Syst 9:249–304

Dezube BJ (2000) New therapies for the treatment of AIDS-related Kaposi's sarcoma. Curr Opin Oncol 12:445–449

Edwards L (2001) The interferons. Dermatol Clin 19:139–146

Eggermont AMM (2001) European Organization for Research and Treatment of Cancer Melanoma Group trial experience with more than 2000 patients, evaluating adjuvant treatment with low or intermediate doses of interferon alpha-2b. Paper presented at the 37th annual meeting of the American Society of Clinical Oncology, 12–15 May, San Francisco, Calif; 2001 Educational Book, pp 88–93

Francis GE, Fisher D, Delgado C, Malik F, Gardiner A, Neale D (1998) PEGylation of cytokines and other therapeutic proteins and peptides: the importance of biological optimisation of coupling techniques. Int J Hematol 68:1–18

Grob JJ, Dreno B, de al Salmoniere P, et al (1998) Randomised trial of interferon alpha-2a as adjuvant therapy in resected primary melanoma thicker than 1.5 mm without clinically detectable node metastases. French Cooperative Group on Melanoma. Lancet 351:1905–1910

Heathcote EJ, Shiffman ML, Cooksley WG, et al (2000) Peginterferon alfa-2a in patients with chronic hepatitis C and cirrhosis. N Engl J Med 343:1673–1680

Kirkwood JM, Strawderman MH, et al (1996) Interferon alfa-2b adjuvant therapy of high-risk resected cutaneous melanoma: the Eastern Cooperative Oncology Group Trial EST 1684. J Clin Oncol 14:7–17

Kirkwood JM, Ibrahim JG, Sondak VK, et al (2000) High- and low-dose interferon alfa-2b in high risk melanoma: first analysis of intergroup trial E1690/S9111/C9190. J Clin Oncol 18:2444–2458

Kirkwood JM, Ibrahim JG, Sosman JA, Sondak VK, et al (2001) High-dose interferon alfa-2b significantly prolongs relapse-free and overall survival compared with the GM2-KLH/QS-21 vaccine in patients with resected stage IIB-III melanoma: results of intergroup trial E1694/S9512/C509801. J Clin Oncol 19:2370–2380

Motzer RJ, Rakhit A, Ginsberg M, et al (2001) Phase I trial of 40-kda branched, pegylated interferon alfa-2a for patients with advanced renal cell carcinoma. J Clin Oncol 19:1312–1319

Pehamberger H, Binder M, Steiner A, Wolff K (1993) In vivo epiluminescence microscopy. Improvement of early diagnosis of melanoma. J Invest Dermatol 100:356–362

Pehamberger H, Soyer H, Steiner A, et al (1998) Adjuvant interferon alfa-2a in resected primary stage II cutaneous melanoma. Austrian Malignant Melanoma Cooperative Group. J Clin Oncol 16:1425–1429

Veronese FM (2001) Peptide and protein PEGylation: a review of its problems and solutions. Biomaterials 22:405–417

Wennberg AM (2000) Basal cell carcinoma – new aspects of diagnosis and treatment. Acta Derm Venereol 209:5–25

Wheatley K, Hancock B, Gore M, Suciu S, Eggermont A (2001) Interferon-$\alpha$ as adjuvant therapy for melanoma: a meta-analysis of the randomised trials. Proceedings of the ASCO, thirty-seventh annual meeting, 12–15 May, San Francisco, Calif., vol 20 (part 1), p 349a (abstract 1394)

Wills RJ (1990) Clinical pharmacokinetics of interferons. Clin Pharmacokinet 19:390–399

Wollina U, Looks A, Meyer J, et al (2001) Treatment of stage II cutaneous T-cell lymphoma with interferon alfa-2a and extracorporeal photochemotherapy: a prospective controlled trial. J Am Acad Dermatol 44:253-260

Zeuzem S, Feinman SV, Rasenack J, et al (2000) Peginterferon alfa-2a in patients with chronic hepatitis C. N Engl J Med 343:1666–1672

# Dendritic Cell Vaccination for the Treatment of Skin Cancer

Frank O. Nestle

## Abstract

Reasons for failure of the immune system to fight cancer include tumor immune escape mechanisms, limited availability of tumor-specific antigens, and failure to deliver tumor antigens in the right immunological context. Progress in molecular biology and immunology has provided technologies that can detect an ever-widening choice of new tumor-specific antigens. One of the most important questions remains the delivery of these tumor antigens in an effective way to the immune system of a cancer patient. This task is performed in normal circumstances by dendritic cells (DCs). DCs are sentinels of the immune system located at sites of antigen entry such as skin. They take up antigen and carry it to secondary lymphoid organs. They are highly specialized antigen-presenting cells (APCs) for the activation of specific effector T cells recirculating in secondary lymphoid organs. In recent years an enormous increase in our understanding of DC biology has opened up new ways of applying these cells for immunotherapy of cancer.

**Abbreviations.**   *APC*, antigen presenting cell; *CR*, complete remission, *CTL*, cytotoxic T-lymphocyte; *DC*, dendritic cell; *DDC*, dermal dendritic cell; *DTH*, delayed-type hypersensitivity; *FLT-3*, fms-like tyrosine kinase 3; *FCS*, fetal calf serum; *GM-CSF*, granulocyte/macrophage-colony stimulating factor; *HLA*, histocompatibility leukocyte antigen; *IFN*, interferon; *CR*, complete response; *IL*, interleukin; *KLH*, keyhole limpet hemocyanin; *LC*, Langerhans cell; *MHC*, major histocompatibility complex; *MoDC*, monocyte derived dendritic cells; *MR*, mixed response; *PBS*, phosphate-buffered saline; *PD*, progressive disease; *PR*, partial response; *SD*, stable disease.

DC are sentinels of the immune system located at sites of antigen entry, such as the skin. They take up antigen and carry it to secondary lymphoid organs. They are highly specialized APCs for the activation of specific effector T cells recirculating in secondary lymphoid organs [1]. In recent years an enormous

Recent Results in Cancer Research, Vol. 160
© Springer-Verlag Berlin Heidelberg 2002

increase in our understanding of DC biology has opened up new ways of applying these cells for immunotherapy of cancer [2]. For a given tumor to be eligible for DC vaccination, tumor antigen has to be available for loading on DC. This might be achieved by loading either defined antigens, such as peptides, or whole antigenic preparations, such as tumor lysate or RNA, on DC [3]. Numerous trials are currently ongoing or planned in the very fast-moving field of DC immunotherapy trials [4]. For the sake of clarity, we will focus in this paper exclusively on published trials in DC vaccination that involve malignant melanoma, renal cell cancer, non-Hodgkin lymphoma, multiple myeloma, and prostate cancer (Table 1). The first preliminary data on the efficiency of APCs, such as GM-CSF-stimulated monocytes, injected intradermally were obtained in melanoma patients. Induction of MAGE-1 MHC class I-restricted peptide-specific CTL were induced by vaccination which also recognized autologous melanoma cells, but in the absence of significant clinical response [5, 6]. A pilot study using idiotypic protein-pulsed DC generated from circulating DC precursors [7] was performed in four patients with malignant B cell lymphoma who had failed conventional chemotherapy. Induction of idiotypic protein-specific immune response was observed, as was complete clinical regression in two of these four patients [8]. One patient remained in complete remission for more than 3 years [4]. The first trial using monocyte-derived dendritic cells pulsed with peptide or tumor lysate in 16 patients with advanced metastatic melanoma reflected our experience with DC vaccination in the planning phase since 1993, with the first patients enrolled in 1996. Objective clinical responses were obtained in 5 of the 16 patients and included 2 complete and 3 partial remissions. Tumor regression occurred in skin, soft tissue, lung, and pancreas, indicating an impact on the clinical course of metastasizing melanoma. In 1 case CR is still ongoing, while the other patient who achieved CR relapsed but has now survived for 42 months. In another case a patient with PR developed CR after repeated vaccination, and this patient has now been alive for 39 months. Induction of immune response was demonstrated by peptide-specific DTH reactions, including proof of recruitment of antigen-specific CTL to the DTH challenge site. In 10 out of 10 HLA A2-positive patients peptide-specific CTL were induced after the first vaccination cycle (paper submitted for publication). Further trials were conducted in advanced melanoma using DC matured in a monocyte-conditioned supernatant. Effective induction of peptide-specific CTL was obtained in the absence of objective clinical response [9]. In a trial in which CD34-derived DC matured with TNF-$\alpha$ was injected i.v. in 14 patients with advanced melanoma, tumor regression was observed in 2 patients, DTH reactions in 4 patients, and expansion of peptide-specific CTL in 1 patient [10]. In another trial to test immature peptide-pulsed DC, 5 out of 16 patients had an immune response to gp100 or tyrosinase, and there was 1 CR [11]. In multiple myeloma patients who had undergone peripheral stem cell rescue following ablative chemotherapy, DCs were loaded with myeloma-specific immunoglobulin idiotypes purified from serum and injected into the patients; 2 out of 12 patients developed an idiotype-specific cellular proliferative immune response, and 1 of 3 patients studied developed a transient but

**Table 1.** Summary of published trials in DC vaccination (*Tulys* tumor lysate, *PAP* prostatic acid phosphatase)

| Reference | Tumor | Source | Antigen | Route | Tu antigen-specific immune response | Objective clinical response |
|---|---|---|---|---|---|---|
| [21] | Melanoma | Monocytes | MelanA, gp100, tyrosinase, Tulys | Intranodal | Yes | Yes |
| [17] | Melanoma | Monocytes | MelanA, gp100, tyrosinase | i.v. | No | Yes |
| [18] | Melanoma | Monocytes | MelanA, gp100 | i.v. | Yes | Yes |
| [9] | Melanoma | Monocytes | MAGE-3 | i.d., i.v. | Yes | No |
| [10] | Melanoma | CD34 | MelanA, gp100, tyrosinase | i.v. | Yes | No |
| [11] | Melanoma | Monocytes | Tyrosinase, gp100 | i.v. | Yes | Yes |
| [20] | RCC | Monocytes | Tulys | i.v. | Yes | No |
| [8] | Lymphoma | DC blood precursors | Idiotype | i.v. | Yes | Yes |
| [13, 14] | Prostate | Monocytes | PSMA | i.v. | Yes | Yes |
| [15] | Prostate | DC blood precursors | PAP-GMCSF fusion protein | i.v. | Yes | Yes |
| [19] | Various | Monocytes | CEA | i.v. | No | No |

idiotype-specific CTL response [12]. Studies in prostate cancer were performed with monocyte-derived DCs pulsed with peptides derived from prostate-specific membrane antigen (PSMA) in combination with radiotherapy and hormonal therapy. Among the 33 patients treated, 6 partial and 2 complete responders were identified by declining serum marker levels and also immunological responses [13, 14]. A further study was conducted in 13 patients suffering from progressive hormone-refractory metastatic prostate carcinoma [15]. DC were generated from circulating blood precursors by a similar method to that introduced by Engleman et al. [7] and pulsed with a fusion protein consisting of human granulocyte/macrophage colony-stimulating factor (GM-CSF) and human prostatic acid phosphatase (PAP). Two injections were given 1 month apart. Circulating prostate-specific antigen levels dropped in 3 patients. T-cells drawn from patients after infusions, but not before, could be stimulated in vitro by PAP.

No significant side effects of DC vaccination have been reported so far. We followed up 30 advanced melanoma patients treated with peptide- or tumor lysate-pulsed DC (M. Gilliet and F. O. Nestle, submitted for publication). In a few patients there was slight fever after vaccination, or painful lymph nodes. Since peptide antigens derived from melanocytic differentiation antigens were used, it was thought that autoimmune-like reactions might occur. Progressive vitiligo, especially in tumor lysate-treated patients, and depigmentation of melanocytic nevi were observed during vaccination. No serious destructive autoimmunity was observed except the rare induction of antithyroid receptor autoantibodies and antinuclear antibodies.

In one study there was an anaphylactoid reaction to bovine proteins in the presence of detectable levels of IgE antibodies [16]. In our study and in others (M. Thurnher, personal communication), no evidence of immediate-type reactions was detected in skin test reactions. IgE-mediated immediate-type reactions might be explained by the use of a special type of DC that induces an IgE favoring a TH-2-type cytokine response.

The brightest future will be in the combination of antigen-specific immunotherapy with target-oriented molecular therapies (e.g., using small molecule inhibitors of signal transduction or cell cycle proteins in tumor cells). The basis will be extensive molecular profiling of tumor cells in a given cancer patient, leading to an individualized and highly effective multitarget therapy with low side effect profiles. Clinically oriented immunotherapists and molecular therapists still have a long way to go before this future comes true.

**Acknowledgements.** Grants from the Cancer League Zurich and the Swiss Cancer League are gratefully acknowledged. We apologize to all our colleagues whose work is not cited because of space limitations.

# References

1. Banchereau J, Briere F, Caux C, et al (2000) Immunobiology of dendritic cells. Annu Rev Immunol 18:767–811
2. Nestle FO, Bancereau J, Hart D (2001) Dendritic cells: on the move from bench to bedside. Nat Med 7:761–765
3. Timmerman JM, Levy R (1999) Dendritic cell vaccines for cancer immunotherapy. Annu Rev Med 50:507–529
4. Fong L, Engleman EG (2000) Dendritic cells in cancer immunotherapy. Annu Rev Immunol 18:245–273
5. Mukherji B, Chakraborty NG, Yamasaki S, et al (1995) Induction of antigen-specific cytolytic T cells in situ in human melanoma by immunization with synthetic peptide-pulsed autologous antigen presenting cells. Proc Natl Acad Sci USA 92:8078–8082
6. Hu X, Chakraborty NG, Sporn JR, et al (1996) Enhancement of cytolytic T lymphocyte precursor frequency in melanoma patients following immunization with the MAGE-1 peptide loaded antigen presenting cell-based vaccine. Cancer Res 56:2479–2483
7. Markowicz S, Engleman EE (1990) Granulocyte-macrophage colony-stimulating factor promotes differentiation and survival of human peripheral blood dendritic cells in-vitro. J Clin Invest 85:955–961
8. Hsu FJ, Benike C, Liles FFTM, et al (1996) Vaccination of patients with B-cell lymphoma using autologous antigen-pulsed dendritic cells. Nat Med 2:52–58
9. Thurner B, Haendle I, Roder C, et al (1999) Vaccination with mage-3A1 peptide-pulsed mature, monocyte-derived dendritic cells expands specific cytotoxic T cells and induces regression of some metastases in advanced stage IV melanoma. J Exp Med 190:1669–1678
10. Mackensen A, Herbst B, Chen JL, et al (2000) Phase I study in melanoma patients of a vaccine with peptide-pulsed dendritic cells generated in vitro from CD34(+) hematopoietic progenitor cells. Int J Cancer 86:385–392
11. Lau R, Wang F, Jeffery G, et al (2001) Phase I trial of intravenous peptide-pulsed dendritic cells in patients with metastatic melanoma. J Immunother 24:66–78
12. Reichardt VL, Okada CY, Liso A, et al (1999) Idiotype vaccination using dendritic cells after autologous peripheral blood stem cell transplantation for multiple myeloma – a feasibility study. Blood 93:2411–2419

13. Lodge PA, Jones LA, Bader RA, Murphy GP, Salgaller ML (2000) Dendritic cell-based immunotherapy of prostate cancer: immune monitoring of a phase II clinical trial. Cancer Res 60:829–833

14. Murphy GP, Tjoa BA, Simmons SJ, et al (1999) Infusion of dendritic cells pulsed with HLA-A2-specific prostate-specific membrane antigen peptides: a phase II prostate cancer vaccine trial involving patients with hormone-refractory metastatic disease. Prostate 38:73–78

15. Burch PA, Breen JK, Buckner JC, et al (2000) Priming tissue-specific cellular immunity in a phase I trial of autologous dendritic cells for prostate cancer (in process citation). Clin Cancer Res 6:2175–2182

16. Mackensen A, Drager R, Schlesier M, Mertelsmann R, Lindemann A (2000) Presence of IgE antibodies to bovine serum albumin in a patient developing anaphylaxis after vaccination with human peptide-pulsed dendritic cells. Cancer Immunol Immunother 49:152–156

17. Lotze MT, Shurin M, et al (2000) Interleukin-2: developing additional cytokine gene therapies using fibroblasts or dendritic cells to enhance tumor immunity. Cancer J Sci Am 6 [Suppl]:S61–66

18. Panelli MC, Wunderlich J, et al (2000) Phase 1 study in patients with metastatic melanoma of immunization with dendritic cells presenting epitopes derived from the melanoma-associated MART-1 and gp100. J Immunother 23:487–498

19. Morse MA, Deng Y, et al (1999) A phase I study of active inmmunotherapy with carcinoembryonic antigen peptide (CAP-1=-pulsed, autologous human cultured dendritic cells in patients with metastatic malignancies expressing carcinoembryonic antigen. Clin Cancer Res 5:1331–1338

20. Holtl L, Rieser C, Papesh C, Ramoner R, Bartsch G, Thurnher M (1998) CD83+ blood dendritic cell as a vaccine for immunotherapy of metastasic renal-cell cancer. Lancet 352:1368

21. Nestle FO, Alijagic S, Gilliet M, Sun Y, Grabbe S, Dummer R, Burg G, Schadendorf D (1998) Vaccination of melanoma patients with peptide- or tumor lysate pulsed dendritic cells. Nature Med 4:328–332

# Gene-based Immunotherapy of Skin Cancers

Yuansheng Sun and Dirk Schadendorf

## Abstract

Skin cancers continue to present a major therapeutic challenge to physicians. Recent advances in molecular genetics and improved understanding of immune responses to tumors have generated an interest in using gene-based immunotherapy for treating these malignancies. Two major forms of gene-based immunotherapy are currently being investigated. One focuses on genetic modification of some target cell populations of the host using immunostimulatory genes such as cytokines, in order to improve tumor immunogenicity and antitumor responses; the other is genetic immunization with the genes coding for melanoma-associated antigens recognized by cytotoxic T cells. This paper reviews these novel strategies and summarizes the most recent data recorded in either experimental studies or clinical trials.

**Abbreviations.** *APC*, antigen-presenting cell; *DC*, dendritic cell; *CTL*, cytotoxic T-lymphocyte; *GM-CSF*, granulocyte-macrophage colony stimulating factor; *HLA*, human histocompatibility leukocyte antigen; *IFN*, interferon; *IL*, interleukin; *MHC*, major histocompatibility complex; *CR*, complete remission; *PR*, partial remission; *SD*, stable disease; *MR*, minor response; *BCG*, bacille Calmette-Guérin; *Th*, T helper; *DTH*, delayed-type hypersensitivity.

## Introduction

Skin cancers are a group of human malignant diseases originally derived from the skin organ. Examples of these diseases include malignant melanoma, the most aggressive skin cancer, with a rapidly rising incidence over recent decades, squamous cell carcinoma of the skin, and basal cell carcinoma, the most common skin cancer in humans. Although these malignancies may be curable when resected at an early stage, metastatic diseases, occurring primarily in malignant melanoma, are highly resistant to standard forms of

Recent Results in Cancer Research, Vol. 160
© Springer-Verlag Berlin Heidelberg 2002

therapy (e.g., surgery, chemotherapy) and cause substantial mortality (Ahmann et al. 1989; Johnson et al. 1995). Given the putative role of the host immune system, and particularly the cell-mediated immunity both in the pathogenesis of melanoma and BCC and in containing tumor growth, many attempts have been made to amplify host antitumor immune responses, such as regional or systemic administration of a variety of biological response modifiers (e.g., BCG, immunostimulatory cytokines, IL-2, IFN-$\alpha$) and the use of various vaccines consisting of intact tumor cells/cell extracts (Berd et al. 1990; Dalgleish 1995; Kirkwood 1991; Oettgen and Old 1991; Rosenberg et al. 1989). Although these treatment modalities induced impressive tumor regression in a subset of selected patients with metastatic melanomas, overall results have been disappointing: none has so far been proven clinically beneficial in terms of patient's overall survival, with the exception that long-term ($\geq 4$ weeks) intramuscular administration of high-dose ($\geq 9$ million units/week) IFN-$\alpha$ might have slightly increased the overall survival of patients with high-risk melanomas (Kirkwood et al. 1996). However, the benefits of this IFN-$\alpha$ treatment regimen are accompanied by the notable side effects. Thus, it is imperative that new approaches – therapeutically effective, but low-toxicity, cancer immunotherapy – continue to be explored.

Recent progress in molecular biology (particularly recombinant DNA technology) and in gene transfer techniques have stimulated considerable interest in the development of gene therapy for the treatment of cancers. One of the most popular approaches currently being developed is so-called immunogene-based therapy, which has thus far involved a large set of cloned functional genes coding for immunostimulatory cytokines and other molecules, such as costimulatory molecules (B7 family), adhesion molecules (ICAM-1), chemokines and foreign MHC antigens. Based on successful animal studies, first clinical trials of this novel approach, particularly with cytokine gene transfer therapy to fight melanoma tumors, have been conducted throughout the world over the last 6 years. Another novel approach to tumor immunotherapy is called genetic immunization, also known as DNA or polynucleotide immunization, which takes advantage of recently cloned genes encoding melanoma-associated antigens recognized by CTL. This approach aims to enhance antigen-specific immune responses of the host to their own tumors by their gene products and is still at the preclinical stage. This paper reviews these novel immunological strategies and summarizes the most recent data observed either in experimental studies or in clinical trials.

## Immunogene-based Therapy – the Concept

Immunogene-based therapy, also known as genetic immunomodulation, is designed to enhance the host antitumor immune response by introducing certain genes (e.g., cytokines, chemokines, costimulatory/accessory molecules or foreign MHC molecules) in some target cell populations of the host, particularly the tumor cells. The conceptional considerations of using gene

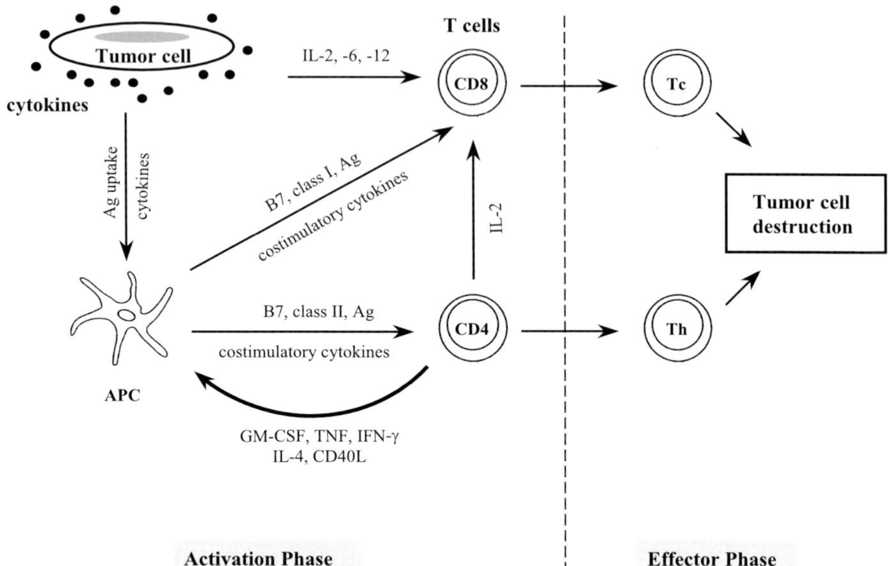



**Fig. 1.** Possible mechanisms of action of cytokine gene transfer in immune modulation. In the T-cell activation phase, gene-transduced cells provide sustained local release of cytokine, leading to CD8$^+$ T-cell priming directly or via activation of accessible bone marrow-derived antigen (*Ag*)-presenting cells (*APC*), such as Langerhans' cells (*LC*) and dermal dendritic cells (*DC*). Activated APCs can take up tumor antigens (e.g., cell debris) stimulating CD4$^+$ T lymphocyte through the class II major histocompatibility complex (*MHC*) pathway. Moreover, CD4$^+$ T-cell activation can further enhance cytotoxic T cell (*CTL*) priming via second cytokine secretion and positive feedback on APC activation, thereby eliciting long-lasting effective antitumor immunity. In the effector phase, circulating CD8$^+$ CTL recognize tumor cells in the context of MHC class I and destroy them. Activated CD4$^+$ T cells may also exert antitumor effects either directly or via activation of other cellular components (e.g., macrophages, eosinophils, neutrophils)

transfer as a means of immune modulation include (1) gene (cytokines, chemokines) transfer into the tumor cell, resulting in sustained local release may avoid apparent systemic effects of toxicity, while producing dramatic local inflammation and immune activation either by transduced cytokines/chemokines, or through second cytokine secretion from activated APC, such as DC or activated CD4$^+$ T cells (Fig. 1); (2) introduction of genes encoding costimulatory molecules (B7 family), adhesion molecules (ICAM-1) or foreign MHC into tumor cells may render them more immunogenic in terms of immune stimulation and/or T-cell activation. Two major strategies are currently being developed for gene transfer – in vivo direct introduction of gene materials into the target cells, and ex vivo gene transfer into explanted cells that are then reimplanted to the patient, by virtue of recombinant viruses or via various physical methods, such as gene gun or liposomes. Both approaches have been applied to cancer patients with the use of various cytokine genes or allogeneic/xenogeneic MHC class I genes.

## Cytokine Gene Transfer Therapies Against Cancers

### Ex Vivo Cytokine Gene Transfer – Preclinical Studies

Cytokines exert important functions in the modulation of host immune responses and display great therapeutic potential for cancer treatment when administered systemically at a high dose. These immune modulators have certainly gained considerable attention in the development of gene-based immunotherapy. One of the first reports, from Tepper et al. (1989), showed that J558L plasmocytoma cells genetically modified with IL-4 gene were rapidly rejected after inoculation in syngeneic animal hosts. Since then, numerous cytokines have demonstrated the ability to reduce tumorigenicity when delivered in such a mode; these include IL-1, IL-2, IL-3, IL-7, IL-12, IFN-$\gamma$, TNF-$\alpha$, and GM-CSF (Avalosse et al. 1995; Gilboa and Lyerly 1994; Pardoll 1995; Vieweg and Gilboa 1995). Importantly, in many instances, cytokine gene-modified tumor cells were also capable of stimulating a systemic protective antitumor immunity, since vaccination of animals with gene-modified tumor cells protected them against a subsequent challenge with parental, unmodified cells at a distant site, and in some cases even eliminated a preexisting tumor. Protection was often found on analysis to be associated with T-cell-mediated responses. Since several studies have used poorly immunogenic or nonimmunogenic tumor models, it was suggested that the protective responses elicited were solely attributable to the transduced cytokine.

### Ex vivo Cytokine Gene Transfer – Clinical Phase I/II Trials

The apparent success in animal studies has fueled considerable interest in the use of cytokine gene-modified cell vaccines to treat cancer patients. We have vaccinated a total of 16 patients with advanced melanomas in two successive phase I trials, one using autologous IL-7 gene-transduced tumor cells in 10 patients (Möller et al. 1998) and the other using IL-12 gene-transduced tumor cells in 6 patients (Sun et al. 1998). Immunizations were performed in weeks 1, 2, 3 and 6, by subcutaneous (s.c.) injection with total numbers of $5\times10^6$ to $3\times10^7$ modified tumor cells. In both trials, treatments were well tolerated and no major toxicity was induced, except for mild fever and flu-like symptoms in some patients vaccinated with IL-12-secreting tumor cells. Although no major clinical responses (CR + PR) were achieved in any trial after the fourth vaccination, in the IL-7 gene trial (Möller et al. 1998) 4 patients showed SD and 2 a mixed response (MR), whereas in the IL-12 gene trial (Sun et al. 1998) 3 patients showed stabilization of the disease, with two still alive for 10+ months. One experienced MR with regression of some cutaneous metastases over 3 months. An extensive immunological evaluation was performed after the fourth vaccination. In the IL-7 gene trial, 4 patients showed increased NK activity and 7 showed an increased LAK response upon vaccination. In 3 of 7 patients evaluated, the frequency of blood tumor-reactive CTLp increased between 2.6- and 28-fold. It is of interest that increased CTL responses were confined exclusively to clinical responders: 2 with a MR and 1 with SD, implying a role of CTL in controlling tumor growth. Moreover, the magnitude of T cell responses induced was closely associated with Karnofsky index and DTH reaction before vaccination, suggesting that patients with minimal tumor load or minimal residual disease may preferentially benefit from such a vaccine. In the IL-12 gene trial (Sun et al. 1998), vaccination induced DTH reactivity against autologous tumor cells in 2 patients, with 1 showing a heavy infiltrate of $CD4^+$ and $CD8^+$ T-cells in a regressing metastasis. The frequency of blood tumor-reactive CTLp was increased (up to 15-fold) in 2 patients after immunization.

Soiffer et al. (1998) immunized 29 melanoma patients with an autologous GM-CSF-secreting tumor vaccine. Immunizations were done in three successive patient cohorts with $10^7$ irradiated tumor cells (each treatment) administered at 28-, 14-, or 7-day intervals for a total of 84 days (total of 3, 6, or 12 vaccinations). One PR, 1 MR, and 3 minor responses were achieved by this treatment. Vaccination elicited substantial erythema and induration at injection sites, characterized histologically by an extensive infiltrate of DC, macrophages, eosinophils and T lymphocytes that extended throughout the dermis and into the subcutaneous fat. In all patients, an initially negative DTH to autologous tumor cells was converted to a strong response after several vaccinations, suggesting an augmented antitumor cellular immunity. In addition, in 7 patients enhanced antimelanoma humoral (IgG-type) immune responses were recorded. Patients were also monitored by biopsy of their distant metastases, with 11 of 16 patients showing a dense infiltrate of both T cells ($CD4^+$ and $CD8^+$) and plasma cells after, but not before, vaccination. In an additional pilot study, Chang et al. (2000) tested autologous GM-CSF-secreting cells as a vaccine to prime draining lymph nodes in 5 melanoma patients. They observed an increased infiltration of DC in the GM-CSF-secreting vaccine sites and a greater number of cells harvested from GM-CSF vaccine-primed lymph node (GM-CSF-VPLNs). Ex vivo propagation of GM-CSF-VPLN cells with anti-CD3 mAb and IL-2 and subsequent adoptive transfer to patients resulted in a durable CR of metastatic tumor in 1 out of 4 patients tested. This suggests the novel use of GM-CSF-secreting vaccine in tumor immunotherapy.

Abdel-Wahab et al. (1997) applied IFN-$\gamma$ gene-transfected autologous tumor cells in escalating doses (2 vaccinations with $2\times10^6$, $6\times10^6$, $18\times10^6$ each) to 20 melanoma patients. No side-effects were noted. Two patients achieved a CR and 2 additional patients showed transient shrinkage of subcutaneous nodular disease. In the immunologic evaluation particular attention was paid to antitumor humoral responses: 8 of 13 accessible patients showed an elevated antimelanoma IgG titer during the course of immunization. The increased antibody response was dominated by IgG2 versus IgG1 isotypes in all 8 responders, suggesting the possible activation of Th type 1 (Th1) cells in these patients. Palmer et al. (1999) conducted a phase II trial to investigate the biological effect of an autologous IL-2-secreting tumor cell vaccine in 12 melanoma patients. Patients were treated with one, two or three administrations of $10^7$ modified tumor cells. No complications were observed. Three patients had stable disease for 7–15+ months and 1, for 17 weeks; the latter developed antitumor DTH after the first vaccination. In 4 patients, including 3 with 7–15+ months disease stabilization, the CTL responses to autologous tumor cells were increased upon vaccination.

Obtaining sufficient numbers of autologous tumor cells for genetic manipulation is sometimes problematic and is time-consuming. Therefore, several studies have used well-characterized, allogeneic melanoma cell lines or fibroblasts as vehicles for cytokine delivery. Arienti et al. (1996) and Belli et al. (1997) first vaccinated 12 melanoma patients with $5 \times 10^7$ or $15 \times 10^7$ IL-2 gene-modified allogeneic melanoma cells. Three of the eight evaluable patients experienced MR. Two patients showed increased reactivity of specific CTL directed against tyrosinase and gp100 melanoma-associated antigens in postvaccination PBL. Two additional patients showed an increased frequency of melanoma-specific CTLp in postvaccination PBL. The same group, in a subsequent study (Arienti et al. 1999), tested IL-4 gene-transduced allogeneic melanoma cells in successive vaccinations in 12 melanoma patients. Both local and systemic toxicities were mild, consisting of transient fever and erythema, swelling and induration at the vaccination site. Two MR were recorded. Of 11 patients tested, antibodies and increased IFN-$\gamma$ responses to allomelanoma cells were documented in 2 and 7 patients, respectively, after vaccination. However, induction of a specific T cell response to autologous tumor cells was obtained in only 1 of 6 cases studied. More recently, in a phase I/II study, Osanto et al. (2000) applied an IL-2-secreting allogeneic melanoma cell line in three successive vaccinations (each $6 \times 10^7$ cells) to 33 melanoma patients. No major side-effects were recorded. Two patients achieved complete or partial regression of subcutaneous metastases. Seven patients had protracted stabilization (4–>46 months) of soft tissue metastases, including 1 who developed vitiligo after vaccination. Immune responses to the vaccine could be detected in 67% of the 27 patients measured. In 2 of 5 patients, the frequency of antiautologous tumor CTLs was significantly increased by vaccination.

Differing from the above-cited studies using genetically modified tumor cells, Veelken et al. (1997), in a pilot study, administered IL-2-secreting allogeneic fibroblasts admixed with autologous tumor cells to 15 patients with advanced malignant tumors, including 6 melanoma patients. No major side-effects were attributable to vaccines. In 2 melanoma patients, a dense infiltrate of both $CD4^+$ and $CD8^+$ T cells at the vaccination sites was demonstrated. T-cell lines generated from biopsies of these vaccination sites exhibited a dominant MHC class I-restricted cytotoxic activity against autologous tumor cells in vitro and had a V-D-J junctional sequence of TCR identical to that of infiltrating lymphocytes obtained from tumor sites of 1 patient. This suggests that the same CTL clone had infiltrated the tumor and circulated in the peripheral blood, and was amplified at the vaccination site (Mackensen et al. 1997).

## In Vivo Cytokine Gene Transfer – Preclinical Results

In addition to ex vivo cytokine gene transfer, a substantial amount of work has recently focused on the direct implantation of the immunogenes in vivo. These have thus far involved the use of a single cytokine alone or various combinations, such as cytokine/cytokine, cytokine/B7.1 costimulatory molecule, or cytokine/chemokines. In different animal models, direct cytokine gene transfer into the tumor cells has been shown to improve the efficacy of the cytokine immunotherapy without the accompanying toxicity. Sun et al. (1995) was the first to show that epidermal administration of human IL-6, TNF-$\alpha$, and murine IFN-$\gamma$ and IL-2 genes (by gene gun) could induce systemic antitumor effects in a renal carcinoma tumor model (Renca). Moreover, IFN-$\gamma$/IL-2 gene cotransfection resulted in eradication of preexisting tumors in 25% of animals. Additional studies by Saffran et al. (1998), using a murine IL-2 expression vector complexed with DMRIE/DOPE lipid, provided further evidence that intratumoral injection of IL-2 gene in Renca-bearing mice induced complete tumor regression, which was mediated by CD8$^+$ T cells. Immunity was systemic, long-lived, and Renca-specific, and further, adoptive, transfer of splenocytes from treated mice protected naive mice against Renca tumor. Subsequent studies have confirmed the antitumor effect in several other animal tumor models induced by intratumoral injection of adenoviral vectors-expressing IL-2 and/or IL-12 (Addison et al. 1998; Emtage et al. 1998, 1999; Lohr et al. 2001; Nasu et al. 1999; Palmer et al. 2001; Pützer et al. 1997; Rakhmilevich et al. 1996; Wang et al. 1999). These studies have shown an important feature for the direct in vivo gene delivery therapy: only combinations of cytokine/cytokine, cytokine/B7.1 costimulatory molecule or cytokine/chemokine (IP-10 or MIG) elicited robust antitumor immunity.


## In Vivo Cytokine Gene Transfer – Clinical Results

Results of first clinical trials at the level of feasibility studies have been appearing in the past few years, with most studies performed on metastatic melanomas. Mastrangelo et al. (1999) constructed a vaccine/GM-CSF recombinant virus and injected it into tumor lesions of seven patients with metastatic melanomas. Clinically, systemic toxicity was infrequent, dose-related, and limited to mild 'flu-like symptoms that resolved within 24 hours. One patient showed PR, with regression of injected and uninjected dermal metastases. Three patients had MR. One patient with only dermal metastases confined to the scalp achieved a CR. Immunohistochemistry studies on biopsy of chronically treated lesions showed a dense infiltration with CD4$^+$ and CD8$^+$ lymphocytes, histiocytes and eosinophils, the last's high enrichment at treatment sites indicating that physiologically significant levels of functional GM-CSF were generated. Thus, these results were very encouraging. In three more phase I/II studies, by Galanis et al. (1999), intratumoral gene transfer of an IL-2 DNA/DMRIE/DOPE lipid complex induced PR (in liver) lasting

16+ months in 1 of the 16 assessable melanoma patients. Three additional patients had SD, the duration of disease stability being 3 months, 17+ months, and 18+ months. Fujii et al. (2000) studied the antitumor effect of IFN-$\gamma$ retroviral vector in 17 patients with advanced melanomas. All patients receiving multiple intratumoral injections either maintained stable disease ($n=5$) or achieved a PR or CR in the injected lesion ($n=3$), whereas of nine patients each receiving a single cycle of treatment, only one had a response. Interestingly, all patients responding to treatment (SD or better) had significantly more elevated antibody responses to a number of melanoma-associated antigens, tyrosinase, gp100, TRP2 and MAGE-A1. Such enhanced antitumor antibody responses to IFN-$\gamma$ retroviral vector treatment were also observed by Nemunaitis et al. (1999), who showed elevated IgG titers in 8 of 17 melanoma patients after intratumoral injection of IFN-$\gamma$ retroviral vector. Thus, this treatment regimen appears to preferentially induce a humoral response to tumor.

In summary, first clinical studies with both ex vivo and in vivo cytokine gene transfer therapy have demonstrated the feasibility, apparent safety, and low toxicity of these novel approaches. Treatment can enhance systemic antitumor cellular and/or humoral responses, or even result in objective tumor regression in a subset of patients with advanced melanoma. Since the magnitude of antitumor responses induced in patients were often correlated with a good clinical performance status, we assume these approaches would exert their most therapeutic effects in patients with low tumor loads.

## Immunogene Transfer Using MHC Class I Genes

### Preclinical Studies

An alternative approach to immunogene-based therapy is to implant allogeneic or xenogeneic class I MHC genes into tumors, in an attempt to trigger responses to tumors. A first report by Hui and Kim (1984) showed that introduction of the class I H-2k gene into H-2d plasmacytoma tumor cells dramatically enhanced immunogenicity, leading to the protection of recipient mice from the parent tumor cell challenge and the generation of specific CTL against the 'wild-type' parental tumor. Since then, many studies have shown a similar effect of an allogeneic class I H-2 gene transfer using other animal tumor models (Gattoni-Celli et al. 1988; Hui et al. 1989; Itaya et al. 1987; Tanaka et al. 1988). In one case, the tumor immunity induced was capable of eradicating the preexisting parental tumors (Hui et al. 1989). Plautz et al. (1993) had first attempted to directly introduce the H-2ks gene into growing CT26 mouse colon adenocarcinoma (H-2kd) or MCA 106 fibrosarcoma (H-2 kb) in mice using either cationic liposomes or retroviral vectors as mediators. In both cases, the H-2ks-treated animals demonstrated retarded tumor growth and, with optimization of the system, increased survival and some complete tumor regressions. Similar results have also been reported recently by Ishida et al. (1999). In their system, direct in vivo gene transfer of H-2 kb DNA-HVJ-liposomes complex into C1300S3 neuroblastomas led to regression of established tumors and prolongation of survival in 50% of treated mice.

## Phase I Clinical Trials

On the basis of successful animal studies, Nabel et al. (1993) first developed a phase I program for the direct injection of HLA-B7 DNA-liposome complexes into melanoma lesions of HLA-B7-negative patients. Complications were not observed, anti-DNA antibodies were not produced, and plasmid DNA was not found in serum, but, together with HLA-B7 protein, could be demonstrated in the tumor tissue in all five patients treated. Immune responses to HLA-B7 and to autologous tumors were demonstrable, and one patient showed regression of injected tumor nodules and distant site tumor. A follow-up report by Nabel et al. (1996) described the results of treating ten patients with stage IV melanoma with the HLA-B7-liposome method. They saw evidence of tumor infiltration by T cells but no increase in the frequency of blood melanoma-specific CTL. Local inhibition of tumor growth was observed in two patients, one achieving complete regression after adoptive transfer treatment with infiltrating lymphocytes derived from the gene-modified tumor. In another phase I study, Stopeck et al. (1997) treated 17 HLA-B7-negative melanoma patients with intralesional gene injections of a lipid-formulated plasmid DNA encoding HLA-B7. Toxicities were related to technical aspects of injections. Seven patients (50%) showed shrinkage of injected tumor nodules by ≥25%. One patient with a single site of disease achieved a complete remission.

In summary, in situ gene therapy of cancers using an allogeneic MHC gene is feasible, safe, and can induce a strong local immune response. Thus, further studies on the mechanism of action, predictors of response, and antitumor efficacy of this approach are warranted.

## Genetic Immunization – DNA-based Vaccines

Genetic immunization or DNA inoculation represents another novel approach in vaccine and active-specific immunotherapy against cancers, and has thus far been evaluated only in animal models. This approach aims to enhance the specific immunological response of hosts to their own tumors by gene products. The concept behind genetic immunization is a simple one: genes encoding antigens are cloned into a plasmid with an appropriate promoter, and the plasmid DNA is administrated to the vaccine recipient. The DNA is taken up by host cells, and the gene is expressed. The resultant 'foreign' protein is produced within the host cell and then processed and presented appropriately to the immune system. This may lead to the induction of a specific CTL response through the MHC class I-restricted pathway. Concurrently, proteins are released extracellularly. It is believed that this exogenously released antigen primes the induction of a humoral response, as well as a helper T lymphocyte (Th) response via MHC class II-restricted antigen presentation by APC that have taken up the foreign antigen (Fig. 2).

The first report of DNA immunization serving as an antigen-specific tumor vaccine was published in early 1996. Zhai et al. (1996) showed that inoculation of C57BL/6 (H-2$^b$) mice with recombinant adenoviruses (Ad2CMV)-delivered plasmid DNA coding for human gp100 tumor antigen induced both anti-gp100 antibody and CTL responses. Importantly, immunization with Ad2CMV-gp100 protected mice from subsequent challenge with murine melanoma B16 in a CD8$^+$ T-cell-dependent manner, indicating that vaccination generated anti-gp100 reactive T cells that were predominantly CD8$^+$ and responsible for tumor protection. Shortly after, several studies demonstrated protective tumor immunity in the B16-C57BL/6 mouse melanoma model by human gp100 DNA inoculation (Hawkins et al. 2000; Mölling et al. 1997; Schreurs et al. 1998; Zhou et al. 1999), independently of the use

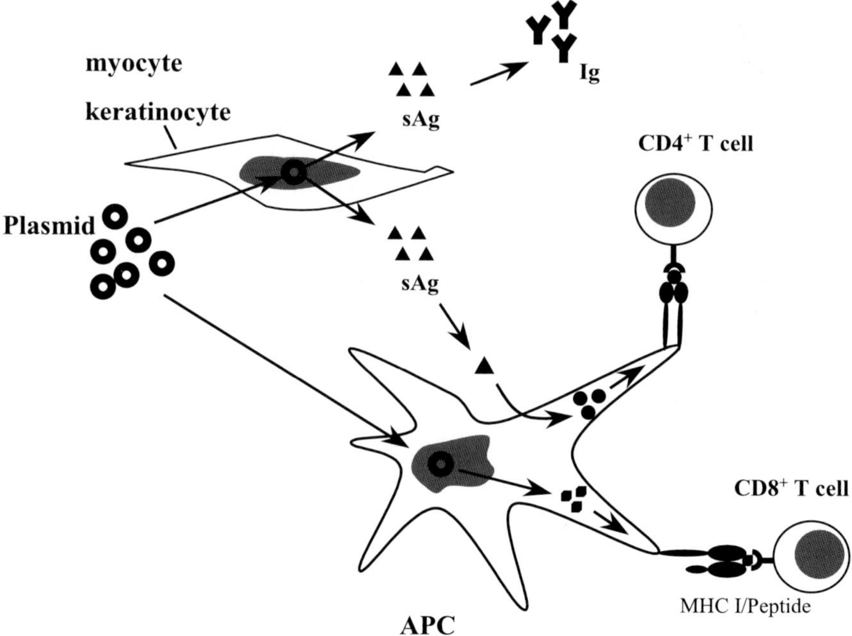


**Fig. 2.** Possible mechanism for the induction of antitumor immunity via genetic immunization. Bone marrow-derived APCs residing in the target tissue may be directly transfected with plasmid DNA, leading to protein production. This protein is processed intracellularly to small peptides, which are then presented in the context of class I MHC molecules to CD8$^+$ T lymphocytes. On the other hand, a tissue-specific cell (e.g., myocyte or keratinocyte) is transfected with plasmid, leading to protein production and secretion. Soluble protein released by transfected cells elicits antibody responses and is taken up by 'professional' APCs, which then stimulate CD4$^+$ T lymphocyte via the MHC class II pathway (*sAg* soluble antigen, *Ig* immunoglobulin)

Gilboa E, Lyerly HK (1994) Specific active immunotherapy of cancer using genetically modified tumor vaccines. In: DeVita VT, Hellman S, Rosenberg SA (eds) Biologic therapy of cancer updates. Lippincott, Philadelphia, pp 1–16

Hawkins WG, Gold JS, Dyall R, Wolchok JD, Hoos A, Bowne WB, Srinivasan R, Houghton AN, Lewis JJ (2000) Immunization with DNA coding for gp100 results in CD4 T-cell independent antitumor immunity. Surgery 128:273–280

Hui KM, Kim BS (1984) Tumor-specific immunity induced by somatic hybrids. IV. Relationship between immunogenicity and expression of surface tumor-associated antigens. Cell Immunol 87:591–600

Hui KM, Sim T, Foo TT, Oei AA (1989) Tumor rejection mediated by transfection with allogeneic class I histocompatibility gene. J Immunol 143:3835–3843

Ishida H, Kaneda Y, Yamane S, Sawada T, Plautz GE, Matsumura T (1999) Allogeneic class I major histocompatibility complex gene transfer in murine neuroblastoma in vivo. Anticancer Res 19:5367–5373

Itaya T, Yamagiwa S, Okada F, Oikawa T, Kuzumaki N, Takeichi N, Hosokawa M, Kobayashi H (1987) Xenogenization of a mouse lung carcinoma (3LL) by transfection with an allogeneic class I major histocompatibility complex gene (H-2Ld). Cancer Res 47:3136–3140

Johnson TM, Smith JW, Nelson BR, Chang A (1995) Current therapy for cutaneous melanoma. J Am Acad Dermatol 32:689–707

Kirkwood JM (1991) Studies of interferons in the therapy of melanoma. Semin Oncol 18:83–90

Kirkwood JM, Strawderman MH, Ernstoff MS, Smith TJ, Borden EC, Blum RH (1996) Interferon alfa-2b adjuvant therapy of high-risk resected cutaneous melanoma: the Eastern Cooperative Oncology Group Trial EST 1684. J Clin Oncol 14:7–17

Lohr F, Lo DY, Zaharoff DA, Hu K, Zhang X, Li Y, Zhao Y, Dewhirst MW, Yuan F, Li CY (2001) Effective tumor therapy with plasmid-encoded cytokines combined with in vivo electroporation. Cancer Res 61:3281–3284

Mackensen A, Vcelken H, Lahn M, Wittnebel S, Becker D, Köhler G, Kulmburg P, Brennscheidt U, Rosenthal F, Franke B, Mertelsmann R, Lindemann A (1997) Induction of tumor-specific cytotoxic T lymphocytes by immunization with autologous tumor cells and interleukin-2 gene transfected fibroblasts. J Mol Med 75:290–296

Mastrangelo MJ, Maguire HC Jr, Eisenlohr LC, Laughlin CE, Monken CE, McCue PA, Kovatich AJ, Lattime EC (1999) Intratumoral recombinant GM-CSF-encoding virus as gene therapy in patients with cutaneous melanoma. Cancer Gene Ther 6:409–422

Mendiratta SK, Thai G, Eslahi NK, Thull NM, Matar M, Bronte V, Pericle F (2001) Therapeutic tumor immunity induced by polyimmunization with melanoma antigens gp100 and TRP-2. Cancer Res 61:859–863

Möller P, Sun Y, Dorbic T, Möller H, Makki A, Jurgovsky K, Schroff M, Henz BM, Wittig B, Schadendorf D (1998) Vaccination with IL-7 gene-modified autologous melanoma cells can enhance the anti-melanoma lytic activity in peripheral blood of patients with a good clinical performance status: a clinical phase I study. Br J Cancer 77:1907–1916

Mölling K, Strack B, Nawrath M, Heinrich J, Döhring C, Wagner SN, Pavlovic J (1997) Development of a DNA vaccine against malignant melanoma. In: Burg G, Dummer RG (eds) Strategies for immunointerventions in dermatology. Springer, Berlin Heidelberg New York, pp 195–206

Nabel GJ, Nabel EG, Yang ZY, Fox BA, Plautz GE, Gao X, Huang L, Shu S, Gordon D, Chang AE (1993) Direct gene transfer with DNA-liposome complexes in melanoma: expression, biologic activity, and lack of toxicity in humans Proc Natl Acad Sci USA 90:11307–11311

Nabel GJ, Gordon D, Bishop DK, Nickoloff BJ, Yang ZY, Aruga A, Cameron MJ, Nabel EG, Chang AE (1996) Immune response in human melanoma after transfer of an allogeneic class I major histocompatibility complex gene with DNA-liposome complexes. Proc Natl Acad Sci USA 93:15388–15393

Nasu Y, Bangma CH, Hull GW, Lee HM, Hu J, Wang J, McCurdy MA, Shimura S, Yang G, Timme TL, Thompson TC (1999) Adenovirus-mediated interleukin-12 gene therapy for prostate cancer: suppression of orthotopic tumor growth and pre-established lung metastases in an orthotopic model. Gene Ther 6:338–349

Nemunaitis J, Fong T, Burrows F, Bruce J, Peters G, Ognoskie N, Meyer W, Wynne D, Kerr R, Pippen J, Oldham F, Ando D (1999) Phase I trial of interferon gamma retroviral vector administered intratumorally with multiple courses in patients with metastatic melanoma. Hum Gene Ther 10:1289–1298

Oettgen HF, Old LJ (1991) The history of cancer immunotherapy. In: DeVita VT, Hellman S, Rosenberg SA (eds) The biologic therapy of cancer: principles and practice. Lippincott, Philadelphia, pp 87–119

Osanto S, Schiphorst PP, Weijl NI, Dijkstra N, Van Wees A, Brouwenstein N, Vaessen N, Van Krieken JH, Hermans J, Cleton FJ, Schrier PI (2000) Vaccination of melanoma patients with an allogeneic, genetically modified interleukin 2-producing melanoma cell line. Hum Gene Ther 11:739–750

Palmer K, Moore J, Everard M, Harris JD, Rodgers S, Rees RC, Murray AK, Mascari R, Kirkwood J, Riches PG, Fisher C, Thomas JM, Harries M, Johnston SR, Collins MK, Gore ME (1999) Gene therapy with autologous, interleukin 2-secreting tumor cells in patients with malignant melanoma. Hum Gene Ther 10:1261–1268

Palmer K, Hitt M, Emtage PC, Gyorffy S, Gauldie J (2001) Combined CXC chemokine and interleukin-12 gene transfer enhances antitumor immunity. Gene Ther 8:282–290

Pardoll DM (1995) Paracrine cytokine adjuvants in cancer immunotherapy. Annu Rev Immunol 13:399–415

Plautz GE, Yang ZY, Wu BY, Gao X, Huang L, Nabel GJ (1993) Immunotherapy of malignancy by in vivo gene transfer into tumors. Proc Natl Acad Sci USA 90:4645–4649

Pützer BM, Hitt M, Muller WJ, Emtage P, Gauldie J, Graham FL (1997) Interleukin 12 and B7–1 costimulatory molecule expressed by an adenovirus vector act synergistically to facilitate tumor regression. Proc Natl Acad Sci USA 94:10889–10894

Rakhmilevich AL, Turner J, Ford MJ, McCabe D, Sun WH, Sondel PM, Grota K, Yang NS (1996) Gene gun-mediated skin transfection with interleukin 12 gene results in regression of established primary and metastatic murine tumors Proc Natl Acad Sci USA 93:6291–6296

Rosenberg SA, Lotze MT, Yang JC, Aebersold PM, Linehan WM, Seipp CA, White DE (1989) Experience with the use of high-dose interleukin-2 in the treatment of 652 cancer patients. Ann Surg 210:474–485

Saffran DC, Horton HM, Yankauckas MA, Anderson D, Barnhart KM, Abai AM, Hobart P, Manthorpe M, Norman JA, Parker SE (1998) Immunotherapy of established tumors in mice by intratumoral injection of interleukin-2 plasmid DNA: induction of CD8$^+$ T-cell immunity. Cancer Gene Ther 5:321–330

Schreurs MW, de Boer AJ, Figdor CG, Adema GJ (1998) Genetic vaccination against the melanocyte lineage-specific antigen gp100 induces cytotoxic T lymphocyte-mediated tumor protection. Cancer Res 58:2509–2514

Soiffer R, Lynch T, Mihm M, Jung K, Rhuda C, Schmollinger JC, Hodi FS, Liebster L, Lam P, Mentzer S, Singer S, Tanabe KK, Cosimi AB, Duda R, Sober A, Bhan A, Daley J, Neuberg D, Parry G, Rokovich J, Richards L, Drayer J, Berns A, Clift S, Cohen LK, Mulligan RC, Dranoff G (1998) Vaccination with irradiated autologous melanoma cells engineered to secrete human granulocyte-macrophage colony-stimulating factor generates potent antitumor immunity in patients with metastatic melanoma. Proc Natl Acad Sci USA 95:13141–13146

Steitz J, Bruck J, Steinbrink K, Enk A, Knop J, Tuting T (2000) Genetic immunization of mice with human tyrosinase-related protein 2: implications for the immunotherapy of melanoma. Int J Cancer 86:89–94

Stopeck AT, Hersh EM, Akporiaye ET, Harris DT, Grogan T, Unger E, Warneke J, Schluter SF, Stahl S (1997) Phase I study of direct gene transfer of an allogeneic histocompatibility antigen, HLA-B7, in patients with metastatic melanoma. J Clin Oncol 15:341–349

Sun WH, Burkholder JK, Sun J, Culp J, Turner J, Lu XG, Pugh TD, Ershler WB, Yang NS (1995) In vivo cytokine gene transfer by gene gun reduces tumor growth in mice. Proc Natl Acad Sci USA 92:2889–2893

Sun Y, Jurgovsky K, Möller P, Alijagic S, Dorbic T, Georgieva J, Wittig B, Schadendorf D (1998) Vaccination with IL-12 gene-modified autologous melanoma cells: preclinical results and a first clinical phase I study. Gene Ther 5:481–490

Tanaka K, Gorelik E, Watanabe M, Hozumi N, Jay G (1988) Rejection of B16 melanoma induced by expression of a transfected major histocompatibility complex class I gene. Mol Cell Biol 8:1857–1861

Tepper RI, Pattengale PK, Leder P (1989) Murine interleukin-4 displays potent antitumor activity in vivo. Cell 57:503–512

Veelken H, Mackensen A, Lahn M, Köhler G, Becker D, Franke B, Brennscheidt U, Kulmburg P, Rosenthal FM, Keller H, Hasse J, Schultze-Seemann W, Farthmann EH, Mertelsmann R, Lindemann A (1997) A phase-I clinical study of autologous tumor cells plus interleukin-2-gene-transfected allogeneic fibroblasts as a vaccine in patients with cancer. Int J Cancer 70:269–277

Vieweg J, Gilboa E (1995) Consideration for the use of cytokine-secreting tumor cell preparations for cancer treatment. Cancer Invest 13:193–201

Wagner SN, Wagner C, Luhrs P, Weimann TK, Kutil R, Goos M, Stingl G, Schneeberger A (2000) Intracutaneous genetic immunization with autologous melanoma-associated antigen Pmel17/gp100 induces T cell-mediated tumor protection in vivo. J Invest Dermatol 115:1082–1087

Wang C, Quevedo ME, Lannutti BJ, Gordon KB, Guo D, Sun W, Paller AS (1999) In vivo gene therapy with interleukin-12 inhibits primary vascular tumor growth and induces apoptosis in a mouse model. J Invest Dermatol 112:775–781

Zhai Y, Yang JC, Kawakami Y, Spiess P, Wadsworth SC, Cardoza LM, Couture LA, Smith AE, Rosenberg SA (1996) Antigen-specific tumor vaccines. Development and characterization of recombinant adenoviruses encoding MART1 or gp100 for cancer therapy. J Immunol 156:700–710

Zhou WZ, Kaneda Y, Huang S, Morishita R, Hoon D (1999) Protective immunization against melanoma by gp100 DNA-HVJ-liposome vaccine. Gene Ther 6:1768–1773

# Cytokine Fusion Protein Treatment

David Schrama, Per thor Straten, Eva-Bettina Bröcker, Ralph A. Reisfeld, and Jürgen C. Becker

## Abstract

Mice suffering from melanoma can be cured by treatment with a recombinant antibody-lymphotoxin-$\alpha$ fusion protein. In order to characterize the involvement of T cells in this syngeneic tumor model, the T cell receptor repertoire was analyzed both quantitatively and qualitatively. In this connection, quantitative analysis of the T cell receptors displayed only a modest overexpression in some of the variable beta chain families over the course of therapy. Clonotypic mapping, however, revealed a marked increase in the number of clonally expanded T cells among the tumor-infiltrating T cells, suggesting a specific activation.

## Introduction

Several tumor-associated antigens have been discovered for tumors in general, and for melanoma in particular (Kirkin et al. 1998). These often elicit detectable antitumor immune responses, which, however, are only able to control tumor growth in rare cases. Thus, much effort is spent on creating antitumor therapy strategies that will enhance the existing T-cell-based immune response. One of these is the genetic fusion of a tumor-specific antibody with a cytokine. This immunocytokine preferentially migrates to the tumor and leads to enrichment of the cytokine in the tumor environment, taking the paracrine working mechanism of cytokines into account. We have previously demonstrated that antibody-mediated targeting of IL-2 to the tumor microenvironment mounts an effective cellular response against murine melanoma (Becker et al. 1996).

This cellular response, however, was shown to be based on boosting of an already existing response without the induction of additional tumor-specific T cells (thor Straten et al. 1998). Because tumor-antigen-specific T cells can be rendered anergic by the tumor (Staveley-O'Carroll et al. 1998), priming of

Recent Results in Cancer Research, Vol. 160
© Springer-Verlag Berlin Heidelberg 2002

additional T cells may be necessary for maintenance of a successful antitumor immune response. Therefore, we examined the effect of targeting a cytokine to the tumor site that plays a major role in lymph node genesis, namely lymphotoxin-$\alpha$ (LT$\alpha$). Moreover, LT$\alpha$ is a potent mediator of proinflammatory activity and itself has tumoricidal activity (De Togni et al. 1994).

Many groups have proven the fundamental function of LT$\alpha$ in lymph node genesis. LT$\alpha_1$/LT$\beta_2$-LT$\beta$R interactions seem to be the most important: disruption of either the *LT$\beta$* or *LT$\beta$R* genes led to the absence of Peyer's patches and most lymph nodes (Koni et al. 1997) with LT$\alpha$–TNFRI interactions probably rescuing some of the lymph node genesis in *LT$\beta$* knock-out mice (Rennert et al. 1996). Thus, in *LT$\alpha$* knock-out mice no lymph nodes were observed at all (De Togni et al. 1994). Furthermore, a lymphoid-like tissue could be induced at the site of expression of *LT$\alpha$* under the control of a rat insulin promoter in transgenic mice. This lymphoid neogenesis, also known as tertiary lymphoid organ, was mediated by LT$\alpha$ through induction of several adhesion molecules and also chemokines in endothelial cells (Ruddle 1999).

Initially, the effect of a tumor-specific antibody–LT$\alpha$ fusion protein was examined in a xenograft melanoma model. This treatment was shown to be effective in eliminating pulmonary metastases (Reisfeld et al. 1996), and analysis of mice with different immune defects demonstrated that this therapeutic effect was not direct but dependent on B lymphocytes and NK cells. These results encouraged us to study the antibody–LT$\alpha$ fusion protein therapy in an autologous murine melanoma model and to analyze the role of T cells in this model.

In this study, we demonstrate that targeted-LT$\alpha$ therapy leads to the eradication of established subcutaneous tumors. Furthermore, our results demonstrate an improved T-cell immune response. Although only slight overexpression of some TCR VB families is observed, TCR clonotype mapping revealed the expansion of new T-cell clones among TIL.

## Materials and Methods

### Animals

The experimental animals were 6-week-old C57BL/6 J mice obtained from Charles River Laboratories (Sulzfeld, Germany). These animals were housed under specific pathogen-free conditions, and all experiments were performed according to National Institute of Health guidelines for care and use of laboratory animals.

## Cell Line and Fusion Proteins

The murine melanoma cell line B78-D14 has been described elsewhere and was derived from B16 melanoma by transfection with genes coding for $\beta$-1,4-$N$-acetylgalactosaminyltransferase and $\alpha$-2,8-sialyltransferase. The resulting cell line constitutively expresses the disialogangliosides GD2 and GD3. B78-D14 melanoma cells were maintained as monolayers in RPMI 1640 medium supplemented with 10% fetal calf serum, 2 mM L-glutamine, 400 µg/ml G418, and 50 µg/ml hygromycin B.

The mouse/human chimeric antibody directed against GD2 (ch14.18) was constructed from the variable region of the murine 14.18 antibody joined to the constant regions of the human $\gamma$1 heavy chain and the $\kappa$ light chain. The ch14.18-LT$\alpha$ fusion protein was constructed by fusion of a synthetic sequence coding for human LT$\alpha$ to the carboxyl end of the human $C\gamma1$ gene (Gillies et al. 1991). The fused genes were inserted into the vector pdHL2, which encodes for the dihydrofolate reductase gene. The resulting expression plasmids were introduced into Sp2/0-Ag14 cells and selected in Dulbecco's modified Eagle's medium supplemented with 10% fetal bovine serum and 100 nM methotrexate. The fusion proteins were purified over a protein A–Sepharose affinity column.

## Treatment Schedule

Soluble LT$\alpha$ or the ch14.18-LT$\alpha$ fusion protein was administered daily by i.v. injection. Therapy was maintained for 7 days.

## RNA Extraction and RT-PCR

RNA was extracted using the Purescript Isolation Kit (Gentra Systems, N.C., USA). Synthesis of cDNA was carried out using 1–3 µg of total RNA, oligo-dT and SuperScript II reverse transcriptase (Invitrogen, Md., USA) in a total volume of 50 µl 1×buffer (Invitrogen) containing 10 mM DTT. Incubations were performed at 42 °C for 50 min and 72 °C for 5 min. Primers used for the quantitative analysis of murine TCR BV regions include 18 primers specific for BV families 1–18 and a constant region primer, BC, as described elsewhere (thor Straten et al. 1998). Prior to analysis, the total amount of TCR cDNA was quantitated by amplification of the constant part of the TCR $\beta$-chain, in order to normalize the amount of TCR cDNA. Amplifications were performed in duplicate by 30 cycles in a Perkin-Elmer GeneAmp PCR System 9600 (Applied Biosystems) using previously described conditions (thor Straten et al. 1998). Negative controls were samples without cDNA. For quantitative PCR analyses the constant region primer (BC) was end-labeled with $^{32}$P. Aliquots (10 µl) of PCR products were electrophoresed in a 2%

NuSieve 3:1 agarose gel (FMC BioProducts, Rockland, Me.), which was subsequently dried under vacuum and exposed to a molecular dynamics storage phosphor screen (Molecular Dynamics, Sunnyvale, Calif.). Quantitation was accomplished using the Imagequant software.

## TCR Clonotype Mapping by Denaturing Gradient Gel Electrophoresis

Denaturing gradient gel electrophoresis (DGGE) analyses for clonotype mapping of the murine TCR BV regions 1–16 have been described elsewhere (thor Straten et al. 1998). In short, all amplified sequences were evaluated using the computer program MELT87, which predicts the melting of a double-stranded DNA molecule on the basis of its base composition. These calculations indicated that the DNA molecules amplified by these primers were suitable for denaturing gradient gel analysis by the attachment of a 50-bp GC-rich sequence (GC clamp) to the 5′-end of the constant region primer BC. For all variable regions the amplified fragments have been functionally analyzed for their ability to resolve in the denaturing gradient gel by the use of cloned transcripts. Likewise, the analyses of polyclonal T-cell population (PBL) were shown to result in a smear in the denaturing gradient gel.

DGGE analysis was done in 6% polyacrylamide gels containing a gradient of urea and formamide from 20% to 80%. Electrophoresis was performed at 160 V for 4.5 h in 1×TAE buffer at a constant temperature of 54 °C. After electrophoresis, the gels were stained with ethidium bromide and photographed under UV transillumination.

## Results

### Therapeutic Effect of Antibody–LT$\alpha$ Fusion Proteins on Subcutaneous Tumors

In preliminary experiments we confirmed the direct cytotoxic effects of the ch14.18–LT$\alpha$ fusion protein against a number of tumor cell lines in vitro and its antigen-specific binding to the disialoganglioside $GD_2$. Additionally, the specific activity of the ch14.18-LT$\alpha$ fusion protein was compared with soluble LT$\alpha$ (sLT$\alpha$) by measuring the number of lysed L929 cells, which was shown to be three logs less for the fusion protein than for an equal amount of protein (data not shown).

Thereafter, we tested the in vivo antitumor effect of this fusion protein in syngeneic C57BL/6J mice upon subcutaneous tumors of B16 melanoma cells that had been genetically engineered to express $GD_2$. Tumors were induced by s.c. injection of $2.5 \times 10^6$ B78-D14 melanoma cells, which resulted in tumors approximately 40 µl in volume within 14 days. Treatment was initiated at day 14 and lasted for 7 consecutive days. In Fig. 1A the mean tumor volumes of three groups of eight mice, one group treated with 10 ng sLT$\alpha$, one with 32 µg antibody-LT$\alpha$ and the third with 64 µg antibody-LT$\alpha$, are dis-

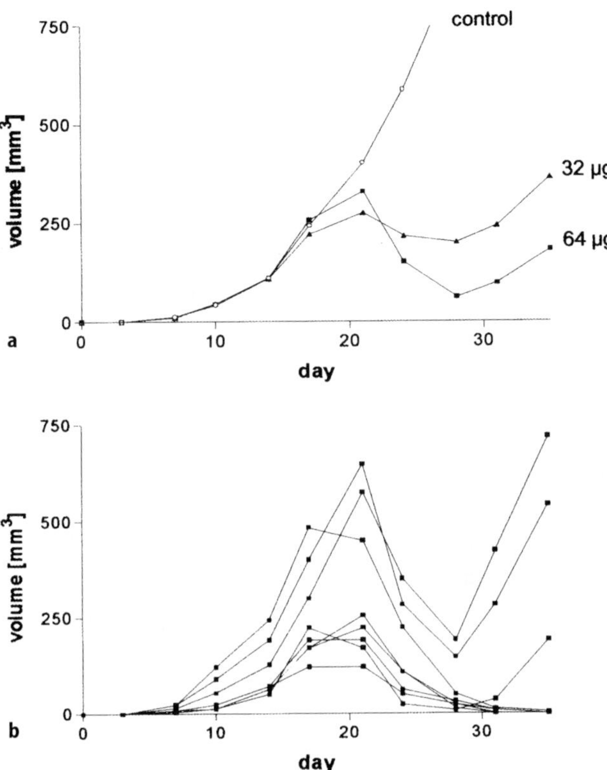

**Fig. 1 a, b.** Therapeutic effect of ch14.18-LT$\alpha$ on subcutaneous tumors. Subcutaneous tumors were induced in C57BL/6 J mice by s.c. injection of $2.5\times10^6$ B78-D14 melanoma cells on day 0. At day 14 therapy was started with either 32 µg or 64 µg ch14.18-LT$\alpha$ for 7 consecutive days. Control animals received 10 ng sLT$\alpha$. **a** Mean tumor volumes of animals ($n=8$) receiving 10 ng sLT$\alpha$ (*open circles*), 32 µg (*closed triangles*) and 64 µg (*closed squares*) ch14.18-LT$\alpha$. **b** The individual tumor volumes of the eight animals treated with 64 µg ch14.18-LT$\alpha$ are depicted

played. The mean tumor volume in the control group receiving sLT$\alpha$ increased constantly over the course of therapy. In contrast, tumor growth in ch14.18-LT$\alpha$ fusion protein-treated mice stagnated after a few days of therapy. Moreover, at day 21 the mean tumor volume started to decrease in these groups, and on day 28 the difference in the reduction of tumor volume between the group treated with 64 µg ch14.18-LT$\alpha$ and the group treated with 10 ng sLT$\alpha$ was highly significant ($P<0.017$). Nevertheless, several days after the treatment was stopped the mean tumor volume started to increase again. However, the individual analysis of tumor sizes of each animal provided a more detailed picture. For example, in five of the eight mice in the group receiving 64 µg ch14.18-LT$\alpha$ the tumor regressed completely and the mice stayed tumor free throughout the observation period of the experiment. In the three remaining mice the tumor volume decreased further for several days before the tumor started to grow again (Fig. 1 B).

## Induction of a Specific T-Cell Response by ch14.18-LT$\alpha$ Therapy

Since we detected a marked infiltration of CD8$^+$ and CD4$^+$ cells by immunohistology (data not shown), we wanted to test the hypothesis that this treatment would change the T-cell response against the tumor. Such a change should translate into variations in the T-cell receptor (TCR) repertoire. Thus, we analyzed the relative expression of all TCR $\beta$-variable (BV) regions prior to and after therapy by semiquantitative PCR, with a specific primer for each of the murine TCR BV family 1–18. Treatment was administered from days 8 through 14. Tumors were excised on days 7, 14, and 21. A representative example is given in Fig. 2 A. Treatment with ch14.18-LT$\alpha$ induced a slight overexpression of TCR BV 5, 8, and 11 on day 21 relative to days 7 and 14. In contrast, analysis of the draining lymph node did not reveal any significant overexpression of any BV region. Furthermore, the control animals also did not display any significant increase in any BV family on day 21 (Fig. 2 B). To test whether the observed quantitative changes were due to clonal expansion of T cells, we performed DGGE-based TCR clonotype mapping for these overexpressed families. This analysis revealed the occurrence of new, prominent bands in the tumor sample obtained on day 21 (lane 3), suggesting that the overexpression of these families was indeed due to the expansion of specific T-cell clones (Fig. 2 A, insert).

## Increase in the Number of T-cell Clones over the Course of Therapy

Since clonal expansion of T cells may also occur in TCR BV regions that are not overexpressed (thor Straten et al. 1999), we analyzed the changes in BV regions 1–16 within the same tumor over the course of ch14.18-LT$\alpha$ therapy. We excluded the variable regions BV 17 and 18, as previous work had shown that they comprised less than 1% of the total TCR transcripts (thor Straten et al. 1998). The subcutaneous tumor was initiated by injection of $2.5 \times 10^6$ B78-D14 melanoma cells and treatment began 8 days after tumor cell inoculation and went on for 7 consecutive days with 64 µg ch14.18-LT$\alpha$ per day. On days 7, 14, and 21 biopsies of the same tumor were obtained. TCR clonotypic maps of BV regions 1–16 were generated by RT-PCR/DGGE analysis. One of those from a ch14.18–LT$\alpha$-treated animal on day 21 is depicted in Fig. 3 A. A polyclonal T cell population is revealed as a smear, whereas an individual T-cell clone is represented by a distinct band in the gel. The number of T cell clones within each TCR BV family is rather heterogeneous, ranging from only one or two clones, such as BV 5, up to seven, e.g. in BV 8. To demonstrate the changes in the occurrence of clones, we provide the total numbers of clones on day 14 and day 21 as percentages of the number on day 7 (Fig. 3 B). Though the occurrence of T-cell clones in control animals was also diverse, the total number of T-cell clones was lower than on day 7. In contrast, the total clone numbers among TIL for ch14.18–LT$\alpha$-treated animals increased during and after therapy. These clones covered the majority of BV regions, but the increase in the number of T-cell clones varied between the BV regions, ranging from 1.25 up to 7 (data not shown).

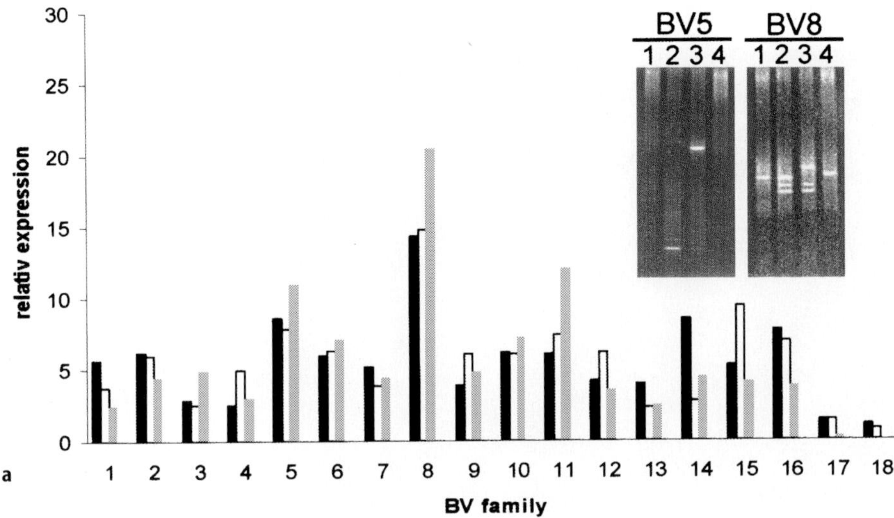


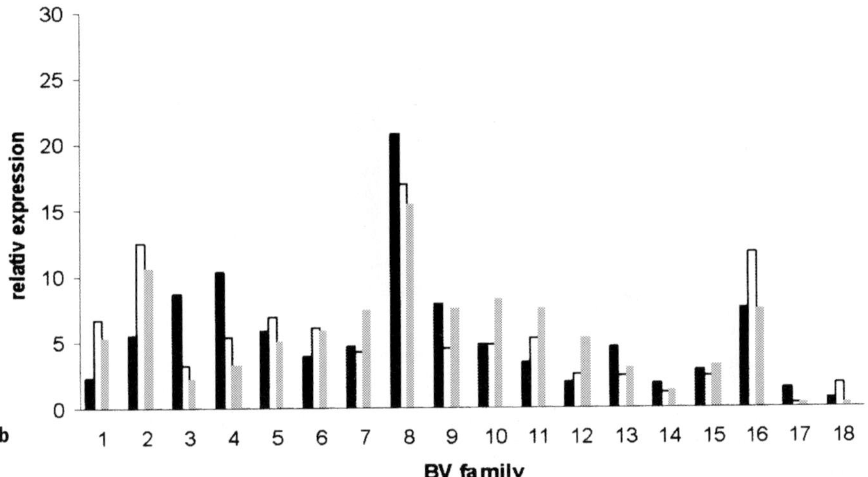

**Fig. 2a, b.** Relative expression of TCR BV regions 1–18 in tissue specimens. Tumors were obtained on days 7 (*black*), 14 (*white*) and 21 (*dark gray*) and lymph node on day 21 (*light gray*) after tumor induction in both ch14.18-LT$\alpha$ treated animals (**a**) and control animals (**b**). Therapy was administered from day 8 through 14. The expression of each BV region was calculated as the percentage of the sum of all BV spots. The *insert* depicts the clonal origin of over-expressed TCR BV families 5 and 8 on day 21 in a ch14.18–LT$\alpha$-treated animal

## Discussion

Cytokines are known to have major roles in the regulation of immune responses. Therefore, many different approaches to their use in anticancer therapies have been investigated. Although systemic administration of some cytokines possessed an antitumor effect, major obstacles resulted because the

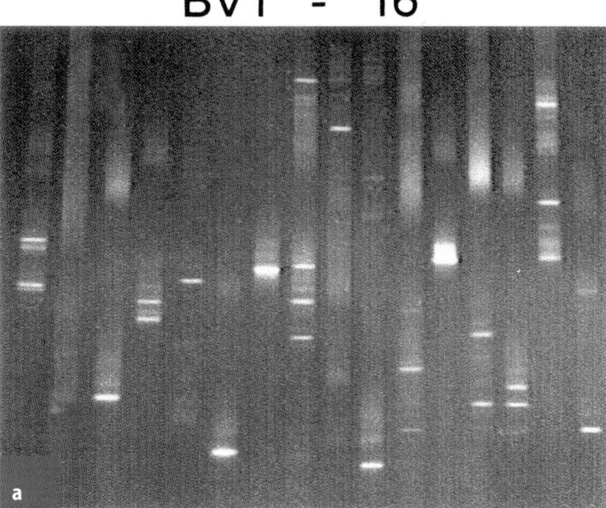



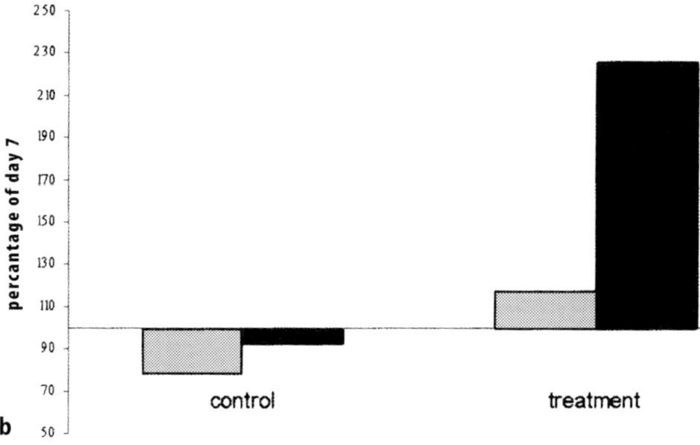



**Fig. 3 a, b.** Clonal alteration of TIL over the course of therapy. Subcutaneous tumors were induced as already described elsewhere. On days 8–14 treatment was administered in the form of 64 μg ch14.18-LT$\alpha$ (**a**, treatment) or 10 ng of sLT$\alpha$ (control). At days 7, 14, and 21 biopsies of tumors were excised and analyzed by TCR clonotype mapping. **a** TCR clonotype map of TIL on day 21 of a ch14.18-LT$\alpha$-treated tumor covering BV regions 1–16. **b** The difference in the number of clonotypic T cells over the course of treatment is shown as a percentage of total number of clones (BV regions 1–16) at days 14 (*gray*) and 21 (*black*), the number on day 7 being used as reference

paracrine working mechanism of cytokines was disregarded. The solution to these problems is the in situ administration of cytokines. Local injection of cytokine into the tumor is an example of such an in situ therapy. This method, however, can only be used for localized and reachable tumors. Another approach to in situ cytokine therapy, based on the idea of Ralph Reisfeld, is an antibody–cytokine fusion protein, i.e., the genetic fusion of a cytokine to a tumor-specific antibody. These immunoconjugates have been shown to possess the binding capacity of the parental antibody as well as the biological activity of the cytokine (Gillies et al. 1991). In vivo they accumulate at the site of antigen expression against which the antibody is directed. An IL-2 fusion protein was one of the first to be tested for antitumor activity. And indeed, antibody-targeted IL2 therapy was effective in eradicating established pulmonary and hepatic melanoma metastases in a syngeneic murine tumor model (Sabzevari et al. 1994). The success of IL-2 in situ therapy depends on T cells. Analysis of the working mechanism revealed that a pre-existing immune response was boosted (thor Straten et al. 1998). To extend this observation to other targeted cytokines we tested targeted LT$\alpha$ therapy. LT$\alpha$ fusion proteins effectively eradicated subcutaneous tumors; this therapeutic effect was dependent on T cells. Although quantitative analysis of the T-cell repertoire revealed only modest differences between control and treated mice, clonotypic mapping displayed a significant increase of T cell clones among TIL during LT$\alpha$ therapy. Moreover, the clonotypic maps over the course of therapy demonstrated the dynamics within TIL with respect to the TCR repertoire usage: some clones vanished, some persisted, and some new ones occurred.

Comparison of the IL-2 and LT$\alpha$ antibody-directed therapies demonstrates that for both, the eradication of melanoma tumors is mediated via clonally expanded T cells rather than via a polyclonal T-cell population. However, the effects of LT$\alpha$ fusion protein differ substantially from the effects of the IL-2 immunoconjugate in that the former allows for recruitment of new T cells, which could be contributed to LT$\alpha$'s role in lymphoid neogenesis.

# References


Becker JC, Pancook JD, Gillies SD, Furukawa K, Reisfeld RA (1996) T cell-mediated eradication of murine metastatic melanoma induced by targeted interleukin 2 therapy. J Exp Med 183:2361–2366

De Togni P, Goellner J, Ruddle NH, Streeter PR, Fick A, Mariathasan S, Smith SC, Carlson R, Shornick LP, Strauss-Schoenberger J (1994) Abnormal development of peripheral lymphoid organs in mice deficient in lymphotoxin. Science 264:703–707

Gillies SD, Young D, Lo KM, Foley SF, Reisfeld RA (1991) Expression of genetically engineered immunoconjugates of lymphotoxin and a chimeric anti-ganglioside GD2 antibody. Hybridoma 10:347–356

Kirkin AF, Dzhandzhugazyan K, Zeuthen J (1998) Melanoma-associated antigens recognized by cytotoxic T lymphocytes. APMIS 106:665–679

Koni PA, Sacca R, Lawton P, Browning JL, Ruddle NH, Flavell RA (1997) Distinct roles in lymphoid organogenesis for lymphotoxins alpha and beta revealed in lymphotoxin beta-deficient mice. Immunity 6:491–500

Reisfeld RA, Gillies SD, Mendelsohn J, Varki NM, Becker JC (1996) Involvement of B lymphocytes in the growth inhibition of human pulmonary melanoma metastases in athymic nu/nu mice by an antibody-lymphotoxin fusion protein. Cancer Res 56:1707–1712

Rennert PD, Browning JL, Mebius R, Mackay F, Hochman PS (1996) Surface lymphotoxin alpha/beta complex is required for the development of peripheral lymphoid organs. J Exp Med 184:1999–2006

Ruddle NH (1999) Lymphoid neo-organogenesis: lymphotoxin's role in inflammation and development. Immunol Res 19:119–125

Sabzevari H, Gillies SD, Mueller BM, Pancook JD, Reisfeld RA (1994) A recombinant antibody-interleukin 2 fusion protein suppresses growth of hepatic human neuroblastoma metastases in severe combined immunodeficiency mice. Proc Natl Acad Sci USA 91: 9626–9630

Staveley-O'Carroll K, Sotomayor E, Montgomery J, Borrello I, Hwang L, Fein S, Pardoll D, Levitsky H (1998) Induction of antigen-specific T cell anergy: an early event in the course of tumor progression. Proc Natl Acad Sci USA 95:1178–1183

thor Straten P, Guldberg P, Seremet T, Reisfeld RA, Zeuthen J, Becker JC (1998) Activation of preexisting T cell clones by targeted interleukin 2 therapy. Proc Natl Acad Sci USA 95:8785–8790

thor Straten P, Guldberg P, Gronbaek K, Hansen MR, Kirkin AF, Seremet T, Zeuthen J, Becker JC (1999) In situ T cell responses against melanoma comprise high numbers of locally expanded T cell clonotypes. J Immunol 163:443–447

# Cytotoxic T-cell Induction in Metastatic Melanoma Patients Undergoing Recombinant Vaccinia Virus-based Immuno-gene Therapy

Giulio C. Spagnoli, Paul Zajac, Walter R. Marti, Daniel Oertli, Elisabetta Padovan, Christoph Noppen, Thomas Kocher, Michel Adamina, and Michael Heberer

## Abstract

In an ongoing phase I/II study, metastatic melanoma patients were treated with a replication-incompetent recombinant vaccinia virus (rVV) encoding Melan-A$_{27-35}$, gp100$_{280-288}$, and tyrosinase$_{1-9}$ HLA-A*201-restricted epitopes together with B7.1 and B7.2 co-stimulatory molecules. rVV was administered in the context of systemic GM-CSF treatment. Boosts were subsequently administered 2 weeks apart with corresponding synthetic nonapeptides and GM-CSF. Two cycles of treatment were administered 2 weeks apart from each other. Specific immune responses were evaluated by quantitative assessment of cytotoxic T-lymphocyte precursor frequency and tetramer staining. By the time the two cycles had been completed, four out of five patients showed significant (greater than threefold) increases in gp100$_{280-288}$-specific and four out of five, in Melan-A$_{27-35}$-specific tetramer staining of CD8+ cells. Frequencies of CTL precursors specific for gp100$_{280-288}$, tyrosinase$_{1-9}$ and Melan-A$_{27-35}$ were also significantly increased in all five, and in four and four of the five patients, respectively, in some cases within 12 days after the first injection of the recombinant vector. Thus, the innovative vector under investigation is able to raise a concurrent and specific cellular immune response against a panel of molecularly defined antigens, thereby increasing the chance of an immune hit against neoplastic cells displaying heterogeneous antigen expression.

## Introduction

The identification of a large number of tumor-associated antigens (TAA) during the past decade (van der Bruggen et al. 1991) has raised wide interest, as it suggests that with appropriate immunization procedures, immune responses targeting cancer cells of potential clinical relevance could be generated. On the other hand, mechanisms inhibiting the induction of immune responses or favoring the escape of tumor cells from the attack of specific ef-

Recent Results in Cancer Research, Vol. 160
© Springer-Verlag Berlin Heidelberg 2002

fectors have started to be clarified (Smyth et al. 2001). The mechanisms include the heterogeneous expression or down-regulation of TAA in clinical neoplastic specimens (Ferrone and Marincola 1995) and the absence of co-stimulation or "danger" signals at the tumor site, resulting in poor T cell activation and ultimately leading to specific tolerance (Fuchs and Matzinger 1996). Clearly, these findings also dictate specific requirements for putative tumor vaccines.

Capitalizing on this background and on our previous "in vitro" studies (Zajac et al. 1997, 1998), we have constructed a recombinant vaccinia virus (rVV) with novel and individual characteristics. It encodes defined antigenic epitopes from multiple melanoma TAA (Cox et al. 1994; Kawakami et al. 1994; Wölfel et al. 1994) under the guidance of leader sequences driving recombinant gene products into the endoplasmic reticulum (ER) and B7.1 and B7.2 co-stimulatory molecules (Azuma et al. 1993; Linsley et al. 1994), thereby inducing high co-receptor expression in infected cells. In addition, it has been rendered replication incompetent, while maintaining a high capacity for transduction and expression of recombinant genes.

With this study, we have addressed the "in vivo" immunogenicity of this reagent, and we report that this novel vaccine is able to stimulate the rapid induction of CTL specific for all three engineered molecularly defined epitopes.

## Materials and Methods

### Vector Construction and Production of Clinical Reagents

The construction of rVV vectors has been described in detail elsewhere (Zajac et al. 1997; Marti et al. 1997). The cDNAs encoding the adenovirus E3/19 k ER signal sequence followed by the sequences specific for HLA-A201-restricted epitopes of Melan-A (27–35), gp100 (280–288) and tyrosinase (1–9), were each separately inserted into one gene locus of the Copenhagen strain of VV. *B7.1* and *B7.2* genes were inserted into two other nonessential viral loci. The virus stock used in this clinical study was produced under GMP conditions by Bioreliance (Stirling, UK).

To enhance its safety, the rVV was rendered replication incompetent by DNA crosslinking using psoralen and limited long-wave UV irradiation, as described elsewhere (Tsung et al. 1996). Following this treatment, rVV was devoid of cytopathic effect, as tested on a monolayer of sensitive BSC-40 cells. The absence of adventitious retrovirus and HIV, HSV, EBV, CMV, HCV, and HBV contamination was demonstrated by the Swiss National Center for Retroviruses (Zurich, Switzerland) and by the Institute of Microbiology of the University of Basel.

## Patients and Vaccination Schedule

HLA-A*201-positive patients who were over 18 years old, had recurrent and/ or advanced stage III or IV malignant melanoma, and were not undergoing chemotherapy, immunotherapy, or other investigational treatments were included in the study, which was approved by the Swiss National Committee on Biological Safety and by the local ethics committee of Basel University Hospital. Two cycles of treatment were administered 2 weeks apart, each including one intradermal injection of the rVV vector ($1 \times 10^7$ PFU in the first and $1 \times 10^8$ PFU in the second cycle) followed after a 14-day interval by two recall injections of Melan/A 27–35, gp100 280–288, and tyrosinase$_{1-9}$ epitope peptides (100 µg each) dissolved in DMSO (Orpegen Therapeutica, Heidelberg, Germany), during systemic treatment with granulocyte-macrophage colony-stimulating factor (GM-CSF) at a daily dose of 5 µg per kg body weight, (Leucomax, Novartis Pharma, Basel, Switzerland).

## Ex Vivo Assessment of Immune Response

At defined time points during the vaccination course, peripheral blood CD8+ cells were isolated and stimulated separately with irradiated autologous CD8– cells pulsed with each of the three epitopes under investigation at 50 µg/ml concentration for 4 h at 37 °C in the presence of $\beta$-2-microglobulin (2.5 µg/ ml). Cultures were set up in bulk or limiting dilution (10 000, 5000, and 2500 cells per well in 32 wells for each cell concentration) conditions. All cultures were restimulated with IL-2 on days 4, 8 (20 U/ml final concentration), and 11 (100 U/ml final concentration) and with the respective soluble peptide (2 µg/ml final concentration) on day 8. On day 15, cells from bulk cultures were stained with tetramer-PE conjugates (courtesy of NIH, Bethesda, Md., 200 ng/sample), together with anti-CD3 PerCP and anti-CD8 FITC mAbs (Becton Dickinson, Basel, Switzerland) in PBS supplemented with 1% FCS, washed, and analyzed by flow cytometry (CellQuest software, Becton Dickinson).

Cytotoxic activity of limiting dilution cultures was tested against $^{51}$Cr-labeled and peptide-pulsed Na-8 cells (courtesy of Dr. F. Jotereau, Nantes, France) at 1000 cells per well, in the presence of a 100-fold excess of unlabeled K562 cells to quench background NK-like activity. For each culture cytotoxicity assays were performed by using, as targets, cells pulsed with specific or control peptides. Data were expressed as percent killing according to the standard formula. Wells were considered positive when their cytolysis exceeded three standard deviations above the value of spontaneous lysis and at least 12% above their respective negative control lysis. Precursor frequencies were calculated on the basis of the number of negative wells and expressed as specific CTL precursors per $10^6$ CD8+ cells.

## Results

Vaccination and GM-CSF treatment did not result in significant modifications of the phenotypic profiles of circulating peripheral lymphocytes in terms of CD3+, CD4+, and CD8+ cell populations, or in the peripheral mobilization of dendritic cells (i.e. $CD11c^+Lin^-$ or $CD123^+Lin^-$).

Percentages of cultured CD8+ cells obtained before vaccination scoring positive for either $gp100_{280-288}$ or $Melan-A_{27-35}$ tetramers ranged between undetectable and 1% (Table 1). Specifically stained CD8+ cells became detectable or increased more than threefold following immunization in all cases, with the exception of $Melan-A_{27-35}$-specific T cells in patient 2 and $gp100_{280-288}$-specific T cells in patient 1. Remarkably, in patient 1 peak $Melan-A_{27-35}$-positive values observed during the treatment accounted for one-fifth of specifically stimulated CD8+ cells.

Limiting dilution analysis (LDA) of cytotoxic precursors addressed the functional properties of these cells. Prior to immunization, $gp100_{280-288}$, $Melan/A_{27-35}$ or $tyrosinase_{1-9}$ cytotoxic precursors were either undetectable or present at concentrations lower than $20/10^6$ CD8+ cells. Upon vaccination, CTL precursors specific for the three epitopes used were detectable or significantly (over twofold) increased in number (Table 2), with the sole exceptions of patient 4 for $Melan/A_{27-35}$ and patient 5 for $tyrosinase_{1-9}$. Remarkably, in several instances, responses could be observed or found to be augmented compared with pretreatment values as early as 12 days after the first rVV injection.

**Table 1.** Tetramer staining of in vitro-stimulated CD8+ cells from treated metastatic melanoma patients[a] (*rVV* recombinant vaccinia virus)

| Patient no. | Pretreatment | After first rVV administration | Peak value |
|---|---|---|---|
| $Melan-A_{27-35}$ tetramers | | | |
| 1 | 1.07 | 1.29 | 21.0 |
| 2 | 0.93 | 0.21 | 0.93 |
| 3 | 0 | 0.42 | 0.54 |
| 4 | 0.21 | 0.92 | 8.25 |
| 5 | 0.18 | 0.04 | 0.67 |
| $gp100_{280-288}$ tetramers | | | |
| 1 | 0.88 | 0.3 | 0.88 |
| 2 | 0.11 | 0.19 | 2.02 |
| 3 | 0.05 | 0.13 | 3.05 |
| 4 | 0.08 | 0 | 1.32 |
| 5 | 0.21 | 0.07 | 1.83 |

[a] CD8+ PBMC were isolated and stimulated in vitro with specific peptides in the presence of autologous APC as described in the "Materials and Methods" section. After 15 days of culture, cells were washed, tetramer stained and analyzed by flow cytometry. Data are reported as percentages of total CD8+ cells

**Table 2.** Cytotoxic T cell precursor frequency in peripheral blood from treated metastatic melanoma patients [a]

| Patient no. | Pretreatment | After first rVV administration | Peak value |
| --- | --- | --- | --- |
| Melan-A$_{27-35}$ specific | | | |
| 1 | 19 | 51 | 51 |
| 2 | 0 | 16 | 39 |
| 3 | 0 | 21 | 56 |
| 4 | 16 | 6 | 17 |
| 5 | 0 | 7 | 53 |
| gp100$_{280-288}$-specific | | | |
| 1 | 6 | 46 | 46 |
| 2 | 0 | 16 | 65 |
| 3 | 0 | 0 | 99 |
| 4 | 0 | 0 | 25 |
| 5 | 0 | 7 | 56 |
| Tyrosinase$_{1-9}$-specific | | | |
| 1 | 0 | 24 | 75 |
| 2 | 0 | 16 | 36 |
| 3 | 0 | 21 | 82 |
| 4 | 0 | 0 | 37 |
| 5 | 17 | 0 | 31 |

[a] CD8+ PBMC were isolated and stimulated in vitro with specific peptides in the presence of autologous APC in limiting dilution conditions, as described in the "Materials and Methods" section. After 15 days of culture, individual wells were split in two and cytotoxicity was evaluated by using, as targets, cells pulsed with control or specific peptides. Data are reported as number of specific CTL precursors per $10^6$ CD8+ cells

## Discussion

Recombinant viruses appear to be of particular interest in the development of TAA-specific immunization procedures, in that their delivery of antigenic transgenes' products closely mimics the physiological endogenous production of class I ligands (Eder et al. 2000; Hörig et al. 2000). Furthermore, and perhaps most importantly, such vectors may per se provide a typical danger signal, possibly activating antigen-presenting cells on the injection site (Fuchs and Matzinger 1996). While these characteristics are common to a number of recombinant reagents currently under clinical investigation, the rVV whose use is described here presents crucial additional characteristics.

Minigenes encoding immunodominant epitopes fused to an endoplasmatic reticulum signal sequence were preferred to full-gene TAA since endogenously produced oligopeptides bound to the signal sequence might bypass discrete antigen-processing steps eventually resulting in enhanced epitope presentation (Bacik et al. 1994). Furthermore, in an attempt to overcome tumor escape from CTL surveillance through down-regulation of individual TAAs, we constructed a reagent containing three immunodominant epitopes from different TAA.

Co-stimulatory molecules play a decisive role in the response to antigenic challenges, steering it towards induction of effector cells instead of tolerance (Schwartz 1990; Linsley et al. 1994). Previous data from our group show that HLA-A*201-positive fibroblasts co-infected with rVV encoding B7.1 or B7.2 and rVV-encoding Melan-A$_{27-35}$ antigen induce an effective CTL response in autologous peripheral blood mononuclear cells from healthy donors (Marti et al. 1997; Zajac et al. 1998). Thus, we inserted both *B7.1* and *B7.2* genes into the rVV currently undergoing clinical evaluation. Finally, we inactivated the viral replication by a psoralen and long-wave UV treatment that does not abrogate the expression of recombinant genes driven by the synthetic early promoters (Marti et al. 1997).

We report here the rapid elicitation of specific CD8+ T cells for Melan/A$_{27-35}$, gp100$_{280-288}$, and tyrosinase$_{1-9}$ upon in vivo gene delivery with this polyepitope and *B7-1-* and *B7-2*-expressing nonreplicating rVV. The immunization was achieved with a relatively easily handled "off-the-shelf" recombinant vector without any ex vivo manipulation of each individual patient's immune cells. The reagents included in this protocol do not require individually tailored generation but are produced in bulk batches under GMP conditions and stored until use, thus enabling economies in terms of production and logistics. These data urge their application in larger clinical trials.

**Acknowledgements.** This study is supported by grants (nos. 4037–055151, 4037–057018, and 31–57473.99) from the Swiss National Science Foundation.

# References

Azuma M, Ito D, Yagita H (1993) B70 antigen: a second ligand for CTLA-4 and CD28. Nature 366:76–79

Bacik I, Cox JH, Anderson R, Yewdell JW, Bennink JR (1994) Transporter associated with antigen processing-independent presentation of endogenously synthesized peptides is enhanced by endoplasmatic reticulum insertion sequences located at the amino but not carboxyl terminus of the peptide. J Immunol 152:381–387

Cox AL, Skipper J, Chen Y, Henderson RA, Darrow TL, Schabanowitz J, Engelhard VH, Hunt DF, Slingluff CL (1994) Identification of a peptide recognized by five melanoma-specific human cytotoxic T cell lines. Science 264:716–719

Eder JP, Kantoff PW, Roper K, Xu GX, Bubley GJ, Boyden J, Gritz L, Mazzara G, Oh WK, Arlen P, Tsang KY, Schlom J, Kufe DW (2000) A phase I trial of a recombinant vaccinia virus expressing prostate-specific antigen in advanced prostate cancer. Clin Cancer Res 6:1632–1638

Ferrone S, Marincola FM (1995) Loss of HLA class I antigens by melanoma cells: molecular mechanisms, functional significance and clinical relevance. Immunol Today 16:487–494

Fuchs EJ, Matzinger P (1996) Is cancer dangerous to the immune system? Semin Immunol 8:271–280

Hörig H, Lee DS, Conkright W, Divito J, Hasson H, LaMare M, Rivera A, Park D, Tine J, Guito K, Tsang KW, Schlom J, Kaufman HL (2000) Phase I clinical trial of a recombinant canarypoxvirus (ALVAC) vaccine expressing human carcinoembryonic antigen and the B7.1 co-stimulatory molecule. Cancer Immunol Immunother 49:504–514

Kawakami Y, Eliyahu S, Delgado CH, Robbins RF, Rivoltini L, Topalian SL, Miki T, Rosenberg SA (1994) Cloning of the gene coding for a shared melanoma antigen recognized by autologous T cells infiltrating into tumor. Proc Natl Acad Sci USA 91:3515–3519

Linsley PS, Greene JL, Brady W, Bajorath J, Ledbetter JA, Peach R (1994) Human B7–1 (CD80) and B7–2 (CD86) bind with similar avidities but distinct kinetics to CD28 and CTLA-4 receptors. Immunity 1:793–801

Marti RW, Zajac P, Spagnoli GC, Heberer M, Oertli D (1997) Non-replicating recombinant Vaccinia virus encoding human B-7 molecules elicits effective costimulation of naïve and memory CD4+ T lymphocytes in vitro. Cell Immunol 179:146–152

Schwarz RH (1990) A cell culture model for T lymphocyte clonal anergy. Science 248:1349–1356

Smyth MJ, Godfrey DI, Trapani JA (2001) A fresh look at tumor immunosurveillance and immunotherapy. Nat Immunol 2:293–299

Tsung K, Yim JH, Marti WR, Buller ML, Norton JA (1996) Gene expression and cytopathic effect of chemically inactivated vaccinia virus. J Virol 70:1265–1271

van der Bruggen P, Traversari C, Chomez P, Lurquin C, De Plaen E, Van den Eynde B, Knuth A, Boon T (1991) A gene encoding an antigen recognized by cytolytic T lymphocytes on a human melanoma. Science 254:1643–1647

Wölfel T, Van Pel A, Brichard V, Scheider J, Seliger B, Meyer zum Bürschenfelde KH, Boon T (1994) Two tyrosinase nonapeptides recognized on HLA-A2 melanomas by autologous cytolytic T lymphocytes. Eur J Immunol 24:759–764

Zajac P, Oertli D, Spagnoli GC, Noppen C, Schaefer C, Heberer M, Marti WR (1997) Generation of tumoricidal cytotoxic T lymphocytes from healthy donors after in vitro stimulation with a replication-incompetent vaccinia virus encoding Mart-1/Melan-A 27–35 epitope. Int J Cancer 71:491–496

Zajac P, Schütz A, Oertli D, Noppen C, Schaefer C, Heberer M, Spagnoli GC, Marti WR (1998) Enhanced generation of cytotoxic T lymphocytes using recombinant vaccinia virus expressing human tumor-associated antigens and B7 costimulatory molecules. Cancer Res 58:4567–4571

# Melanoma 3

Pathogenesis
Epidemiology
Diagnostic
Therapy
**Follow-up**

# A Rational Approach to the Follow-up
# of Melanoma Patients

Claus Garbe

## Abstract

There are no generally accepted guidelines for the follow-up of cutaneous melanoma (CM), and there is an ongoing debate about the value of follow-up examinations. Some authors doubt whether early detection has any beneficial effect on patient survival and suggest that it may only prolong the patient's period of suffering from the knowledge of having metastasis. A systematic review of the literature on early detection and resection of CM metastasis shows the following picture: (1) In in-transit metastasis and in regional node metastasis, the tumour volume of the metastatic nodules at the time of diagnosis is prognostically significant. Either the number of nodes involved in regional metastasis or the diameter of the largest node showed prognostic impact in different studies. Therefore, early detection seems to affect the cure rate in this stage of disease. (2) In distant metastasis, surgical resection of all recognisable metastases prolongs survival. This is true as long as only one organ system is involved and particularly if complete resection of all metastases can be achieved. Therefore, early detection contributes to prolongation of survival. We performed a follow-up study in 2008 prospectively documented consecutive patients with stage I–III cutaneous melanoma who presented for follow-up examination at the Department of Dermatology of the University of Tübingen from August 1996 to August 1998. Stage-appropriate follow-up examinations were carried out according to the German Society of Dermatology guidelines. A total of 3800 clinical examinations and 12 398 imaging techniques were documented: 62 second primary melanomas were detected in 46 patients and 233 disease recurrences in 112 patients during this time. Physical examination was responsible for the discovery of 50% of all recurrences, with the patient initially detecting the metastasis on self-examination in 17% of these cases. Technical examinations were responsible for the detection of the remaining 50%. In the primary tumour stages, 21% of all recurrences were discovered by lymph node sonography, the majority being classified as early detection. Among the recurrences, 48% were classified as early

Recent Results in Cancer Research, Vol. 160
© Springer-Verlag Berlin Heidelberg 2002

detection, and these patients had a significantly more favourable probability of recurrence-free survival than those with recurrences classified as late detection. The results of our study suggest that a follow-up schedule elaborated for cutaneous melanoma is suitable for the early detection of second primary melanomas and of early recurrences in approximately 5% of patients during a 2-year follow-up period.

## Epidemiological Developments and New Demands of Follow-up

Epidemiology of cutaneous melanoma has been shaped mainly by two trends during the last two decades. The first trend to be observed is an increased incidence in the industrial nations with white populations, which is more pronounced than the increase in the incidence of any other kind of tumour [16, 39]. The incidence of cutaneous melanomas in German-speaking countries is about 12 cases per 100 000 inhabitants per year. In the Scandinavian countries and the USA, it is higher by 50–100%, and the highest incidence rates are reported from Australia, where figures of 50 cases per 100 000 inhabitants and year are sometimes exceeded (for a review see [16]). In the decades to come, an increase in incidence rates is to be expected for Germany and for most of the other Western industrialized countries. About 10 000 new cases of malignant melanoma are being diagnosed in Germany per year.

The second important trend concerning the malignant melanoma is a significant improvement in the rate of early detection in the German-speaking area, which is reflected in a considerable decrease in tumour thickness [16, 17]. From the beginning of the 1980s to today, the median tumour thickness has decreased from about 1.5 mm to 0.75 mm. About 50% of all patients with a malignant melanoma who come for a first diagnosis now have a tumour thickness less than 0.75 mm. The patients who have thinner melanomas have an excellent prognosis, with a 10-year survival rate of about 95%. All newly diagnosed melanoma patients have a survival rate of 75–80%.

These two impressive developments in the epidemiology of cutaneous melanoma have a considerable effect on follow-up. A fast increase in patient numbers has been registered. Each year about 2000 patients present for follow-up examinations in the University Department of Dermatology in Tübingen. There are also more than 400 new melanoma patients annually. Some of the patients are in the stage of progressive disease, and increasingly extensive screening and therapy concepts are realised for them. The follow-up of melanoma patients has reached and even by far exceeded the clinical capacities. The University Department of Dermatology in Tübingen has started a cooperative model, in which physicians in private practice have an integral role in the follow-up examination schedule. Patients with thin melanomas are examined once a year in the clinic, and any interim follow-up examinations are conducted by physicians in private practice.

Another important development is that an increasing number of patients with low-risk melanomas are followed up. This study shows, as could be expected from the epidemiological development, that more than 50% of all patients in follow-up have tumours ≤0.75 mm thick and their prognosis is extremely favourable. For these patients, too, the guidelines of the German Society of Dermatology recommend four physical examinations a year and an annual hi-tech examination. It seems evident that cutbacks in the expenditure are indicated. About 75% of all patients in clinical follow-up have a clinical stage I melanoma with a favourable prognosis of about 90% survival rate. Precisely for this group, a modification of the follow-up strategy should be considered.

## Relevance of Early Detection of Recurrences to Prognosis of Malignant Melanoma

In 70% of cases, first recurrences of primary melanomas are found in the loco-regional area. First metastases are found in distant sites in about 30% of cases.

It is known that the extent of the tumour mass has a considerable influence on the prognosis in the case of loco-regional metastases, especially lymph node metastases. In the TNM classification, a distinction is made between diameters smaller (N1) and larger (N2) than 3 cm for the largest lymph node affected [47]. Studies have revealed that the number of lymph nodes affected in the stage of regional metastasis is a prognostic feature [42]. Unpublished evaluations performed by us show that during the period of an intensive follow-up strategy the occurrence of several affected lymph nodes is rare and that the volume of the first lymph node affected is a relevant prognostic feature. The probability of a 5-year survival with lymph node metastasis varies between 20% and 40%. This means that early detection in this group can double the survival expectancy.

This situation is less clear in the stage of distant metastasis. In two very well-documented patient groups in Tübingen and Berlin it was noted which patients with distant metastases survived for 2 years and more. During the first examination it turned out that these patients either became tumour free with surgery in the stage of distant metastasis or had a complete remission brought about by systemic therapy [15]. A second study in patients in Tübingen revealed that the significant factor was the possibility of removing all tumour masses by surgery. However, no decisive systemic therapies were performed in these cases. According to experience so far, the response of malignant melanoma to chemotherapy also depends on the existing tumour mass. No response can be expected as soon as a certain mass size is exceeded. The early detection of recurrences, in the stage of distant metastases, also seems to be of relevance for the survival expectancy of patients.

## Follow-up Strategies for Malignant Melanomas

There are different recommendations on follow-up strategy in various countries. The German Society of Dermatology, like the Swiss Society, recommends regular chest X-ray examinations, abdominal sonography and lymph node sonography, in addition to blood tests. The recommendations of the two societies differ hardly at all [34, 40]. In France and The Netherlands no technical examinations are recommended for follow-up examinations of patients treated for primary malignant melanomas; only clinical examinations are proposed [1, 2, 37]. A consensus conference of the National Institute of Health (NIH) about melanomas with a tumour thickness up to 1 mm was held in the USA in 1992. Examinations directed at the staging of these tumours were not recommended [32, 33]; clinical follow-up examinations of the patients were considered reasonable. There were differing views on the roles of blood tests and imaging techniques [27].

Provost et al. published a study in 1997, in which 30 world surgical and dermatological experts on malignant melanoma were questioned on their approaches to staging and follow-up. Most (23) of these experts came from the USA, 2 from Australia, and 5 from Europe. The enquiry revealed different management strategies. Only about half of the persons questioned perform initial staging for melanomas with a tumour thickness of 0.75 mm or less. Technical examinations in the group of patients with low-risk tumours were only performed by one-third of the persons questioned. Initial staging was performed for tumours 0.76–1.5 mm thick by about 80% of the persons questioned. Blood tests and imaging techniques were used during follow-up by 50–80%. The percentage of experts who perform imaging examinations during follow-up increased with the thickness of the tumours [36]. This enquiry does not only show that the recommendations differ from country to country, but also that the practical procedure adopted for follow-up examinations differs even within the same country. In fact, there are not many data that could support the various management strategies in malignant melanoma: it is essential that the database be improved.

## The Value of Technical Examinations in Detecting Metastases

During the aforementioned study on the methods followed by 30 experts for melanoma follow-up, the chest X-ray examination was the most frequently applied imaging technique. The few systematic examinations of the value of chest X-ray examination have shown that few metastases can be detected by this means. Weiss et al. analysed the data of 261 patients with melanomas with a tumour thickness of more than 1.7 mm, some of whom also had regional lymph node metastases, and found that 145 of them developed tumour recurrences: 68% were diagnosed on the basis of their case history, 26% on a physical examination, and only 6% on the grounds of a chest X-ray examination [46]. A similarly designed study showed that the recurrences in 47 out of 49 patients were found by examination of their history or on a physical examination, and only 2 (5%) from a chest X-ray examination. The number of positive findings on abdominal sonography was similarly low [3].

A French study evaluated the results of the follow-up examinations of 528 patients with primary melanomas who had been examined twice by chest X-ray and abdominal sonography: 115 of the 528 patients developed recurrences, 30 of them distant metastases; 6 distant metastases were detected by chest X-ray examination and 6 by abdominal sonography. With the high number of examinations in mind, the authors regard the ratio between the cost of such examinations and the benefit to the patients as unfavourable [4].

The staging procedure for detecting metastases of primary melanomas at the time of diagnosis must also be questioned. The chest X-ray examinations of 876 consecutive, asymptomatic patients with stage I and II primary cutaneous melanomas were also evaluated. True-positive metastases were found in 1 patient (0.1%) [44]. Three hundred and ninety-three patients with stage I and II primary melanomas were examined for the predictive value of a routine staging test battery including blood tests and chest X-ray examination, and also CT and liver and bone scintigraphy in some of the patients. Metastases were detected in only 9 patients, and in 8 of them it was the physical examination that revealed them. The metastasis of only 1 patient was detected by imaging techniques. In contrast, 15 false-positive diagnoses were indicated by imaging techniques [28]. Examinations in smaller groups have yielded similar results.

Lymph node sonography had a more favourable result. This technique revealed a lymph node metastasis in about one-third of all cases before palpation was possible [8, 35]. As 70% of primary tumour metastases are loco-regional [22], lymph node sonography has a high relative value among the technical examinations available. The study described was the first in which the value of lymph node sonography was investigated in a large group of patients.

CT turned out to be less suitable for primary staging of malignant melanomas, as positive findings were accurate in only a low number of cases. Thus, they were not helpful in identifying patients who would develop a metastasis later. Moreover, they led to false-positive results in 17% of cases, meaning that further, sometimes costly, examinations were needed later for clarification [9]. In patients with regional lymph node metastasis, the rate of true-positive results was only 7%. In contrast, false-positive results requiring clarification by means of other examinations or control examination were found on whole-body CT in 22% of the patients. CT was recommended by the authors for patients with loco-regional metastases [10]. With the aid of CT, metastases can also be detected in patients with primary tumour metastases, but the rate is only 0.5% [20]. In patients with a primary tumour, the rate of false-positive to true-positive results was found to be especially high [30]. From a study of 788 CT examinations in patients with loco-regional metastases, Kuvshinoff et al. report 4.2% true-positive and 8.4% false-positive results [31]. In a similar study with CT of 127 patients with loco-regional metastases, Johnson et al. found 16% true-positive and 12% false-positive results. Obviously, CT examinations are best suited to early detection of metastases in the stage of loco-regional metastasis [5].

## Value of Blood Tests for Diagnosis of Metastases

LDH has been reported as a suitable marker for detecting liver metastases [14], although its increased level is not very specific for this kind of metastasis. Khansur et al. found an increased serum LDH value in most patients with distant metastases [30]. However, an increase in LDH can also be prompted by other disease entities or by an operation. An increase in LDH was found to be the first hint of a metastasis in up to 12% of the cases [14]. Altogether, LDH determination is an examination method with a low sensitivity in detection of distant metastases.

Examinations of the blood parameters give hardly any indication of developing metastases [25, 46]. Biochemical examinations for 5-$S$-cysteinyl-dopa, 6-hydroxy-5-methoxyindol-2-carboxylacid, L-dopa, and alpha-MSH have not been found to be suitable markers for detecting metastases in the blood.

## New Diagnostic Developments

Positron emission tomography (PET) is one of the most interesting imaging techniques for diagnosing metastases. This technique allows scanning of the whole body during a single examination session [43]. The sensitivity during the first examinations was given as 91–93%, but the specificity was under 80%. As patients are referred for a PET examination only after preliminary imaging technique examinations, it is to be expected that if PET were to be used as the primary examination method the sensitivity would decrease considerably. Within the scope of follow-up examinations, the diagnostic "hit score" on PET examination was between 55% and 77% [38]. In the case of lymph node metastases, PET examinations seem to be inferior to sonography [7, 38]. However, lymph node metastases that are not yet palpable can be detected by PET [45].

During recent years, increasing efforts have been made to develop tumour markers for malignant melanoma. The protein S100 seems to be an interesting marker, which can become positive especially in patients with disseminated disease [21, 24, 26]. Examinations of melanoma patients in various stages of the disease have shown that the number of positive findings increases in more advanced stages. So far, no studies have examined how suitable the marker is for early detection of metastases.

More recent examination techniques involve using the polymerase chain reaction (PCR) to detect circulating tumour cells in the blood. This method exploits the fact that melanoma cells normally express genes that are required for pigment synthesis and are not expressed in other blood cells.

With the aid of reverse transcriptase (RT), the mRNA of the key enzyme tyrosinase is transcribed to cDNA and amplified by the PCR. Positive findings indicate circulating melanoma cells in the blood [12]. In the meantime, the same technique is also used to detect micrometastases in the lymph nodes [6, 41]. In more recent studies, findings were positive with RT-PCR examinations in about half of all patients who had a known disseminated metastasis [19]. Even some of the patients with earlier tumour stages showed positive findings, which may possibly have a prognostic significance. Recently, an attempt was made to combine several markers for this examination [23]. Parallel proof of the tyrosinase gene and of MAR1/Melan A turned out to be a highly specific combination with increased sensitivity [11, 13]. However, whether RT-PCR diagnosis in the blood is suitable for monitoring patients in follow-up has not yet been determined.

## Follow-up Study of the Central Malignant Melanoma Registry in Germany

This study was conducted with the aim of a descriptive analysis of the existing follow-up strategy for malignant melanoma. In particular, it was aimed at finding out by what means and how early disease recurrences could be detected. It also examined by whom second melanomas were detected.

Within this prospective, single-centre study, all follow-up examinations carried out in the University Department of Dermatology in Tübingen from August 1996 to August 1998 were documented. With the aid of a specially developed computer program, the results of all physical examinations, blood tests, and imaging techniques were documented in a standardised manner. New tumour recurrences were analysed in a detailed way. The statistical evaluation was carried out with the "Statistical Package for Social Sciences" and "S-Plus" computer programs.

In all, 3800 clinical examinations, about 3000 blood tests, and about 9400 examinations with imaging techniques were carried out in 2008 patients. During the specified period, 233 tumour recurrences were found in 112 patients and 62 second melanomas were detected. In 84% of cases, the tumour recurrences were diagnosed during the follow-up examinations for the first time. In 17% of all cases it was the patient who recognised the occurrence of a metastasis. About half of them were detected during clinical examinations. In the primary tumour stage about 20% of the recurrences were detected on lymph node sonography. Within the stages of metastasis, CT was definitely the most valuable of the imaging techniques, revealing about 28% of the recurrences. Only 4 recurrences were detected by 1981 chest X-ray examinations of primary tumours, and 1 recurrence was found in 2034 abdominal sonographies. About 50% of all recurrences were detected in an early stage of growth. In consequence, these patients had a prognostic advantage. The remaining 50% were not detected until late in the course, despite the time consuming and costly follow-up examinations. This holds especially true for distant metastases and for the findings on chest X-ray examinations, abdominal sonography, and CT. The group in whom recurrences were detected early had a median survival of 18 months, while the group with late detection had a median survival of 12 months ($P < 0.01$). Stages I and II had 2-year survival rates for the two subgroups (earlier and later diagnosis) of 80% and 30%, respectively.

This study is by far the largest investigation conducted into follow-up examinations for malignant melanoma. The largest examinations published before this one involved not more than about 500 patients, and much lower numbers of clinical and technical examinations were evaluated [3, 4, 29, 46]. The study described in this chapter was based on the follow-up recommendations of the German Society of Dermatology [18, 34]. These recommendations are based on the experience of experts rather than on systematic examinations. All patients attended for clinical examinations four times or twice a year. In the case of a stage I or II primary tumour a technical examination was conducted once a year. In the stage of loco-regional metastasis, technical examinations were performed twice a year. The results of the clinical and technical examinations performed in this study were evaluated. A record was made of whether recurrences were detected by physicians with their own practices outside the hospital or by physicians in the Tübingen clinic. The examinations that revealed the recurrences were also documented.

With the aid of this follow-up strategy, second melanomas were detected in about 2% of the patients. Early detection of developing metastases was also recorded in about half the cases. The effectiveness of the follow-up strategy was made clear by the fact that 84% of recurrences were detected during follow-up examination. Lymph node sonography contributed to the detection of tumour recurrences from stage II onward, while the remaining imaging techniques led to an increasing number of detected tumour recurrences from stage III on. The results obtained suggest that the follow-up strategy for malignant melanoma should be modified, with the following focus: (a) reduction of the number of hi-tech examinations with imaging techniques in the early stages of melanoma, (b) enhanced patient responsibility, to be achieved

**Table 1.** Modified follow-up schedule for malignant melanoma: proposal for a comparative study. Figures show time between examinations in months (*TD* tumour diameter)

| Stage | Clinical examination 1st–5th years | Clinical examination 6th–10th years | Lymph node sonography 1st–10th years | Blood tests[a] 1st–10th years | Technical examinations[b] 1st–10th years |
|---|---|---|---|---|---|
| I <1 mm TD | 6 | 12 | None | None | None |
| I+II >1 mm TD | 3 | 6 | 6 | 6 | None |
| III | 3 | 6 | 3–6 | 3–6 | 6 |
| IV | Individually decided | | | | |

[a] LDH, alkaline phosphatase, blood parameters, BSG, protein S100
[b] X-ray, abdominal sonography or computed tomography

by training in self-examination and intensive education on the objects of follow-up, (c) shifting of examinations of patients with low risk of recurrence from the clinic to physicians in private practice, and (d) intensification of the follow-up examinations for patients with an increased risk of recurrence. On the basis of the study results presented, a modified follow-up schedule for malignant melanoma was suggested (see Table 1). This follow-up schedule is to be compared with the existing one in a newly activated comparative study.

## References


1. Anonymous (1995a) Conférence de consensus. Suivi des patients opérés d'un mélanome de stade I. Ann Dermatol Venereol 122:250–258
2. Anonymous (1995b) Conférence de consensus. Suivi des patients opérés d'un mélanome de stade I. Paris, France, 30 March 1995. Ann Dermatol Venereol 122:250–391
3. Ardizzoni A, Grimaldi A, Repetto L, Bruzzone M, Sertoli MR, Rosso R (1987) Stage I–II melanoma: the value of metastatic work-up. Oncology 44:87–89
4. Basseres N, Grob JJ, Richard MA, Thirion X, Zarour H, Noe C, Collet VA, Lota I, Bonerandi JJ (1995) Cost-effectiveness of surveillance of stage I melanoma. A retrospective appraisal based on a 10-year experience in a dermatology department in France. Dermatology 191:199–203
5. Berman C, Reintgen D (1993) Radiologic imaging in malignant melanoma: a review. Semin Surg Oncol 9:232–238
6. Blaheta HJ, Schittek B, Breuninger H, Maczey E, Kroeber S, Sotlar K, Ellwanger U, Thelen MH, Rassner G, Bultmann B, Garbe C (1998) Lymph node micrometastases of cutaneous melanoma: increased sensitivity of molecular diagnosis in comparison to immunohistochemistry. Int J Cancer 79:318–323
7. Blessing C, Feine U, Geiger L, Carl M, Rassner G, Fierlbeck G (1995) Positron emission tomography and ultrasonography. A comparative retrospective study assessing the diagnostic validity in lymph node metastases of malignant melanoma. Arch Dermatol 131:1394–1398
8. Blum A, Dill-Müller D (1998) Ultrasound of lymph nodes and the subcutis in dermatology. Hautarzt 49:942–949
9. Buzaid AC, Sandler AB, Mani S, Curtis AM, Poo WJ, Bolognia JL, Ariyan S (1993) Role of computed tomography in the staging of primary melanoma. J Clin Oncol 11:638–643
10. Buzaid AC, Tinoco L, Ross MI, Legha SS, Benjamin RS (1995) Role of computed tomography in the staging of patients with local-regional metastases of melanoma. J Clin Oncol 13:2104–2108
11. Curry BJ, Smith MJ, Hersey P (1996) Detection and quantitation of melanoma cells in the circulation of patients. Melanoma Res 6:45–54
12. Curry BJ, Myers K, Hersey P (1998) Polymerase chain reaction detection of melanoma cells in the circulation: relation to clinical stage, surgical treatment, and recurrence from melanoma. J Clin Oncol 16:1760–1769
13. Farthmann B, Eberle J, Krasagakis K, Gstottner M, Wang N, Bisson S, Orfanos CE (1998) RT-PCR for tyrosinase-mRNA-positive cells in peripheral blood: evaluation strategy and correlation with known prognostic markers in 123 melanoma patients. J Invest Dermatol 110:263–267
14. Finck SJ, Giuliano AE, Morton DL (1983) LDH and melanoma. Cancer 51:840–843
15. Garbe C (1996) Verlängertes Überleben bei fernmetastasiertem Melanom und der Einfluss von Behandlungen: Analyse des Krankheitsverlaufs von 22 Patienten mit einer Überlebenszeit von zwei Jahren und länger. Hautarzt 47:35–43
16. Garbe C (1997) Epidemiologie des Hautkrebses. In: Garbe C, Dummer R, Kaufmann R, Tilgen W (eds) Dermatologische Onkologie. Springer, Berlin, Heidelberg, New York, pp 40–56

17. Garbe C, Büttner P, Ellwanger U, Bröcker EB, Jung EG, Orfanos CE, Rassner G, Wolff HH (1995) Das Zentralregister Malignes Melanom der Deutschen Dermatologischen Gesellschaft in den Jahren 1983–1993. Epidemiologische Entwicklungen und aktuelle therapeutische Versorgung des malignen Melanoms der Haut. Hautarzt 46:683–692
18. Garbe C, Reusch M, Breuninger H, Dummer R, Hauschild A, Kaufmann R, Mensing HO, Meyer, Panizzon R, Schmöckel C, Schöfer H, Sebastian G, Soyer HP, Sterry W, Tilgen W, Volkenandt M (1998) Diagnostische und therapeutische Standards in der dermatologischen Onkologie. Hautarzt 48 [Suppl 1]:S13–S55
19. Gläser R, Rass K, Seiter S, Hauschild A, Christophers E, Tilgen W (1997) Detection of circulating melanoma cells by specific amplification of tyrosinase complementary DNA is not a reliable tumor marker in melanoma patients: a clinical two-center study. J Clin Oncol 15:2818–2825
20. Goerz G, Schulte BR, Roder K, Schoppe WD, Munchhoff C, Jungblut RM (1986) Malignes Melanom. Welche Untersuchungen sind fur Staging und Verlaufskontrollen sinnvoll? Dtsch Med Wochenschr 111:1230–1233
21. Guo HB, Stoffel WB, Bierwirth T, Mezger J, Klingmüller D (1995) Clinical significance of serum S100 in metastatic malignant melanoma. Eur J Cancer [A] 31:1898–1902
22. Häffner AC, Garbe C, Burg G, Büttner P, Orfanos CE, Rassner G (1992) The prognosis of primary and metastasising melanoma. An evaluation of the TNM classification in 2,495 patients. Br J Cancer 66:856–861
23. Hanekom GS, Johnson CA, Kidson SH (1997) An improved and combined reverse transcription-polymerase chain reaction assay for reliable detection of metastatic melanoma cells in peripheral blood. Melanoma Res 7:111–116
24. Hauschild A, Engel G, Brenner W, Gläser R, Mönig H, Henze E, Christophers E (1999) S100B protein detection in serum is a significant prognostic factor in metastatic melanoma. Oncology 56:338–344
25. Hauschild A, Michaelsen J, Brenner W, Rudolph P, Gläser R, Henze E, Christophers E (1999) Prognostic significance of serum S100B detection compared with routine blood parameters in advanced metastatic melanoma patients. Melanoma Res 9:155–161
26. Henze G, Dummer R, Joller JH, Böni R, Burg G (1997) Serum S100 – a marker for disease monitoring in metastatic melanoma. Dermatology 194:208–212
27. Huang CL, Provost N, Marghoob AA, Kopf AW, Levin L, Bart RS (1998) Laboratory tests and imaging studies in patients with cutaneous malignant melanoma. J Am Acad Dermatol 39:451–463
28. Iscoe N, Kersey P, Gapski J, Osoba D, From L, DeBoer G, Quirt I (1987) Predictive value of staging investigations in patients with clinical stage I malignant melanoma. Plast Reconstr Surg 80:233–239
29. Kersey PA, Iscoe NA, Gapski JA, Osoba D, From L, DeBoer G, Quirt IC (1985) The value of staging and serial follow-up investigations in patients with completely resected, primary, cutaneous malignant melanoma. Br J Surg 72:614–617
30. Khansur T, Sanders J, Das SK (1989) Evaluation of staging workup in malignant melanoma. Arch Surg 124:847–849
31. Kuvshinoff BW, Kurtz C, Coit DG (1997) Computed tomography in evaluation of patients with stage III melanoma. Ann Surg Oncol 4:252–258
32. National Institutes of Health (1992) Diagnosis and treatment of early melanoma. NIH Consensus Development Conference, 27–29 January 1992. Consensus Statement 10:1–25
33. National Institutes of Health (1992) NIH Consensus conference. Diagnosis and treatment of early melanoma. JAMA 268:1314–1319
34. Orfanos CE, Jung EG, Rassner G, Wolff HH, Garbe C (1994) Stellungnahme und Empfehlungen der Kommission malignes Melanom der Deutschen Dermatologischen Gesellschaft zur Diagnostik, Behandlung und Nachsorge des malignen Melanoms der Haut. Stand 1993/94. Hautarzt 45:285–291
35. Prayer L, Winkelbauer H, Gritzmann N, Winkelbauer F, Helmer M, Pehamberger H (1990) Sonography versus palpation in the detection of regional lymph-node metastases in patients with malignant melanoma. Eur J Cancer 26:827–830

36. Provost N, Marghoob AA, Kopf AW, DeDavid M, Wasti Q, Bart RS (1997) Laboratory tests and imaging studies in patients with cutaneous malignant melanomas: a survey of experienced physicians. J Am Acad Dermatol 36:711–720
37. Rümke P, van-Everdingen JE (1992) Consensus on the management of melanoma of the skin in The Netherlands. Dutch Melanoma Working Party. Eur J Cancer 28:600–604
38. Rinne D, Baum RP, Hor G, Kaufmann R (1998) Primary staging and follow-up of high risk melanoma patients with whole-body 18F-fluorodeoxyglucose positron emission tomography: results of a prospective study of 100 patients. Cancer 82:1664–1671
39. Salopek TG, Marghoob AA, Slade JM, Rao B, Rigel DS, Kopf AW, Bart RS (1995) An estimate of the incidence of malignant melanoma in the United States. Based on a survey of members of the American Academy of Dermatology. Dermatol Surg 21:301–305
40. Schweizerische Gesellschaft für Dermatologie und Venerologie (1993) Das primäre maligne Melanom der Haut. Bull Med Suisse 74:1021–1024
41. Shivers SC, Wang X, Li W, Joseph E, Messina J, Glass LF, DeConti R, Cruse CW, Berman C, Fenske NA, Lyman GH, Reintgen DS (1998) Molecular staging of malignant melanoma: correlation with clinical outcome. JAMA 280:1410–1415
42. Stadelmann WK, Rapaport DP, Soong SJ, Reintgen DS, Buzaid AC, Balch CM (1998) Prognostic clinical and pathologic features. In: Balch CM, Houghton AN, Sober AJ, Soong SJ (eds) Cutaneous melanoma. Quality Medical Publishing, St Louis, pp 11–50
43. Steinert HC, Huch BR, Buck A, Böni R, Berthold T, Marincek B, Burg G, von-Schulthess GK (1995) Malignant melanoma: staging with whole-body positron emission tomography and 2-[F-18]-fluoro-2-deoxy-d-glucose. Radiology 195:705–709
44. Terhune MH, Swanson N, Johnson TM (1998) Use of chest radiography in the initial evaluation of patients with localized melanoma. Arch Dermatol 134:569–572
45. Wagner JD, Schauwecker D, Hutchins G, Coleman JJ (1997) Initial assessment of positron emission tomography for detection of nonpalpable regional lymphatic metastases in melanoma. J Surg Oncol 64:181–189
46. Weiss M, Loprinzi CL, Creagan ET, Dalton RJ, Novotny P, O'Fallon JR (1995) Utility of follow-up tests for detecting recurrent disease in patients with malignant melanomas. JAMA 274:1703–1705
47. Wittekind C, Wagner G (1997) TNM Klassifikation maligner Tumoren, 5th edn. Springer, Berlin Heidelberg New York

# Epithelial Skin Tumours **4**

## Therapy

# Micrographic Surgery of Basal Cell Carcinomas of the Head

Birgit Woerle, Marc Heckmann, and Birger Konz

## Abstract

Basal cell carcinoma (BCC) is a locally invasive malignant cutaneous tumour with a rising incidence. This tumour can be treated successfully by a variety of techniques, including local excision, radiation, cryotherapy, curettage, electrodessication and laser obliteration. Micrographic surgery is a specialised type of minimal marginal surgery that offers higher cure rates than do other options in the treatment of contiguous skin cancers in selected settings. The horizontal frozen histological sections of the excised tumour permit complete microscopic examination of the surgical margin. Maximum sparing of tumour-free adjacent tissue is achieved with histological mapping of the tumour boundaries, and subsequent wound reconstruction is optimised. Data on topographical distribution, histopathological subtype, subclinical tumour extension, therapeutic procedures required for complete eradication, and recurrence rates were recorded in 3065 BCC of the head. Micrographic surgery is the treatment of choice for large or invasive primary BCC with uncertain clinical boundaries, especially in difficult anatomical regions, for recurrent or re-recurrent BCC, and for tumours with an aggressive histopathological pattern.

## Introduction

Basal cell carcinoma (BCC) is the most common nonmelanoma skin cancer in the world, and its incidence is rising (Wennberg 2000). This tumour developes from the basal cell layer of the epidermis and the epidermal appendages and requires a stroma for proper growth. The malignant character of this skin tumour depends on its destructive growth. It rarely metastasises (Lo et al. 1991). The treatment modalities most frequently used are surgical excision, cryosurgery, curettage, electrodessication, laser obliteration, immunotherapy and radiation (Thissen et al. 1999). Surgical excision has been the

Recent Results in Cancer Research, Vol. 160
© Springer-Verlag Berlin Heidelberg 2002

treatment of choice, especially for BCC located in difficult anatomical regions, for example in the face, the preferred location of this tumour, ever since Frederic E. Mohs developed the method of micrographic surgery (Mohs 1941). Originally this technique required in situ tissue fixation with zinc chloride before excision of the tumour. The fresh tissue technique has generally been used since the early 1970s, the first to have used it being Theodore A. Tromovitch (Brodland et al. 2000). Horizontal frozen histological sections of the excised BCC permit more complete microscopic examination of the surgical margin than traditional methods. Malignant extensions of the tumour are pursued with staged excisions until the whole tumour is removed. A maximum sparing of tumour-free adjacent tissue is achieved with histological mapping of the tumour boundaries (Shriner et al. 1998). Therefore, the subsequent wound reconstruction is optimised (Dobke and Miller 1997). In the last 25 years the method of micrographic surgery has been further developed and modified. There are now three different fresh tissue micrographic techniques available: the Mohs method, the margin strip method ("Tübinger Torte") and the "Munich" method (Kopke and Konz 1995). These methods all have the same goal of radical tumour resection with optimal sparing of tumour-free adjacent tissue, but differ in the technique of tumour excision, the preparation of the histological specimens, and the interpretation of the slides. Our report summarizes the data on 3065 BCC of the head in 2795 patients treated by the "Munich" method of micrographic surgery.

## Methods

In the Department of Dermatology, Ludwig-Maximilians-University of Munich, Germany, about 2795 patients with BCC located on the head were treated by micrographic surgery in the years 1979–1994. The clinical diagnosis of BCC was confirmed histopathological prior to or at the time of excision of the tumour. Microscopically controlled surgery was carried out using three-dimensional tumour evaluation based on cryostat sections as described above (Kopke and Konz 1995).

The following data were recorded: date of birth, age at the time of diagnosis, sex, histopathological subtype of BCC, previous therapeutic efforts, whether primary or recurrent BCC, number of surgical excisions until complete tumour removal, tumour extension in the case of incomplete first excision and exact localization of the tumour. The last two were documented graphically on a schematic drawing (scale 1:1). Likewise tumour residuals, if extending to one of the edges of the excised tissue, were documented graphically, vertical and/or horizontal tumour extension being distinguished in one, two, three or all four quadrants of the specimen.

Standard anatomical regions of the face were chosen to group the BCC within particular areas and were defined in further detail according to their topographical idiosyncrasies; for example the nasolabial fold was defined as an individual region. Furthermore the periorbital region was differentiated into upper and lower lid, medial and lateral angle, and the nasal region was subdivided into root, dorsum, ala and apex of the nose. The auricular region was differentiated into conchal, retro- and preauricular areas.

Statistical analysis of all data was performed using Excel and SPSS (Microsoft, worldwide) computer software. The Chi-square test was used to calculate the level of significance.


## Results


This study involved 2795 patients with a total of 3065 BCC on the head. At the time of diagnosis 297 patients (10.6%) had more than 1 BCC in the face. Male patients were slightly more prevalent, accounting for 53% of the total patient population. The youngest of our patients was 20 years old and the oldest patient, 101 years; the mean (SD) age of the patients at the time of diagnosis was 63.2 (±12.9) years. The incidence of BCC increased steadily up to the 8th decade. There was no sex difference in age at time of diagnosis.

The most frequent localization of BCC was the nose, 1373 of 3065 BCC (44.8%) being found in this region. The second most common site was the periorbital (12.6%), followed by the auricular (8.7%), the frontal (6.9%), the temporal (6.7%) and the nasolabial (6.4%) regions. The buccal and the infra-orbital regions were each affected in 4.6% of cases. Least affected were the mental (1.5%) and the perioral regions (0.2%). With respect to their hetero-geneous topographical characteristics, the periorbital, nasal and auricular re-gions were differentiated and analysed in further detail. Most strikingly with-in the periorbital region, BCC occurred almost ten times as frequently in the medial corner of the eye as in the lateral corner. The alar part of the nose was affected almost twice as frequently as its apex. In the auricular region there was no significant difference between the pre- and the retroauricular part. BCC was found in 24% in the conchal part of the ear. The patient's age at the time of diagnosis had no influence on the pattern of occurrence within particular anatomical regions.

Depending on their histopathological features, all BCC were categorised as solid ($n=1514$), morphea-like ($n=1149$), or adenoid-cystic ($n=402$). Most (928) of the morphea-like BCC displayed this feature exclusively, while the re-maining 221 tumours were composed of solid tumour islands mixed with morphea-like features. Comparison of the histopathological subtypes of BCC in the different regions of the face revealed relatively high percentages of this morphea-like type, in descending order of frequency in the buccal, temporal, perioral and frontal regions, exceeding the percentage of the solid type. Comparison of histopathological types in both sexes revealed that the solid type of BCC was 1.2 times as frequent in men than in women, while mor-phea-like BCC were 1.3 times as frequent in women ($P<0.0001$). The ade-noid-cystic type of BCC was only marginally more frequent in women ($P=0.085$).

The number of BCC previously treated by other methods, i.e. of recurrences prior to the introduction of micrographic surgery, was 831 (27%). In this group female (51%) and male (49%) patients were affected equally. Histopathological differentiation into subtypes revealed a relative increase of morphea-like BCC in recurrences (34.9%) although solid BCC was still the most frequent subtype (43.0%).

The clinical extension of the BCC was evaluated under the lamps in the operating room prior to excision. Safety margins of at least 2 mm beyond visible tumour extension were observed. Tumours with diameters greater than 10 mm were excised with 4-mm safety margins, and tumours measuring more than 20 mm, with about 8-mm safety margins. The first excision removed 53.3% of all BCC treated by micrographic surgery in this study (tumour-free tissue at all edges of the specimen). Another 36.9% of lesions were free of BCC after the second excision, while 9.8% of the tumours required more than two excisions to be removed totally. On average, 1.6 excision steps were required to achieve complete tumour removal. The tumour residuals after the first excision affected one quadrant in 33.5% and two quadrants in 46.5% in the horizontal spread, whereas in the vertical spread only 11.0% of the tumours were not removed. Horizontal and vertical spread residuals of BCC were found after the first excision in 9.0% of cases. Influences of the different histopathological subtypes on the number of excisions necessary for complete removal of the BCC were calculated. One-step excision was sufficient in about 80% of adenoid-cystic BCC, in over 50% of solid BCC and in 43% of morphea-like BCC. Four or even more excision steps were required in about 6% of morphea-like BCC, in 2% of solid BCC and in under 1% of adenoid-cystic BCC.

The follow-up period over more than 5 years showed recurrences of BCC in 41 of the 1604 patients (2.6%). Thirty-six percent of these recurrent BCC were re-recurrent tumours; 64% of these tumours were initially primary BCC. The rate of the histopathological subtypes of BCC in the group of patients with recurrent tumours was 41.5% for the solid and also for the morphea-like type. The cure rate of BCC was 97.4% (75% primary BCC/25% recurrent BCC).

There are prognostic factors in recurrences of BCC of the face, including the history of tumour growth, histopathological subtype, tumour size and localization, and previous treatment. So-called "high-risk" localizations are situated in the middle of the face. More than 80% of the patients included in our study had BCC in a "high-risk" localization. BCC were found in various "low-risk" localizations: the periorbital region (5.4%) and the buccal (4.8%), the auricular (2.0%), the perioral (1.8%) and other (4.9%) regions; in all, these accounted for 18.9% of the BCC. History of tumour growth for longer than 1 year, morphea-like subtype of BCC, tumour diameter greater than 20 mm, and previous treatments are further indicators of a poor prognosis, i.e., "high-risk" factors.

## Discussion

The only rational principle in surgical therapy of BCC is attempted complete removal of the tumour (Lawrence 1999). Leaving residual tumour leads to tumour recurrence in the vast majority of cases. BCC spread by continuous growth. Because of unpredicted asymmetrical and subclinical spread of BCC, even radical safety margins might not be sufficient to ensure complete excision (Breuninger and Dietz 1991; Breuninger et al. 1989). On the other hand, uninvolved skin might be unnecessarily excised. The technique of micrographic surgery allows sparing of a maximum of tumour-free adjacent tissue and optimisation of the subsequent wound reconstruction, especially in difficult anatomical regions (Shriner et al. 1998). Especially in the face, a tissue-sparing approach is necessary if cosmetically and functionally acceptable results of wound reconstruction are to be achieved (Konz 1975). Our data show that complete tumour removal was achieved by micrographic surgery in one excision step in only 53.3% of BCC. A second excision step was sufficient in more than 90% of cases. Nearly 10% of the tumours required more than two excisions to be removed completely. In this study, morphea-like BCC involved the highest risk of tumour residuals after the first excision (43%), and this subtype required four or even more excisions to achieve tumour-free edges more often than the other types. Among recurrent BCC treated prior to micrographic surgery, the morphea-like type was only relatively more frequent (35%, as against 28% among primaries), while the solid subtype was predominant in both groups. Therefore, even in the absence of morphea-like histopathological features micrographic surgery is still justified. The 5-year cure rate of our cases, including those with locally recurrent disease only, is about 97.4%. This result fits in with other reports of local recurrences after micrographic surgery (Hruza 1994).

## References

Breuninger H, Dietz K (1991) Prediction of subclinical tumor infiltration in basal cell carcinoma. J Dermatol Surg Oncol 17:574–578

Breuninger H, Schippert W, Black B, Rassner G (1989) Untersuchungen zum Sicherheitsabstand und zur Exzisionstiefe in der operativen Behandlung von Basaliomen. Hautarzt 40:693–700

Brodland DG, Amonette R, Hanke W, Robins P (2000) The history and evolution of Mohs micrographic surgery. Dermatol Surg 26:303–307

Dobke MK, Miller SH (1997) Tissue repair after Mohs surgery. A plastic surgeon's view. Dermatol Surg 23:1061–1066

Hruza GJ (1994) Mohs micrographic surgery local recurrences. J Dermatol Surg Oncol 20:573–577

Konz B (1975) Use of skin flaps in dermatologic surgery of the face. J Dermatol Surg 3:25–30

Kopke LFF, Konz B (1995) Mikrographische Chirugie. Eine methodische Bestandsaufnahme. Hautarzt 46:607–614

Lawrence CM (1999) Mohs' micrographic surgery for basal cell carcinoma. Clin Exp Dermatol 24:130–133

Lo JS, Snow SN, Reizner GT, Mohs FE, Larson PO, Hruza GJ (1991) Metastatic basal cell carcinoma: report of twelve cases with a review of the literature. J Am Acad Dermatol 24:715–719

Mohs FE (1941) Chemosurgery: a microscopically controlled method of cancer excision. Arch Surg 42:279–295

Shriner DL, McCoy DK, Goldberg DJ, Wagner RF (1998) Mohs micrographic surgery. J Am Acad Dermatol 39:79–97

Thissen MRTM, Neumann MHA, Schouten LJ (1999) A systematic review of treatment modalities for primary basal cell carcinomas. Arch Dermatol 135:1177–1183

Wennberg A-M (2000) Basal cell carcinoma – new aspects of diagnosis and treatment. Acta Derm Venereol Suppl 209:5–25

# Repair of Cutaneous Defects After Skin Cancer Surgery

Monika Hess Schmid, Claudia Meuli-Simmen, and Jürg Hafner

## Abstract

The goal of this chapter is to present an overview of the main clinical applications of surgical repair in the various anatomical regions of the head. Special consideration will be given to the areas that require reconstruction and to possible problems and complications. Although the skin lesion often dictates the type of incision made, there are various options. The biggest advantage of flaps is the excellent aesthetic result; this is feasible because the skin is similar in color and texture to that being replaced, and moreover no contracture occurs. On the other hand, a flap requires additional incisions and tissue movement, which increases the risks of postoperative complications. The range of flaps that can be used is discussed in detail. Full-thickness skin grafts are an important and necessary tissue source for reconstructive surgery in the face. They must meet the functional and aesthetic challenge posed by the surgical defect and are usually chosen because of the lack of adjacent tissue. Whenever possible, the skin grafts should resemble the surrounding skin in texture, color and thickness.

## Introduction

In this chapter we would like to present an overview of the main clinical applications of surgical repair in the various anatomical regions of the head. Special consideration will be given to the areas that require reconstruction and to possible problems and complications.

Although the skin lesion often dictates the type of incision, there are various options. The resultant scars should be sited in natural skin creases or wrinkles or at the junction of anatomical landmarks [2]. Facial movement will show up these creases even in young patients.

Recent Results in Cancer Research, Vol. 160
© Springer-Verlag Berlin Heidelberg 2002

The biggest advantage of flaps is that, because the skin is similar in color and texture to that being replaced, they allow the best possible result in aesthetic terms and no contracture occurs. For effective use of local flaps excess skin must be available; therefore the flap that makes the best use of skin laxity should always be selected. On the other hand, a flap requires additional incisions and tissue movement, which increases the risks of postoperative complications.

Full-thickness skin grafts are an important and necessary tissue source for reconstructive surgery in the face. They must meet the functional and aesthetic challenge posed by the surgical defect and are usually chosen because of the lack of adjacent tissue [15]. Whenever possible, the skin grafts should resemble the surrounding skin in texture, color, and thickness.

## Nose

The nose is subdivided into many aesthetic units, the main four areas being the medial canthal region, the side of the nose, the nasal tip and the columella. The nasal skin varies in these different areas in texture, color and appearance. The incisions should be vertical in the glabellar area or along the nasolabial fold; nasal obstruction and asymmetry of the nose and nostrils must be avoided. In male patients the hair-bearing skin of the cheek should not be transposed to the tip of the nose [3, 10].

In the nasal area the use of flaps is more demanding, but they are extremely functional. Since flaps have their own blood supply, they can be placed over poorly vascularized structures (e.g. bone or cartilage). A finger flap is a midline transposition flap and is the method of choice for closure of a defect on the medial canthus; it is also very suitable for the reconstruction of defects on the side of the nose. The flap design is simple, and the donor site can easily be closed [3]. The rhomboid flap is also suitable for use on the side of the nose (Fig. 1a–c), but is limited by the amount of skin available on the nose and is a little more difficult to design. The bilobed flap [5] is a very good solution for the medial canthal area, the side of the nose, and the nasal tip [20]. Large defects can be closed in this way. Another very good flap for reconstruction of defects of the lateral tip that do not involve the ala nasi is an advancement flap. This flap can be moved into place along the alar crease. The U-plasty [9] can be advanced directly downward to close nasal tip defects. It provides a similar type of skin, but it is not always possible to achieve sufficient advancement; necrosis of the distal end of the flap can then result. The perialar crescentic advancement flap is an excellent flap for closure of even quite large defects in the alar base-nasolabial region [16]. Triangles are excised above and below the defect along the nasolabial fold, and the skin of the cheek is undermined to obtain enough advancement.

A defect on the nasal tip is a good indication for a full-thickness skin graft. It is a simple way of closing a defect, and the aesthetic results are satisfactory. Enlargement of some lesions may be indicated in order to allow

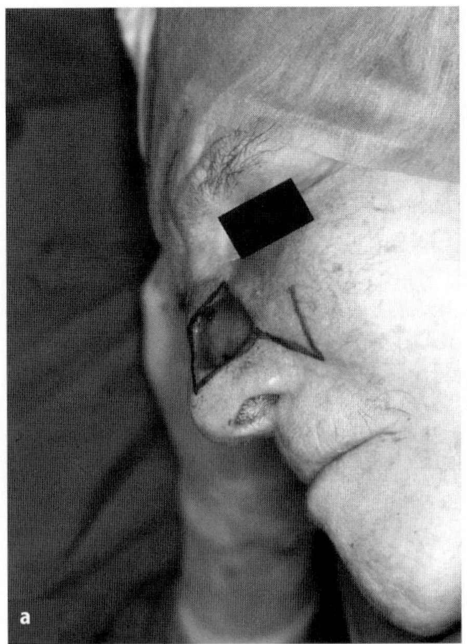

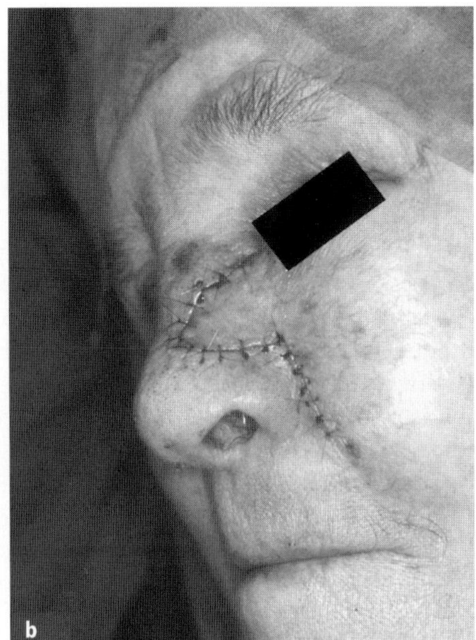

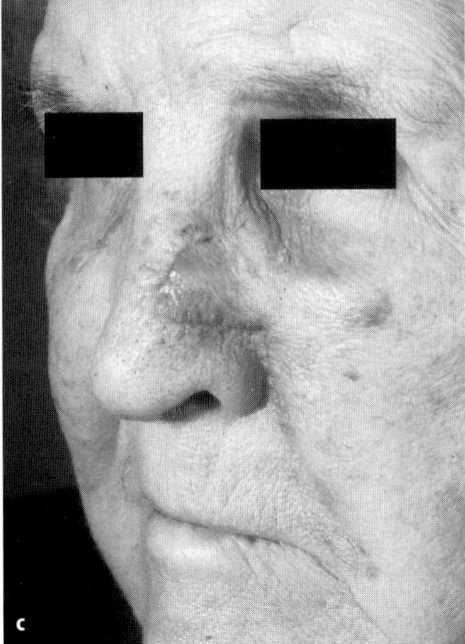

**Fig. 1. a** Defect after excision and planned rhomboid flap (Limberg). **b** Limberg flap sutured in place. **c** Healing after 10 days

placement of the graft on a contour line, and the possibility of contraction of the graft must be considered and allowed for. In addition, it must be borne in mind that bare cartilage will not sustain a graft.

## Ear

The structure of the ear is very complex, with a variety of convexities and concavities and varying thickness of cartilage, subcutaneous tissue, and skin. An important complication is perichondritis. If untreated, the risk of a permanent deformity of the ear is very high. If incisions are made across concavities, scar contracture will cause deformity. Therefore, incisions should be made within folds. The main areas are the helix, the concha, the lobule and the posterior ear.

For closure of a small defect of the rim and concha a simple wedge excision and direct closure [17] can be performed. Subcutaneous sutures should be used to approximate the auricular cartilage. Simple wedges should only be small, because approximation of the cartilage tends to push the ear outwards. To avoid this, secondary wedges can be removed; various geometrical patterns can be designed with this technique [10, 14]. For larger defects a rim advancement flap is very helpful, the rim being advanced upward to close the defect. Lesions arising on the anterior skin of the concha can be closed very well with a full-thickness graft [14] providing it is not necessary to remove the perichondrium. If the cartilage is exposed, small punch holes can be made so that granulation tissue can grow through them [6]. One major advantage of flaps in auricular reconstruction [11] is that they are suitable for patients who wear glasses, as flaps are more resistant to pressure than full-thickness grafts. The most useful flap for closure of a defect on the posterior ear is the transposition flap [17].

## Lips

Each of the upper and lower lips is a symmetrical structure, and together they form an anatomical unit. In the midline of the upper lip the philtrum emphasizes the symmetry. The main areas are the vermilion, the upper and lower lip and the philtrum. To ensure perfect realignment of the two cut edges of the vermilion borders during repairs, it is helpful to mark the border between skin and vermilion prior to surgery. A primary closure should not be performed if the tumor is larger than one-third of the lip, as it would lead to the problem of a narrowed oral aperture.

Defects of the vermilion can be reconstructed with flaps and grafts. If a large part of the vermilion has to be excised, vermilionectomy (lip shave) is a very good solution. After horizontal excision of the vermilion the oral mucosa has to be undermined, and the denuded surface can be covered with the advanced mucosa [7, 8]. In general, if the defect is less than one-third of

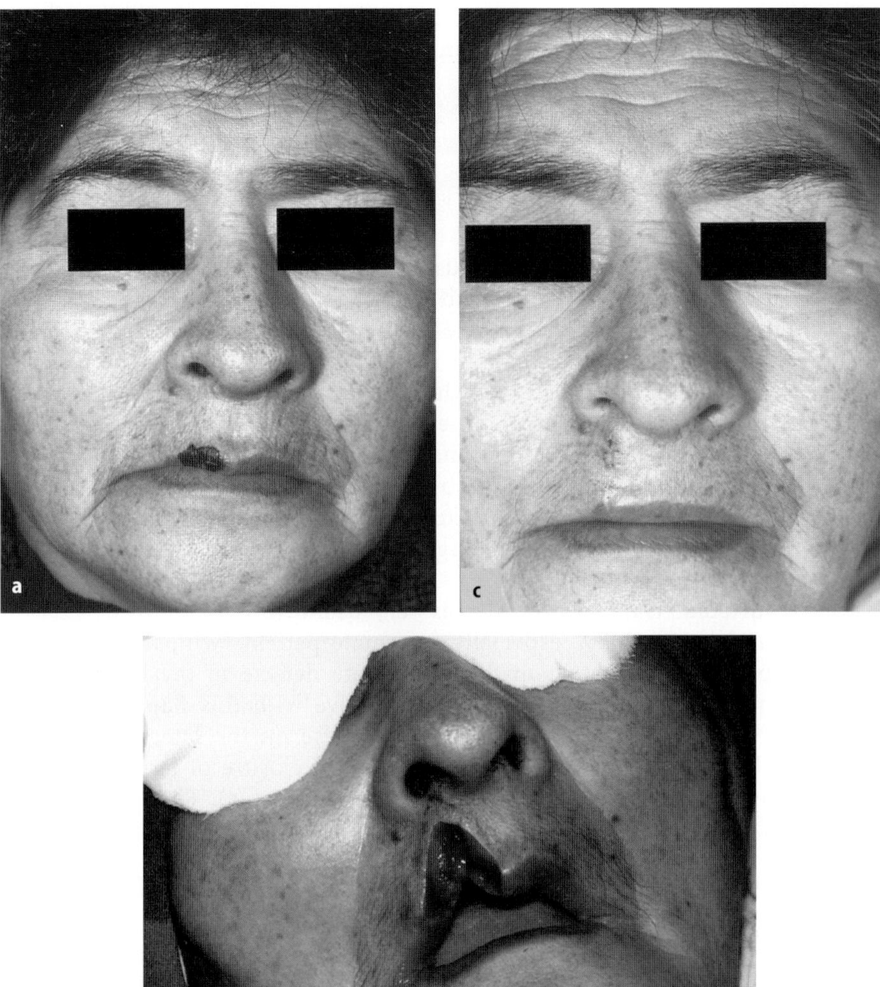

**Fig. 2. a** Melanoma before excision. **b** Defect after excision. **c** Healing after 1 week

the lip a full-thickness wedge excision (Fig. 2a–c) can be performed and closed directly [18]. On the lower lip the wedge should not extend below the horizontal chin crease. The Abbé-Estlander flap can be used for repairs of both the upper and the lower lip. The tumor is excised in a wedge-shaped fashion, but the defect is closed with a wedge-shaped transposition flap from the opposing lip, which is served by the labial artery and vein. The vascular pedicle must be separated after 2–3 weeks [1]. This flap can be used to reconstruct more than one-third of the lip. It offers immediate replacement of the total lip anatomy. The step technique can be used for defects affecting up to two-thirds of the lower lip by moving the advancement flaps in a stepwise fashion to bridge the defect [4, 12].

## Cheek

Because of the variations in color and texture of the skin it is possible to get a poor skin match when a flap is used. Closure of larger defects of the cheeks may cause facial asymmetry if the nasolabial fold or other creases and wrinkles are significantly flattened [14]. Transposition of hair-bearing skin to regions where the natural skin is not hair bearing can cause unsatisfactory cosmetic results. Especially when defects in the supramedial cheek are reconstructed, flaps may cause an ectropion of the lower eyelid, which is an unacceptable result in both functional and aesthetic terms.

In some cases a direct closure can be performed, and the aesthetic results are often very good. Care must be taken to avoid tension on important free margins and to avoid excessively long straight incisions, as otherwise the scars are obvious [14].

The preauricular transposition flap is very useful for closure of defects on the lateral and lower cheek, especially in female patients with fair skin. The bilobed flap can be used for small to moderate defects of the lateral cheek and malar region, but scarring is more extensive with this flap. The rhomboid flap can be used for similar defects to these on the lateral and lower cheek. The lateral cheek rotation flap is useful for closure of large defects in the malar region and in the supramedial cheek (Fig. 3 a–c). The loose skin of the preauricular area and lower face and neck is advanced to close a medial defect. The flap has to be designed to be large enough, as otherwise ectropion of the lower eyelid can occur. The inferior rotation flap is advanced upward along the nasolabial fold, and a Burow triangle must be excised from the caudal end of the incision. This flap is well suited to the closure of defects in the supramedial cheek region. The incision line lies in the nasolabial fold, so that scars are not very obvious later. However, ectropion of the lower eyelid is known to be a problem. The subcutaneous pedicle flap can be used in the supramedial cheek area and in the alar base-nasolabial region. The flap is mobilized on its subcutaneous pedicle until the required amount of cranial/medial movement can be achieved. A V-Y closure is performed, and the incision line should be along the nasolabial fold.

On the cheek, skin grafts are almost always less satisfactory than flaps.

## Forehead

The forehead, as one of the major cosmetic or aesthetic units of the face, presents certain challenges for the reconstructive surgeon [13]. The skin texture on the forehead is uniform. The main four areas are main forehead area,

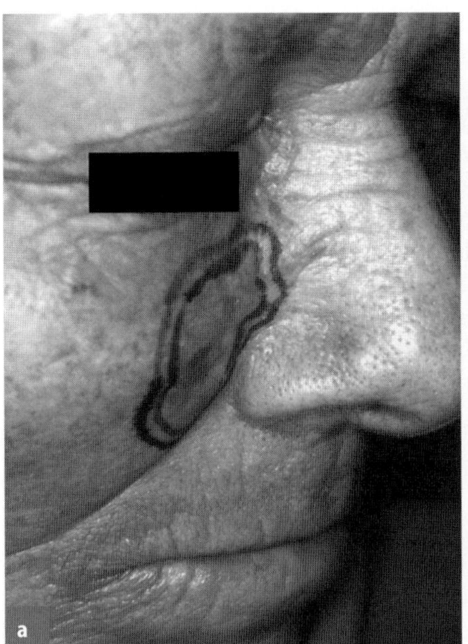
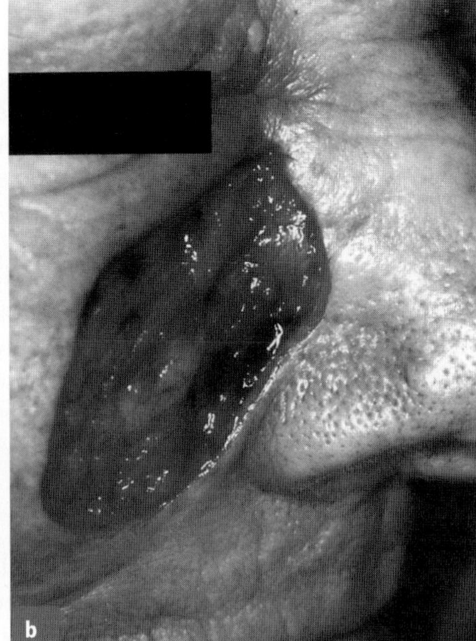
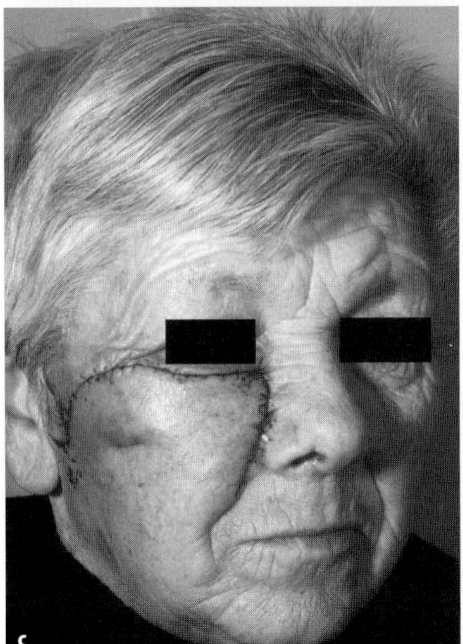

**Fig. 3. a** Basalioma before excision. **b** Defect after excision. **c** Lateral cheek rotation flap sutured in place

supra-eyebrow area, temporal region, and glabellar region. The lines in the main forehead area are transverse and those in the glabellar area, vertical. The forehead does not provide much excess skin. Therefore, skin tension occurs after many reconstructions, and flap necrosis may occur. It is important not to alter the hairline or the eyebrows. The facial nerve should be preserved in the temporal region.

The H-plasty is the most common bilateral advancement flap and is very suitable even for quite large median lesions. It maximizes horizontal incisions and minimizes vertical incisions, thus ensuring that scars are placed in the expected forehead lines [14]. Rhomboid flaps can provide an ideal solution when defects in the temporal region or glabella have to be closed.

The area above the eyebrow and the temples are also good places for full-thickness skin grafts, as the differences in structure are not very obvious.

## Scalp

Primary closure of wounds is often difficult on the scalp. The skin is thick and is attached to the skull. In some cases, especially in elderly patients, healing by secondary intention [19] can be advisable.

The best flap for use on the skull is a rotation flap. It should be mobilized at the level of the galea, as this allows easier movement. However, there are no ideal lines on the scalp, so scars are always visible, especially in bald men. Another method of closing defects is to use an advancement flap; Burow triangles may have to be excised.

Full-thickness skin grafts can also be applied to the scalp. They are indicated especially in elderly multimorbid patients with large defects.

## References


1. Estlander JA (1872) Eine Methode, aus der einer Lippe Substanzverluste der anderen zu ersetzen. Arch Klin Chir 14:622–631
2. Fratila A (1999) Bedeutung ästhetischer Regionen für die Rekonstruktion von Tumorexzisionsdefekten-Leitstrukturen bei lokalen Lappenplastiken. Springer, Berlin Heidelberg New York, pp 99–110
3. Jackson IT (1985) Local flaps in head and neck reconstruction. Mosby, St Louis
4. Johanson B A-E, Breine U, Holmström H (1974) Surgical treatment of non-traumatic lower lip lesions with special reference to the step technique. Scand J Plast Reconstr Surg 8:232–240
5. McGregor JC S-D (1981) A critical assessment of the bilobed flap. Br J Plast Surg 34:197
6. Mellette JR (1991) Ear reconstruction with local flaps. J Dermatol Surg Oncol 16:1102–1105
7. Petres J H-M, Hagedorn M (1977) Unterlippenkarzinome und deren operative Behandlung. Springer, Berlin Heidelberg New York, pp 137–144
8. Petres JR-R, Robins P (1996) Dermatologic surgery: textbook and atlas. Springer, Berlin Heidelberg New York
9. Rintala AE A-S-S (1969) Reconstruction of the midline skin defects of the nose. Scand J Plast Reconstr Surg 3:105

10. Roenigk RK R-H (1996) Dermatologic surgery: principles and practice, 2nd edn. Dekker, New York
11. Rompel R P-J (1993) Reconstructive techniques in oncologic dermatosurgery of the auricular region. FACE 2:171–177
12. Sebastian G (1988) Spätergebnisse nach operativer Behandlung von Unterlippentumoren, vol 4. Springer, Berlin Heidelberg New York, pp 108–121
13. Siegle RJ (1991) Forehead reconstruction. J Dermatol Surg Oncol 17:200–204
14. Summers BK S-R (1993) Facial cutaneous reconstructive surgery: facial flaps. J Am Acad Dermatol 29:917–941
15. Summers BK S-R (1993) Facial cutaneous reconstructive surgery: general aesthetic principles. J Am Acad Dermatol 29:669–681
16. Webster JP (1944) Crescentic peri-alar cheek excision for upper lip flap advancement with a short history of upper lip repair. Plast Reconstr Surg 16:434
17. Weerda H (1984) Probleme der operativen Therapie der Ohrmuschel-Malignome, vol 1. Springer, Berlin Heidelberg New York, pp 197–204
18. Wheeland RG (1991) Reconstruction of the lower lip and chin using local and random pattern flaps. J Dermatol Surg Oncol 17:605–615
19. Zitelli JA (1984) Secondary intention healing: an alternative to surgical repair. Clin Dermatol 2:92–106
20. Zitelli JA F-M (1991) Reconstruction of the nose with local flaps. J Dermatol Surg Oncol 17:184–189

# Radiotherapy of Skin Tumors

R. G. Panizzon


## Abstract

The incidence of cancers of the skin is increasing, as is life expectancy among most of the population. Besides surgery, all skin cancers can be treated with radiotherapy, with excellent results. Unfortunately, both less training and less equipment are available than earlier, which means that dermatologists also have less experience in this field. We would like to propose radiotherapy for medium-sized or larger lesions, especially on the face in elderly people. Good indications are keratoacanthomas, extensive actinic keratoses, Bowen's disease including erythroplasia of Queyrat, basal cell and squamous cell carcinomas, but also lentigo maligna and lentigo maligna melanomas. These tumors can be treated in a curative way. Excellent results of palliative X-ray therapy are achieved in Kaposi's sarcoma and in lymphomas, and also in Merkel cell tumors. After 100 years of treatment of skin cancers by radiotherapy, dermatologists should not forget that if appropriate principles are followed and precautions are taken, X-ray treatment is still a safe and effective method.


Carcinoma of the skin is the most accessible cancer, and basal cell carcinoma (BCC) is the most frequently occurring cancer overall in Caucasians. The diagnosis is readily made, and the limits of the lesion are usually easy to define. There is no single treatment method that is best for all cancers of the skin. Careless application of any method can produce a poor cosmetic effect or result in a recurrence. If the sole criterion of success is eradication of the lesion, surgery and radiotherapy lead to similar results. Most cutaneous cancers, especially BCC and squamous cell carcinoma (SCC), are sufficiently sensitive to radiation to be eradicated by doses that are well tolerated by the surrounding normal tissue [7]. If appropriate principles are followed and precautions are taken, X-irradiation is a safe and effective method of therapy [12, 18].


Recent Results in Cancer Research, Vol. 160
© Springer-Verlag Berlin Heidelberg 2002

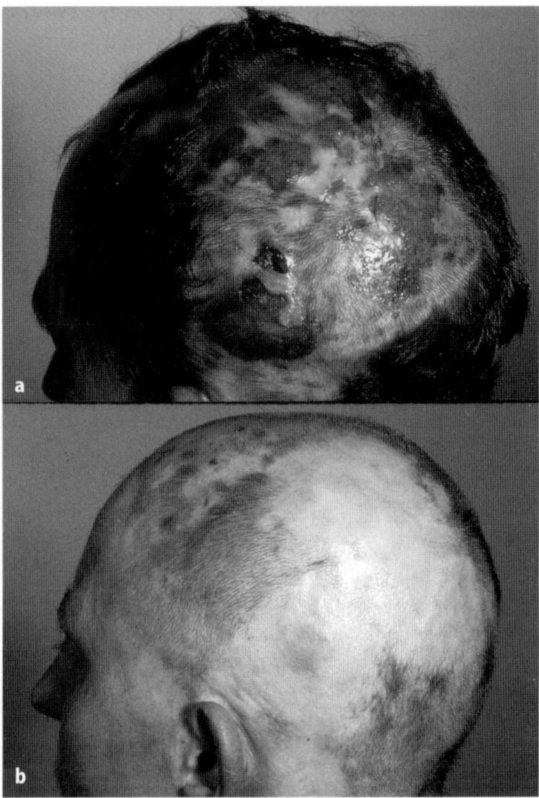

**Fig. 1. a** Mycosis fungoides in a 45-year-old woman before radiotherapy. **b** The same patient 1 month after radiation treatment with a total dose of 8 Gy in four fractions, 40 kV

Modern dermatological radiotherapy is still an indispensable primary or alternative modality for the treatment of skin cancers. Typically, radiotherapy is still indicated in medium-sized tumors of the face in elderly persons, i.e. patients over 60 years old and up to 90 years old or even older [11]. The types of radiotherapy mostly used in dermatology are Grenz rays, contact therapy, superficial X-rays, supervoltage or megavoltage therapy, electron beam therapy, and irradiation from implanted radioactive isotopes [9]. Theoretically, nearly all cutaneous cancers anywhere on the body can be treated successfully with X-rays. However, experience has shown that the cosmetic results of radiotherapy are less satisfactory on the trunk and extremities [7, 12]. Adequate treatment requires that a margin of skin with a normal appearance be included. In certain anatomical regions this may pose a problem for the surgeon, but not for the radiotherapist. Therefore, preferred localizations for radiotherapy are the eyelids, the ears, the nose and the lips [7, 12]. In these areas, radiotherapy may be the treatment of choice because the cosmetic and/or functional results are excellent. In elderly patients there is less danger of late radiation dermatitis. X-ray therapy is not traumatic, can be done on an outpatient basis, is painless and ideal for the physically or psychologically handicapped patient, and is mostly independent of any medication [12]. Before radiotherapy is started, the diagnosis must be confirmed by histological examination. This gives information on the type and the depth of the tumor, but also its radiosensitivity; finally, it can exclude an error.

Radiotherapy is not generally indicated at localizations where the tumor might be intraoral or extend into the nostrils or in the case of tumors that have originated in scars of osteomyelitis, chronic ulcers or burns [7]. In general, a second radiation therapy for a skin cancer is not recommended at the same localization or for tumors originating in chronic radiodermatitis. Other contraindications are proneness of any patient to multiple carcinomas, as in patients with xeroderma pigmentosum or basal cell nevus syndrome, for in these patients X-ray radiation can even induce new neoplasms. Superficial X-ray therapy is not indicated for the treatment of tumors that are invading cartilage or bone.

We recommend, as rule of thumb, that radiation qualities with a D 1/2 corresponding to the depth of the tumor be selected. Most of the radiation will then be absorbed in the pathologic tissue so the likelihood of undesirable radiation effects on underlying uninvolved tissue will be markedly reduced [7]. The biopsy specimen can be used to measure the exact depth of the tumor.

If the tumors are larger and deeper more penetrating radiation qualities are required, and the 80% depth dose is then more appropriate than the D 1/2 con-

**Table 1.** Recommended doses for the treatment of skin tumors with soft X-rays

| Diagnosis | Dose (kV) | Field (Ø, cm) | Fractionation (Gy) | Total dose (Gy) | Time interval (days) |
|---|---|---|---|---|---|
| Lentigo maligna | 12 | <2 | 5–6×20 | 100–120 | 4–7 |
|  |  | >2 | or 10–12×10 | 100–120 | 3–4 |
| Bowen's disease/Queyrat's | | <2 | 3–4×8 | 24–32 | 4–7 |
| erythroplasia | 20 | >2 | 8–10×4 | 32–40 | 3–4 |
| Keratosis, senile | 12 | <2 | 5–7×8 | 40–56 | 4–7 |
|  | 20 |  | 2–3×8 | 16–24 | 4–7 |
|  |  | >2 | 5–7×4 | 20–28 | 3–4 |
| Basal cell carcinoma/squamous cell | | <2 | 5–6×8 | 40–48 | 4–7 |
| carcinoma | 20–50 | 2–5 | 10–12×4 | 40–48 | 3–4 |
|  |  | >5 | 26–28×2 | 52–56 | daily |
| Mycosis fungoides/other malignant | 20–50 | | 3–7×2 | 6–14 | 3–4 |
| lymphomas/leukemic infiltrates | teleroentgen | | 4–10×1 | 4–10 | 3–7 |
| Lentigo maligna melanoma/melanoma metastases | 20–50 | | 7–9×6 | 42–54 | 4–7 |
| Kaposi's sarcoma | 20–50 | <2 | 3–5×8 | 24–40 | 4–7 |
|  |  | >2 | 5–10×4 | 20–40 | 3–4 |

cept. In the treatment of most cutaneous cancers it has been established that better clinical results can be obtained by spreading the total treatment over a period of 2–6 weeks: once a day on 5 days of each week, 3 times each week or only once a week. The total dose might change from 34 to 60 Gy. The higher the individual doses, the smaller the total dose. Small lesions up to 2 cm in diameter can be irradiated with 8 Gy in five fractions once or twice a week, medium-sized lesions (mostly 2–4 cm) with 4 Gy/fraction in 12 fractions three times a week, large lesions (over 4 cm) with 2 Gy/fraction in at least 26 fractions given daily. The total dose is mostly between 40 Gy and 52 Gy, respectively. This schedule is mostly suited for the most frequent skin cancers (see Table 1), i.e. BCCs or SCCs. In a series of 300 BCCs we found a recurrence rate of only 5%. The only condition is that these BCCs are histologically of the nodular type. The recurrence rate is much higher if the histopathology shows a BCC of the sclerosing type [12].

The same dose schedule can be used for SCCs, but we propose a higher fractionation rate for these, since in general they grow faster. Sometimes higher single doses or total doses might also be required [7, 12]. Exophytic tumors can be treated in two ways: (1) shaving before radiotherapy and (2) radiotherapy from the beginning and adaptation of the radiation penetration during the course of the treatment. As mentioned above, tumors invading cartilage or bone or originating in damaged skin, e.g. in burns, scars, or in chronic inflammatory diseases are not indicated for a superficial X-ray therapy.

Radiotherapy is also possible for tumors that have previously been incompletely excised or treated inadequately with curettage and/or electrodesiccation [7]. In radiotherapy of other cutaneous tumors, e.g., keratoacanthoma, the general therapeutic approach is not different from that described for SCCs. There is always the possibility of therapy in fast-growing keratoacanthomas, and there is therefore a threat to cosmetically important areas. In these cases we would not feel justified in waiting for a spontaneous regression and immediate and appropriate treatment is recommended [2].

Radiotherapy is an excellent modality in extensive actinic keratoses and has a longer lasting effect than most other techniques [7, 12].

Bowen's disease and its special form of erythroplasia of Queyrat are in situ carcinomas and are suitable for Grenz ray or superficial X-ray treatment. In these cases a higher total dose is recommended. The treatment results are excellent [12]. The same is true for lentigo maligna and lentigo maligna melanoma; for these two entities irradiation also has a definitive role as a curative treatment [5, 13, 16]. The results show that the techniques utilizing higher doses per fraction are preferred and effective [13, 16]. Again, medium-sized or large lesions in the face, such as those typical for lentigo maligna or lentigo maligna melanoma (LMM), are excellent indications for a radiation treatment. A study comparing an irradiated group and a surgically treated group of LMM patients matched for tumor thickness and tumor levels found no statistically significant difference between the two treatment modalities [13]. Even as a palliative treatment, radiotherapy is successful in cases of melanoma metastases to lymph nodes, bone, or central nervous system [6, 17].

Palliative X-ray treatment with excellent results is well known to dermatologists in Kaposi's sarcoma of the classic type [7, 12, 18]. Especially painful tumors, infected tumors, or rapidly growing or disfiguring tumors are good indications. The AIDS-associated type of Kaposi's sarcoma is also radiosensitive, especially the facial lesions, but also those of the foot. Kaposi's sarcoma is a relatively radiosensitive tumor, and small total doses of radiation can be used to keep this tumor under control.

Other indications for palliative X-ray therapy are cutaneous T-cell lymphomas, especially mycosis fungoides, and certain B-cell lymphomas [1, 8, 15]. Extensive plaques and tumors of T-cell lymphomas are highly radiosensitive and respond to low doses of radiation; a few sessions with 2 Gy per session are effective [12, 18]. It has been shown that in the erythrodermic type of mycosis fungoides the addition of total skin electron beam therapy to extracorporal photopheresis improves survival [20].

Other studies have shown that the combination of photon beams or nitrogen mustard and total skin electron beam irradiation is beneficial for the advanced stages of mycosis fungoides [3, 10]. The combination of radiotherapy and hyperthermia has also proved to be an effective treatment for recurrent lymphomas [4].

Merkel cell tumor has a very characteristic clinical and histopathological appearance. This tumor tends to frequent recurrences. For this reason a surgical approach together with radiation therapy is often recommended [19].

Chronic radiodermatitis can follow radiotherapy of skin tumors. Following standard treatment of these cutaneous cancers with total doses of 40–60 Gy, oozing and sloughing of the irradiated skin occurs, which is accompanied by intense erythema but rarely associated with pain. This acute radiodermatitis heals gradually within 3–6 weeks. In most cases, the irradiated area looks inconspicuous for many years, especially if it is in the face [14]. However, some patients develop progressive atrophy after 3–24 months, often associated with irregular areas of hypopigmentation or hyperpigmentation, telangiectasias, and increased sensitivity to minor symptoms. This type of radiodermatitis may also occur after treatment of internal malignancies or following treatment of benign skin lesions. Because of the cell-killing effect, radiation-induced skin carcinomas are rarely seen in radiodermatitis caused by the high total doses used for skin tumors, but rather in multiple series of radiation treatment administered in former times for benign skin diseases [14].

# References


1. Bekkenk MW, Vermeer MH, Geerts ML, Noordijk EM, Heule F, van Voorst Vader PC, van Vloten WA, Meijer CJ, Willemze R (1999) Treatment of multifocal primary cutaneous B-cell lymphoma: a clinical follow-up study of 29 patients. J Clin Oncol 17:2471–2478
2. Caccialanza M, Sopelama N (1988) Radiation therapy of kerato-acanthomas: results in 55 patients. Int J Radiat Oncol Biol Phys 16:475–477

3. Chinn DM, Chow S, Kim YH, Hoppe RT (1999) Total skin electron beam therapy with or without adjuvant topical nitrogen mustard or nitrogen mustard alone as initial treatment of T2 and T3 mycosis fungoides. Int J Radiat Oncol Biol Phys 43:951–958

4. Donato V, Zurlo A, Nappa M, Capua A, Banelli E, Martelli M, Gabriele P, Amichetti M, Biagini C (1997) Multicentre experience with combined hyperthermia and radiation therapy in the treatment of superficially located non-Hodgkin's lymphomas. J Exp Clin Cancer Res 16:87–90

5. Gaspar ZS, Dawber RP (1997) Treatment of lentigo maligna. Australas J Dermatol 38:1–6; quiz 7–8

6. Geara FB, Ang KK (1996) Radiation therapy for malignant melanoma. Surg Clin North Am 76:1383–1398

7. Goldschmidt H (1991) Radiation therapy of cutaneous carcinomas. In: Goldschmidt H, Panizzon RG (eds) Modern dermatologic radiation therapy. Springer, Berlin Heidelberg New York, pp 65–131

8. Kirova YM, Piedbois Y, Le Bourgeois JP (1999) Radiotherapy in the management of cutaneous B-cell lymphoma. Our experience in 25 cases. Radiother Oncol 52:15–18

9. Kohler-Brock A, Prager W, Pohlmann S, Kunze S (1999) The indications for and results of HDR afterloading therapy in diseases of the skin and mucosa with standardized surface applicators (the Leipzig applicator). Strahlenther Onkol 175:170–174

10. Maingon P, Truc G, Dalac S, Barillot I, Lambert D, Petrella T, Naudy S, Horiot JC (2000) Radiotherapy of advanced mycosis fungoides: indications and results of total skin electron beam and photon beam irradiation. Radiother Oncol 54:73–78

11. Mitsuhashi N, Hayakawa K, Yamakawa M, Sakurai H, Saito Y, Hasegawa M, Akimoto T, Hayakawa K, Niibe H (1999) Cancer in patients aged 90 years or older: radiation therapy. Radiology 211:829–833

12. Panizzon RG (1993) Roentgen therapy of malignant skin tumors. Ther Umsch 50:835–840

13. Panizzon RG (1999) Radiotherapy of lentigo maligna and lentigo maligna melanoma. Skin Cancer 14:203–207

14. Panizzon RG (1991) Radiation reactions and sequels. In: Goldschmidt H, Panizzon RG (eds) Modern dermatologic radiation therapy. Springer, Berlin Heidelberg New York, pp 25–36

15. Pimpinelli N, Santucci M (2000) The skin-associated lymphoid tissue-related B-cell lymphomas. Semin Cutan Med Surg 19:124–129

16. Schmid-Wendtner MH, Brunner B, Konz B, Kaudewitz P, Wendtner CM, Peter RU, Plewig G, Volkenandt M (2000) Fractionated radiotherapy of lentigo maligna and lentigo maligna melanoma in 64 patients. J Am Acad Dermatol 43:477–482

17. Seegenschmiedt MH, Keilholz L, Altendorf-Hofmann A, Urban A, Schell H, Hohenberger W, Sauer R (1999) Palliative radiotherapy for recurrent and metastatic malignant melanoma: prognostic factors for tumor response and long-term outcome: a 20-year experience. Int J Radiat Oncol Biol Phys 44:607–618

18. Voss N, Kim-Sing C (1998) Radiotherapy in the treatment of dermatologic malignancies. Dermatol Clin 16:313–320

19. Weymuller EA Jr, Marks M, Ridge D (1991) Merkel cell carcinoma of the ear. Head Neck 13:68–71

20. Wilson LD, Jones GW, Kim D, Rosenthal D, Christensen IR, Edelson RL, Heald PW, Kacinski BM (2000) Experience with total skin electron beam therapy in combination with extracorporeal photopheresis in the management of patients with erythrodermic (T4) mycosis fungoides. J Am Acad Dermatol 43:54–60

# Photodynamic Therapy and Fluorescence Diagnosis of Skin Cancers

Rolf-Markus Szeimies and Michael Landthaler

## Abstract

In several countries throughout the world the photosensitizer porfimer-sodium has been approved for systemic photodynamic therapy (PDT) for different oncological indications. However, owing to the prolonged photosensitization entailed, the use of this porphyrin derivative is restricted. Currently, the most promising sensitizers in dermatology that can be applied topically are 5-aminolevulinic acid (ALA) or ester derivatives that are precursors of heme biosynthesis. ALA has shown good clinical and excellent cosmetic results in superficial skin cancer and precancerous conditions, e.g. superficial basal cell carcinoma (BCC), or actinic keratoses (AK): phase III studies have demonstrated its efficacy especially in Bowen's disease and AK. ALA-PDT for AK was therefore approved by the FDA in late 1999, and the corresponding registration process is currently in train in Europe. Besides its usefulness in oncological therapy, ALA also has a unique feature that can be exploited for diagnostic purposes: after topical or systemic application protoporphyrin IX is induced rather selectively in epithelial tumors, with a high tumor-to-surrounding tissue ratio, which can be visualized after excitation with light. By using a CCD camera system together with digital imaging, the contrast of the acquired fluorescence images can be significantly enhanced and allows the determination of a threshold, which can be utilized either for a directed biopsy or for preoperative planning when Mohs' surgery is scheduled. At present, the routine employment of such systems is being assessed in prospective studies.

## Introduction

As long ago as at the beginning of the last century, photodynamic therapy (PDT) was already being used for the treatment of cutaneous malignancies (von Tappeiner and Jesionek 1903). In a cooperation between the pharmacol-

Recent Results in Cancer Research, Vol. 160
© Springer-Verlag Berlin Heidelberg 2002

ogist von Tappeiner and A. Jesionek in the Department of Dermatology at the University of Munich, facial skin tumors, mostly basal cell carcinomas, in six patients were treated over a period of 2–8 weeks with different dyes, such as eosin solution (1–5%). The dye was painted directly onto the tumor, and patients were afterwards exposed either to sunlight or carbon arc light. With this first topical PDT protocol four patients were cured. Since then the efficacy of PDT for skin tumors has been demonstrated in various reports (Dougherty et al. 1978; Kennedy et al. 1990; Morton et al. 2001; Szeimies et al. 1996; Wolf et al. 1993).

## Photosensitizers

The intravenous administration of hematoporphyrin derivatives (HpD) or the purified form porfimer-sodium and subsequent irradiation with red light from a laser was the first approved sensitizer in the early 1990s. So far it is approved worldwide only for such indications as esophageal or lung cancer and not for dermatological purposes. The main disadvantage of i.v.-administered porfimer-sodium (Photofrin) is the subsequent prolonged cutaneous photosensitivity, which can last for some weeks (Landthaler et al. 1993; Szeimies et al. 2001). This severe side effect makes systemic PDT with porfimer-sodium unsuitable for small, single cancers of the skin, although its results are excellent in terms of scarring.

Topical administration would exclude this side effect, but owing to its high molecular weight and polarity, porfimer-sodium does not penetrate the skin in significant amounts. In contrast, 5-aminolevulinic acid (ALA) and its derivative ALA-methyl ester are able to penetrate parakeratotic horn, which overlies the lesions to be treated (Kennedy et al. 1990). ALA, a precursor of heme, is transformed to photosensitizing porphyrins, mainly protoporphyrin IX after topical application.

## Fluorescence Diagnosis of Tumors

The synthesis of porphyrins is selective in such fast-proliferating tissues as basal cell carcinomas and squamous cell carcinomas, but also in psoriasis plaques (Fritsch et al. 1999). Epithelial tumors can therefore be visualized by fluorescence utilizing the ALA-induced selective porphyrin accumulation. For this purpose an area where tumor is suspected is covered with ALA and then illuminated with blue light matching the highest absorption peak of the porphyrins (the so-called Soret band). Emitted pink-red fluorescence, which is restricted to the areas where porphyrin synthesis takes place, is then easily detected (Fig. 1). Light sources for fluorescence diagnosis can be conventional Wood's light or, preferably, specific computerized detection systems, which are able to enhance the contrast by digital-image analysis (Ackermann et al. 2000). Fluorescence diagnosis is suitable for detection of occult cancer

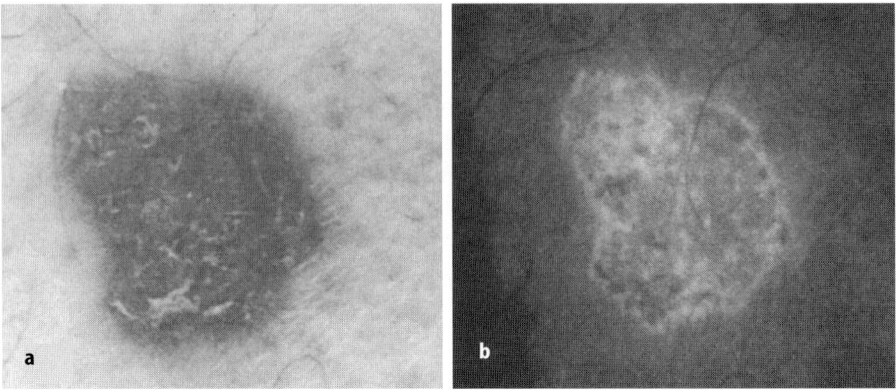

**Fig. 1. a** Clinical and **b** fluorescence image of a basal cell carcinoma after topical application of 5-aminolevulinic acid

in pretreated areas with scarring and pigmentary changes (following surgery, cryotherapy, or radiotherapy) and can also be done as an adjunct to Mohs' surgery, to look for tumor-free resection margins even during the surgical procedure.

## Light Sources for PDT

The penetration depth of light into skin increases up to $\lambda = 1100$ nm (infrared) (Anderson and Parrish 1981). The last absorption maximum of the porphyrins is at about 630 nm, which is therefore used for irradiation. At 630 nm the penetration depth of light is about 3 mm, which limits the thickness of tumors that can be treated to that. So far, dye laser systems have been used for irradiation, but high acquisition and maintenance costs have prevented their widespread distribution in dermatology departments and practices. However, for surface illumination incoherent light sources can also be used where fiber coupling is not necessary.

Meanwhile a variety of incoherent light sources are available for dermatological purposes, covering areas 5–20 cm in diameter. The only point it is crucial to match is the light uniformity over the area to be treated, to avoid underdosage mainly at the rims of the exposure field.

## Mechanism of Action

The PDT-induced destruction of skin tumors is mediated by photo-oxidative reactions inducing the generation of mainly singlet oxygen. The biological effects can be divided into *primary, cellular* and *secondary, vascular* damage (see Table 1) (Szeimies et al. 2001). Depending on the subcellular localization

**Table 1.** In vitro and in vivo effects of photodynamic therapy (*NT* normal tissue, *TT* tumor tissue)

| Primary cytotoxicity (cellular effects in vitro and in vivo) | Secondary cytotoxicity (vascular effects in vivo) |
| --- | --- |
| Damage of cell organelles | Vasoconstriction of arterioles (NT) |
| Membrane damage | Accumulation of leukocytes (NT) |
| Cell swelling | Perivascular edema (NT + TT) |
|  | Thrombosis (TT) |

of the photosensitizer, different cell organelles, such as mitochondria or lysosomes, are damaged, resulting in tumor cell necrosis. After topical PDT necrosis of tumor tissue leads in addition to the release of such inflammation mediators as histamine or arachidonic acid metabolites, which contribute to deleterious effects. In contrast is the damage to the tumor vasculature and the induction of tumor ischemia that are crucial for the success of PDT after systemic administration of photosensitizers (Dellian et al. 1995).

With either route of drug administration, after 2–3 days clinically obvious necrosis occurs, which is sharply restricted to the diseased tissue, resulting in complete healing within 14 days with an excellent cosmetic outcome.

## PDT for Oncological Indications in Dermatology

An overview of the suitable indications for PDT in dermatology is given in Table 2. So far most data in dermatology have been recorded after treatment with hematoporphyrin derivatives or the purified form, porfimer-sodium. Both BCC and SCC have already been treated with systemically administered HpD or porfimer-sodium. However, owing to the prolonged cutaneous photosensitization it causes, this procedure should be limited to tumors of large extent and/or patients in whom classic therapeutic procedures, such as surgery or radiotherapy, are not possible.

In contrast, topical PDT will soon be added to the therapeutic armamentarium of the dermatologist. ALA-PDT was approved for the treatment of actinic keratoses in combination with blue light in the USA in December 1999 (Levulan Kerastick) and the corresponding registration process for its use in Europe is currently in train. ALA-methyl ester combined with red light has also been approved for BCC and actinic keratoses in Europe.

**Table 2.** Oncological indications for photodynamic therapy with 5-aminolevulinic acid

| Precancerous lesions | Tumors (not exceeding 2 mm in tumor thickness) |
| --- | --- |
| Actinic keratoses (including arsenic-induced) | Superficial basal cell carcinoma |
| Bowen's disease | Initial squamous cell carcinoma |
|  | Gorlin-Goltz syndrome |
|  | Mycosis fungoides |

The experience with treatment of epithelial cancers and precancerous conditions with PDT so far reported in the literature suggest that actinic keratoses (Szeimies et al. 1996; Jeffes et al. 1997; Karrer et al. 1999; Kurwa et al. 1999), Bowen's disease (Morton et al. 1996) and superficial BCCs (Haller et al. 2000; Wang et al. 2001) and initial SCCs (tumor thickness less than 2 mm) are the only tumors that are suitable indications for topical ALA-PDT with curative intent. For this purpose ALA is applied topically using 20% in proprietary cream base formulations with occlusion for 4–6 h. Afterwards light is applied; using red light, the light intensity is in the range of 100–150 mW/cm$^2$ and the fluence 100–150 J/cm$^2$. PDT is not suitable for treatment of very crusty lesions or pigmented tumors, since hemorrhagic crusts or melanin prevent the penetration of light.

The only reported side effect of ALA-PDT is a burning sensation closely related to the period of irradiation, which can vary widely between different patients and requires strong analgesics in some cases.

The advantages of topical PDT are that it is a noninvasive procedure that can be used repeatedly with excellent cosmetic results. Moreover, it seems that, unlike many other forms of phototherapy, PDT mediates its effects by causing membrane damage, and to a much lesser extent by causing DNA damage, so that it involves a lower risk for mutations and carcinogenesis (Moan 1986). Nevertheless, the limitations, such as the depth of penetration of light and the penetration of the photosensitizer into the skin, should be taken carefully into account and should be individualized for each patient.

## References


Ackermann G, Abels C, Karrer S, Bäumler W, Landthaler M, Szeimies RM (2000) Fluoreszenzgestützte Biopsie von Basalzellkarzinomen. Hautarzt 51:920–924

Anderson RR, Parrish JA (1981) The optics of human skin. J Invest Dermatol 77:13–19

Dellian M, Abels C, Kuhnle GE, Goetz AE (1995) Effects of photodynamic therapy on leucocyte-endothelium interaction: differences between normal and tumour tissue. Br J Cancer 72:1125–1130

Dougherty TJ, Kaufman JE, Goldfarb A, Weishaupt KR, Boyle D, Mittleman A (1978) Photoradiation therapy for the treatment of malignant tumors. Cancer Res 38:2628–2635

Fritsch C, Lehmann P, Stahl W, Schulte KW, Blohm E, Lang K, Sies H, Ruzicka T (1999) Optimum porphyrin accumulation in epithelial skin tumours and psoriatic lesions after topical application of $\delta$-aminolaevulinic acid. Br J Cancer 79:1603–1608

Haller JC, Cairnduff F, Slack G, Schofield J, Whitehurst C, Tunstall R, Brown SB, Roberts DJH (2000) Routine double treatments of superficial basal cell carcinomas using aminolaevulinic acid-based photodynamic therapy. Br J Dermatol 143:1270–1274

Jeffes EW, McCullough JL, Weinstein GD, Fergin PE, Nelson JS, Shull TF, Simpson KR, Bukaty LM, Hoffman WL, Fong NL (1997) Photodynamic therapy of actinic keratosis with topical 5-aminolevulinic acid. Arch Dermatol 133:727–732

Karrer S, Bäumler W, Abels C, Hohenleutner U, Landthaler M, Szeimies RM (1999) Long pulse dye laser for photodynamic therapy – investigations in vitro and in vivo. Lasers Surg Med 25:51–59

Kennedy JC, Pottier RH, Pross DC (1990) Photodynamic therapy with endogenous protoporphyrin IX: basic principles and present clinical experience. J Photochem Photobiol B 6:143–148

Kurwa HA, Yong-Gee SA, Seed PT, Markey AC, Barlow RJ (1999) A randomized paired comparison of photodynamic therapy and topical 5-fluorouracil in the treatment of actinic keratoses. J Am Acad Dermatol 41:414–418

Landthaler M, Rück A, Szeimies RM (1993) Photodynamische Therapie von Tumoren der Haut. Hautarzt 44:69–74

Moan J (1986) Porphyrin photosensitization and phototherapy. Photochem Photobiol 43:681–690

Morton CA, Whitehurst C, Moseley H, McColl JH, Moore JV, Mackie RM (1996) Comparison of photodynamic therapy with cryotherapy in the treatment of Bowen's disease. Br J Dermatol 135:766–771

Morton CA, Whitehurst C, McColl JH, Moore JV, MacKie RM (2001) Photodynamic therapy for large or multiple patches of Bowen disease and basal cell carcinoma. Arch Dermatol 137:319–324

Szeimies RM, Karrer S, Sauerwald A, Landthaler M (1996) Topical photodynamic therapy with 5-aminolevulinic acid in the treatment of actinic keratoses: a first clinical study. Dermatology 192:246–251

Szeimies RM, Karrer S, Abels C, Landthaler M, Elmets CA (2001) Photodynamic therapy in dermatology. In: Krutmann J, Hönigsmann H, Elmets CA, Bergstresser PR (eds) Dermatological phototherapy and photodiagnostic methods. Springer, Berlin Heidelberg New York, pp 209–247

von Tappeiner H, Jesionek A (1903) Therapeutische Versuche mit fluorescierenden Stoffen. Münch Med Wochenschr 47:2042–2044

Wang I, Bendsoe N, Klinteberg CAF, Enejder AMK, Andersson-Engels S, Svanberg S, Svanberg K (2001) Photodynamic therapy vs. cryosurgery of basal cell carcinomas: results of a phase III clinical trial. Br J Dermatol 144:832–840

Wolf P, Rieger E, Kerl H (1993) Topical photodynamic therapy with endogenous porphyrins after application of 5-aminolevulinic acid. J Am Acad Dermatol 28:17–21

# Intralesional Interferon in Basal Cell Carcinoma: How Does It Work?

Stanislaw Buechner, Marion Wernli, Felix Bachmann, Thomas Harr, and Peter Erb

## Abstract

Basal cell carcinoma (BCC) is the most common skin cancer among Caucasians, and its incidence is increasing. Intralesional injection of interferon alpha (IFN alpha) has been shown to provide a safe and effective treatment for BCCs. The predominant mechanism for the effect of IFN alpha on BCC has been partially identified. We have shown that in untreated patients, BCC cells constitutively express CD95 ligand (CD95L), but not the receptor. BCC cells make use of the CD95 ligand to escape from a local immune response by averting the attack from activated CD95 receptor-positive CD4$^+$ T cells. The CD95L of BCC cells is functional as CD95$^+$ target cells incubated on BCC cryosections become apoptotic and are lysed. In IFN alpha-treated patients BCC cells express not only CD95L but also CD95 receptor, and regress by committing suicide or fratricide through apoptosis induction via CD95 receptor-CD95L interaction. Peritumoral infiltrating cells, predominantly CD4$^+$ T cells, may support regression of BCC by the secretion of cytokines such as IFN gamma or interleukin-2 which may also be responsible for the up-regulation of CD95 on BCC cells.

## Introduction

Basal cell carcinoma (BCC) is by far the most common skin malignancy throughout the world, accounting for about 75% of nonmelanoma skin cancers (Strom and Yamamura 1997). Estimates of the incidence of BCC in the United States alone approach 1 million cases each year (Strom and Yamamura 1997; Lear and Smith 1997). The incidence of this cancer seems to be increasing worldwide. In Australia, the incidence of BCC increased by 11% between 1985 and 1990 (Lear and Smith 1997). In New Hampshire (USA), between 1979–1980 and 1993–1994 the incidence rates of BCC rose from 170 to 310 per 100 000 in men and from 91 to 166 per 100 000 in women, represent-

Recent Results in Cancer Research, Vol. 160
© Springer-Verlag Berlin Heidelberg 2002

ing increases of 82% in both men and women (Karagas et al. 1999). BCC is believed to arise from the hair follicle or pluripotent cells in the basal layer of the epidermis. The most significant etiological factor is chronic exposure to ultraviolet light, so that exposed areas, such as the head and neck, are the sites most commonly involved (Miller 1995). However, an increased frequency of BCCs was found in areas that are relatively well protected from light, such as the trunk and lower limbs. BCC is a slow-growing tumor and very rarely a life-threatening condition, but it does cause progressive local tissue destruction. The most common clinical presentation of BCC is as a smooth skin-colored indurated nodule with a telangiectatic surface and a raised border (Lear and Smith 1997). The majority of BCCs begin as small lesions typically less than 1 cm in diameter and can be successfully treated in a variety of ways. Treatment goals focus on complete tumor removal and minimization of cosmetic and functional defects. Effective methods of treatment include excisional surgery, curettage and electrodesiccation, cryosurgery, radiotherapy, and Moh's micrographic surgery (Telfer et al. 1999). However, many BCCs present considerable therapeutic difficulties because of the location and size of the tumor and the age of the patient. Especially, large and recurrent tumors usually require extensive resection with rotation of tissue, or free or composite grafts. Recently, results from several clinical trials have shown that intralesional interferon (IFN) is an effective treatment modality for BCC (Buechner 1991; Chimenti et al. 1995; Cornell et al. 1990; Greenway et al. 1986; Ikic et al. 1991; Thestrup-Pedersen et al. 1990). Interferons are a group of naturally occurring glycoproteins that possess multiple biological effects, including the control of cell growth and differentiation, regulation of cell surface antigen expression, and modulation of humoral and cellular immune responses (Gresser 1990; Ucar et al. 1995). Although the effectiveness of intralesional IFN therapy in BCC has been established in a number of clinical trials, the duration and dosing of IFN alpha in the treatment of BCC are still controversial. There is evidence to suggest that the cure rate decreases if lower doses of IFN and fewer injections are used. Most frequently, dosages of $1.5–3.0\times10^{6}$ IU of IFN alpha have been injected intralesionally three times a week for 3 weeks. Using intralesional IFN alpha over a 3-week period the overall success rate in most clinical trials was between 70% and 100%. The reasons for the various responses may include different histological type, anatomical site, and size of tumors, tumor weight variability, and inadequate distribution of IFN within the lesion. In most studies reported, primary surgical resection of BCC is associated with a 95% cure rate (Telfer et al. 1999). With the use of cryosurgery for primary BCC, 5-year cure rates ranging from 94% to 99% have been reported. Although intralesional therapy with IFN does not offer such high cure rates as the more conventional treatments, it is a promising new therapy for BCC and may find a role particularly for patients desiring a more favorable cosmetic result and who want to avoid a surgical procedure.

## How Does IFN Alpha Work in BCC? Possible Mechanism of Action

The rationale for the use of IFNs for the treatment of BCCs rests primarily on their ability to control cell growth and differentiation (Gresser 1990). There is also increasing evidence that IFNs act indirectly on tumor cells by inducing a variety of immune effects (Gresser 1990; Ucar et al. 1995). The fact that a considerable increase in the number of CD4[+] T cells infiltrating the dermis and surrounding the BCC nests was observed after intralesional IFN alpha therapy has been interpreted as indicating that this T cell subset is involved in triggering the immune response against tumor cells (Buechner 1991; Buechner et al. 1997; Mozzanica et al. 1990). The major mechanism by which cytolytic CD4[+] and CD8[+] T cell subsets kill target cells, including tumor cells, is by inducing apoptosis. CD4[+] cytotoxic T cells preferentially induce apoptosis in their target cells via CD95 receptor–CD95L interaction (Ashkenazi and Dixit 1998; Hahn et al. 1995). CD95 (or Fas) receptor, a cell surface molecule belonging to the tumor necrosis factor receptor superfamily, is expressed on a variety of cell types (Wehrli et al. 2000). CD95 expression has been found on the membrane of basal and suprabasal keratinocytes in normal human epidermis, whereas BCC tumor cells have low to undetectable levels of CD95 expression (Buechner et al. 1997; Gutierrez-Steil et al. 1998; Lee et al. 1998; Oishi et al. 1994). CD95L is expressed on activated T cells, BCC and squamous cell carcinoma cells (Buechner et al. 1997; Wehrli et al. 2000). In addition, CD95L is expressed on the basal cells and keratinocytes in the spinous layer of the normal human epidermis (Buechner et al. 1997; Lee et al. 1998).

Using the terminal deoxynucleotidyl transferase-mediated dUDP nick end labeling (TUNEL) technique, no apoptotic cells were found in BCCs. In contrast, numerous single apoptotic cells were identified within the tumor masses in patients with BCC treated with intralesional injections of IFN alpha (Buechner et al. 1997). IFN-treated BCCs revealed a dense dermal lymphoid infiltrate surrounding the tumor nests. The majority of the peritumoral infiltrate were CD4[+] T cells. However, few T cells were found within the tumor nodules. On immunohistochemistry, BCC cells of untreated patients were seen to be completely CD95 negative, but were strongly CD95L positive. Upon treatment with IFN alpha the BCC cells expressed not only CD95L, but also CD95 receptor (Buechner et al. 1997). To evaluate whether the CD95L expressed by BCC from patients treated or not treated with IFN alpha is functional, CD95-positive cells (A20.2 J, a B lymphoma) were incubated on BCC cryosections, and apoptosis and lysis were measured. FACS analysis after propidium iodide staining showed an increase in the amount of apoptosis of A20.2 J added for 6 h onto BCC from both IFN alpha-treated and IFN alpha-untreated patients. Normal skin also induced a small amount of apoptosis, which is not surprising since keratinocytes are CD95L positive. Moreover, the A20.2 J cells incubated on BCC cryosections for 24 h were lysed as demonstrated in the more sensitive $^{51}$Cr release assay, regardless of whether the BCC originated from IFN alpha-treated or IFN alpha-untreated patients.

Normal skin also induced some lysis of A20.2 J, again reflecting CD95L expression of the keratinocytes (Buechner et al. 1997). Our study shows that apoptosis is the major mechanism of tumor cell death in regressing BCC after intralesional IFN alpha treatment. Since the BCCs of untreated patients express CD95L, the tumor cells may lyse, attacking CD95-expressing effector T cells via their CD95L. These data suggest that the expression of CD95L on BCC cells may play a significant part in the tumor progression. In keeping with the findings that CD95L may be involved in the formation of immune privilege in some organs, such as the eye and the testis (Griffith et al. 1995; Nagata 1996), BCC tumor cells can evade immune destruction. Therefore, we propose that the up-regulation of CD95L is a defensive strategy of BCC cells attempting to escape from immune surveillance. The concomitant expression of both CD95 and CD95L in IFN alpha-treated BCC induces apoptosis within the tumor cells, eventually leading to cell death by suicide or fratricide. The presence of large numbers of CD4$^+$ T cells around BCCs after intralesional IFN alpha injections supports the hypothesis that IFN alpha may also provoke the enhanced recruitment of infiltrating lymphoid cells, and especially of IFN gamma-producing CD4$^+$ T cells (Brinkmann et al. 1993). Recently, it has been shown that spontaneous regression of BCCs is associated with a significantly increased level of the Th1 type cytokine IFN gamma (Wong et al. 2000). In addition, it has been demonstrated that BCC regression induced by intralesional IFN alpha is accompanied by the elevation of IL2 expression (Wong et al. 2000). It is well established that CD95 expression can be induced by IL2 or IFN gamma (Nagata and Goldstein 1995). Thus, it is likely that infiltrating peritumoral T cells up-regulate CD95 on BCC cells by secreting these cytokines, and thus indirectly contribute to the CD95L-based cytotoxicity. In summary, the apoptotic cell death in BCC upon intralesional IFN alpha treatment, as identified by DNA fragmentation and followed by tumor regression, results from specific CD95–CD95L interactions.

## References


Ashkenazi A, Dixit V (1998) Death receptors: signaling and modulation. Science 281:1305–1308

Brinkmann V, Geiger T, Alkan S, Heusser CH (1993) Interferon-alpha increases the frequency of interferon-gamma-producing human CD4+ T-cells. J Exp Med 178:1655–1663

Buechner SA (1991) Intralesional interferon alfa-2b in the treatment of basal cell carcinoma. J Am Acad Dermatol 24:731–734

Buechner SA, Wernli M, Harr T, Hahn S, Itin P, Erb P (1997) Regression of basal cell carcinoma by intralesional interferon alpha-treatment is mediated by CD95 (APO-1/FAS)-CD95-ligand induced suicide. J Clin Invest 100:2691–2692

Chimenti S, Peris K, Di Cristofaro S, Fargnoli MC, Torlone G (1995) Use of recombinant interferon alfa-2b in the treatment of basal cell carcinoma. Dermatology 190:214–217

Cornell RC, Greenway HT, Tucker SB, Edwards L, Ashworth S, Vance JC, Tanner DJ, Taylor EL, Smiles KA, Peets E (1990) Intralesional interferon therapy for basal cell carcinoma. J Am Acad Dermatol 23:694–700

Greenway HT, Cornell RC, Tanner DJ, Peets E, Bordin GM, Nagi C (1986) Treatment of basal cell carcinoma with intralesional interferon. J Am Acad Dermatol 15:437–443

Gresser I (1990) Biologic effects of interferons. J Invest Dermatol 95:66S–71S

Griffith TS, Brunner T, Fletcher SM, Green DR, Ferguson TA (1995) Fas ligand-induced apoptosis as a mechanism of immune privilege. Science 270:1189–1192

Gutierrez-Steil C, Wrone-Smith T, Sun X, Krueger J, Coven T, Nickoloff B (1998) Sunlight-induced basal cell carcinoma tumor cells and ultraviolet-B-irradiated psoriatic plaques express Fas ligand (CD95L). J Clin Invest 101:33–39

Hahn S, Gehri R, Erb P (1995) Mechanism and biological significance of CD4-mediated cytotoxicity. Immunol Rev 146:57–79

Ikic D, Padovan I, Pipic N, Knezevic M, Djakovic N, Rode B, Kosutic I, Belicza M (1991) Basal cell carcinoma treated with interferon. Int J Dermatol 30:734–737

Karagas MR, Greenberg ER, Spencer SK, Stukel TA, Mott LA (1999) Increase in incidence rates of basal cell and squamous cell skin cancer in New Hampshire, USA. New Hampshire Skin Cancer Study Group. Int J Cancer 81:555–559

Lear JT, Smith AG (1997) Basal cell carcinoma. Postgrad Med J 73:538–542

Lee S, Jang J, Lee J, Kim S, Park W, Shin M, Dong S, Na E, Kim K, Kim C, Kim S, Yoo N (1998) Fas ligand is expressed in normal skin and in some cutaneous malignancies. Br J Dermatol 139:186–191

Miller SJ (1995) Etiology and pathogenesis of basal cell carcinoma. Clin Dermatol 13:527–536

Mozzanica N, Cattaneo A, Boneschi V, Brambilla L, Melotti E, Finzi AF (1990) Immunohistological evaluation of basal cell carcinoma immunoinfiltrate during intralesional treatment with alpha-2-interferon. Arch Dermatol Res 282:311–317

Nagata S (1996) Fas ligand and immune evasion. Nat Med 2:1306–1307

Nagata S, Golstein P (1995) The Fas death factor. Science 267:1449–1456

Oishi M, Maeda K, Sugiyama S (1994) Distribution of apoptosis-mediating Fas antigen in human skin and effects of anti-Fas monoclonal antibody on human epidermal keratinocyte and squamous cell carcinoma cell lines. Arch Dermatol Res 286:396–407

Strom SS, Yamamura Y (2001) Epidemiology of nonmelanoma skin cancer. Clin Plast Surg 24:627–636

Telfer NR, Colver GB, Bowers PW (1999) Guidelines for the management of basal cell carcinoma. British Association of Dermatologists. Br J Dermatol 141:415–423

Thestrup-Pedersen K, Jacobsen IE, Frentz G (1990) Intralesional interferon-alpha 2b treatment of basal cell carcinoma. Acta Derm Venereol (Stockh) 70:512–514

Ucar R, Sanwo M, Ucar K, Beall G (1995) Interferons: their role in clinical practice. Ann Allergy 75:377–386

Wehrli P, Viard I, Bullani R, Tschopp J, French LE (2000) Death receptors in cutaneous biology and disease. J Invest Dermatol 115:141–148

Wong DA, Bishop GA, Lowes MA, Cooke B, Barnetson RSC, Halliday GM (2000) Cytokine profiles in spontaneously regressing basal cell carcinomas. Br J Dermatol 143:91–98

# Epithelial Malignancies in Organ Transplant Patients: Clinical Presentation and New Methods of Treatment

E. Stockfleth, C. Ulrich, T. Meyer, and E. Christophers

## Abstract

Transplantation of solid organs has been well established as a mode of therapy for the treatment of various end-stage organ diseases for many years. Up to now, it has benefited more than 1 million patients worldwide. The long-term success of organ transplantation depends particularly on the prevention of allograft rejection. Various regimens have been used to suppress hosts' cellular immune responsiveness to the grafted organs. Nowadays immunosuppressive therapies consist mainly in prednisolone, azathioprine, cyclosporine, anti-T-lymphocyte-globulin (ATG), anti-CD 3 antibody (OKT3) and substances of a new generation, such as tacrolimus or mycophenolic acid. However, not only the patient's reactivity to the graft is impaired, but also that to infectious organisms. Chronically altered immune responsiveness is especially associated with a dramatically increased risk of malignancy, most frequently non-Hodgkin's lymphoma and skin cancer. Within the first 5 years of immunosuppression 40% of transplant recipients experience premalignant skin tumors such as actinic keratoses and Bowen's disease, and also such skin cancers as squamous cell carcinomas and basal cell carcinomas. Quite often these have an aggressive biology and an uncommon morphology. Cancer is now responsible for a mortality rate of 5–8% in organ transplant patients.

Various risk factors, such as exposure to sun and infections with oncogenic viruses (e.g. HPV) contribute to the already increased risk of dysplasia when lifelong immunosuppression is required. Prophylactic strategies therefore include the development of virus-like particles (VLPs) as anticancer vaccines, which might become a very interesting approach to preventing HPV-associated cancer. The prevention of precancerous conditions and mature skin cancers in grafted patients includes protective clothing and adequate protection of UV-exposed skin regions, including lips, from sunlight with appropriate sunscreen. Close dermatological surveillance through a specialized outpatient department should be ensured to detect potentially fatal skin ma-

Recent Results in Cancer Research, Vol. 160
© Springer-Verlag Berlin Heidelberg 2002

lignancies at an early stage. Early treatment of precancerous lesions includes topical retinoids, such as tretionin, tazarotene or adapalene. A 5% fluorouracil cream is widely used but shows variable effects on manifest actinic keratoses. As cellular immunity seems to play the major part in the prevention and cure of malignant and premalignant cutaneous neoplasias as well as viral infections, a specific enhancement of the local immunity would be desirable. Imiquimod is one of a class of agents known as immune response modifiers. The drug has been shown to have both antiviral and antitumor activity. Application of immune response activators or modifiers such as imiquimod might be premising in the case of transplant recipients.

## Skin Cancer in Organ Transplant Patients

Accounting as it does for almost 50% of all malignancies in transplant patients, skin cancer is by far the most common neoplasm diagnosed in this group of patients. Studies on heart- and kidney-grafted patients show that they have a significantly increased risk of nonmelanoma skin cancer. The cancers in transplant patients tend to be squamous cell carcinomas (SCC), which is a point of difference from the general population, in whom basal cell carcinoma (BCC) outnumbers SCC by 5 to 1.6 [1–4].

Emphasizing these findings, the incidence of premalignant lesions such as actinic keratoses has also been shown to be increased in transplant patients [5]. Data from the dermatological outpatient department of the University of Kiel indicate that 40% of the organ-grafted patients have premalignant or malignant lesions on their first visit. Later on, 22% develop SCC, 17% BCC, 12% Bowen's disease, and nearly 5% malignant melanoma. Actinic keratoses are found in 43% of these patients. As already reported by other groups, 66% of the lesions are located on sun-exposed areas of the skin [6].

The incidence of skin cancer rises in parallel with the time survived after transplantation. In Australian studies, 7% of the grafted patients show first malignant lesions after just 12 months of immunosuppression. After 20 years the incidence rises to 70% [2]. Comparable studies from The Netherlands show a cumulative rate of skin cancer of 0.2% after the 1st year and 41% after 20 years from transplantation [2]. Data recorded in a Canadian study on kidney-grafted patients show a latency of 8 years to the onset of skin cancer [7], whereas the average time in Australian and Spanish transplant patients is less than 3 years [4, 8].

In parallel with the increase in the risk of nonmelanoma skin cancer, in kidney-grafted patients the incidence of malignant melanoma is 2–9 times that in the general population [9, 10] and that of Merkel cell carcinoma is 50 times that in the general population [11].

However, skin cancer is not only increased in its incidence but appears to behave more aggressively than comparable tumors in nonimmunosuppressed patients.

Among patients documented in the Cincinnati Transplant Tumor Registry (CTTR), 5.7% had lymphogenous metastases at the time of their first diagnosis of skin cancer. In contrast to the situation in immunocompetent patients, 74% of these metastases had originated from SCC and only 17% were metastases from malignant melanomas. The mortality rate of skin cancer in organ transplant patients is around 5% [12].

## Mechanisms and Risk Factors in Skin Cancerogenesis in Organ Transplant Patients

In the face of the dramatically increased incidence and the aggressive behavior of skin cancers in grafted patients, a careful analysis of cancerogenic risk factors is necessary. In addition to the impairment of the host immune system, ultraviolet radiation is known to be a key pathogenic factor in the induction and promotion of neoplastic cells. Other groups emphasize the role of potentially oncogenic viruses, such as the human papillomaviruses (HPV). A more detailed analysis of known risk factors is given in the overview below.

### Immunosuppressive Treatment

Lifelong immunosuppression plays a key part in the pathogenesis of de novo skin cancer after transplantation. Prednisolone, azathioprine, cyclosporin A, mycophenolic acids and tacrolimus are widely used and are frequently supplemented by anti-T-lymphocyte serum or anti-CD3 antibodies (OKT 3) during the initial induction or cortisone-resistant graft rejection.

The significance of the different modes of immunosuppressive therapies concerning induction and promotion of cutaneous skin malignancies is frequently discussed. In studies on kidney-grafted patients Jensen (1999) reported that the risk of SCC in the cyclosporine-treated group was 2.8 times that in a comparable group of patients treated with prednisolone and azathioprine. The highest incidence was detected in the group of patients treated with a triple therapy composed of cyclosporine, azathioprine and prednisolone [1]. Other studies showed a frequency of skin malignancies ranging between zero and 11% in patients treated with cyclosporine [13], compared with 0.5–15.6% in a series of patients with no cyclosporine treatment at all [5]. Other authors found no significant differences in the oncogenic potency of different groups of immunosuppressants.

However, it has even been suggested that cyclosporine can be directly responsible for cancer progression by way of a cell-autonomous mechanism. Hojo (1999) described tumor growth factor (TGF) beta-related cancer progression in immunodeficient SCID mice treated with cyclosporin A [14].

## Ultraviolet Radiation

Exposure to sunlight is known to be a major risk factor in nonmelanoma skin cancer overall. Both precancerous and cancerous lesions are located mainly on sun-exposed areas of the skin in organ transplant patients. There is evidence for the significance of UV irradiation in the induction and promotion of skin cancer, especially in subjects whose immunological surveillance is already suppressed [15]. A striking correlation between an increasing incidence of skin cancer and decreasing nearness to the Equator is frequently described. The incidence of skin cancer is dramatically increased in transplant patients living in sunny countries, such as Australia (45% after 11 years) or Spain (43% after 7 years) [2, 3]. However, whereas patients with Anglo-Celtic backgrounds and those living close to the Equator were found to have a significantly increased cancer risk in Australian studies on grafted patients, others with an Aboriginal background had a substantially reduced risk of developing skin cancer [16]. Chronic sunlight exposure even before organ transplantation seems to be another determinant and a predictable risk factor. Ong (1999) found a direct correlation between age at the time of transplantation and the later incidence of skin cancer [5, 16]. Studies on kidney-grafted patients reveal a close correlation between sun exposure prior to the age of 30 and the incidence of skin cancer [3]. The local immunosuppressive effect of ultraviolet radiation (290–320 nm) seems to be related to the increased incidence of cutaneous malignancies, actinic keratoses and viral lesions.

## Human Papillomavirus Infection

In addition to immunosuppression and UV-radiation, HPV infection may also be involved in the development of nonmelanoma skin cancer. The association between HPV infection and the development of cutaneous SCCs was first described in patients with epidermodysplasia verruciformis (EV). EV is a rare hereditary cutaneous disorder characterized by infection with a particular subset of HPV types (EV-associated HPV types). These HPVs induce extensive flat polymorphous warts that progress into malignant lesions within 25 years in about 30% of these patients [17, 18].

The majority of EV-associated skin cancers represent SCCs that predominantly contain HPV 5 and HPV 8 [19]. EV is associated with a deficiency of cellular immunity, probably both disposing for HPV-infection and impairing the elimination of neoplastic cells. In addition, UV radiation seems to be involved in tumorigenesis, since skin cancers of EV patients develop predominantly in sun-exposed skin areas. Thus, EV-associated skin cancers suggest a multifactorial etiology of skin cancer.

Typical HPV-associated skin lesions in the general population are represented by verrucae vulgares. These common warts are mainly caused by other cutaneous HPV types. Over 90% of transplant recipients have been reported to develop common viral warts [15]. With increasing duration of immunosuppressive treatment, atypical flat warts, predominantly located on sun-exposed skin areas, appear. The progression of these warts to dysplastic lesions and SCCs has been shown in both clinical and histological studies [20]. In contrast to the course in nonimmunosuppressed patients, spontaneous regression is seen rarely in transplanted patients. Thus, viral warts, which are usually considered benign lesions in immunocompetent patients, have a different prognostic importance in immunosuppressed patients.

In earlier studies on HPV detection in nonmelanoma skin cancer biopsies from non-EV patients, viral DNA was detected with varying frequencies [21]. These discrepant findings most probably relate to methodical differences. In general, the HPV detection rate was higher in recent studies using consensus PCRs that encompass broad ranges of HPV types [22]. But even in these PCR studies, the frequency and spectrum of HPV types is influenced by the primer sets and amplification conditions used [23]. In transplant recipients the rate of HPV-positive premalignant and malignant skin lesions is higher than in nonimmunosuppressed patients [22, 23]. The combined results of two PCR assays with different systems of degenerate primers showed that HPV DNA was detected in 91% of SCC from transplanted patients [24]. These findings indicate a general association of HPV infection with SCC in transplanted patients.

Besides the high prevalence of HPV DNA in tumor biopsies, the possible role of HPV in skin cancerogenesis is also supported by the persistence of HPV infections in benign, premalignant and malignant skin lesions of renal transplant recipients [22]. The E6 protein of some EV-HPV types has been shown to prevent infected cells from apoptosis [25]. Furthermore, UV-responsive elements were identified in the promoter region of several HPV types [26]. Thus, UV-induced viral proteins such as E6 may interfere with the cell proliferation by inhibiting apoptosis.

On the other hand, HPV DNA is detected in significant numbers of normal skin biopsies and plugged hairs [26, 27]. In addition, viral DNA is usually detected in DNA extracts of skin tissues when there is no information about the intracellular localization. In most of the specimens HPV-positive results are obtained only after nested PCR, indicating rather low amounts of viral DNA. Indeed, HPV DNA (RTRX7) could not be detected by Southern blot hybridization with a homologous probe in a PCR-positive SCC, indicating that the DNA concentration was below 1 copy per 10 cells in the investigated tissue specimen [28, 29].

In summary, the role of HPV in the development of cutaneous malignancies under immunosuppression is not clear at present and needs to be clarified in future studies. Large-scale epidemiological studies are necessary to characterize the risk of HPV infection in the development of skin cancer in transplant recipients.

## Treatment and Prevention of Skin Tumors in Organ Transplant Patients

Although the exact role of HPV in the development of cutaneous malignancies under immunosuppression is still not clear at present, viral infection provides an important basis for preventive and therapeutic strategies against skin tumors. Currently applied treatment modalities for HPV-associated tumors are based mainly on the destruction of affected skin areas. These include surgical excision by cryotherapy or electrocautery and the use of such keratinolytic or cytotoxic drugs as 5′-fluorouracil (5-FU) or podophyllotoxin. All these conventional therapies are highly irritative and painful for the patient. In addition, a relatively high rate of relapse has been described after these treatments. Interferon-$\alpha$ (IFN$\alpha$) has also been used for the treatment of skin tumors [30]. Its clinical use is limited by severe side effects. However, since it was shown to be effective for actinic keratoses and BCCs, the development of other immunomodulatory agents with less severe side effects seems promising.

Imiquimod is an immune response modifier. The drug has been shown to have both antiviral and antitumor activity. The mode of action probably involves stimulation of the production of several cytokines and enhancement of cell-mediated cytolysis [31, 32]. Early experience with imiquimod in the treatment of cutaneous lesions involved topical application in particular cases of different skin tumors. According to these preliminary studies, imiquimod has proved effective in the resolution of verrucae vulgares, stucco keratosis, actinic keratosis, BCCs and epidermodysplasia verruciformis [33, 34].

Most importantly, no severe side effects were observed during this treatment. As a minor side effect, the development of erythema was a common finding, which is due to the local immune activation by imiquimod. On the other hand, the appearance of erythema is a useful indicator of treatment response and thus may be considered a desirable skin reaction rather than an unwanted side effect.

At first sight, the application of immune response activators or modifiers such as imiquimod might seem paradoxical in the case of transplant recipients requiring immunosuppressive treatment. However, since the local application of imiquimod does not cause systemic side effects, it is very interesting for the treatment of skin tumors in transplant patients.

In addition to improvement of treatment options, strategies to counteract HPV-associated skin tumors also include measures to prevent tumor formation. The development of virus-like particles (VLPs) as anticancer vaccines has become a very interesting approach to preventing HPV-induced cancer [35]. VLPs induce neutralizing antibodies against the HPV capsid proteins and thus primarily protect against primary infection. Using chimeric VLPs consisting of fusion proteins of the viral structural proteins (L1) and oncogene products (E7), it was possible to prevent the growth of virus-transformed cells and even to treat pre-existing HPV-induced tumors in animal models [36, 37].

Although these effective animal studies look promising, there may be some difficulties in applying HPV vaccination in organ transplant patients.

Owing to the constant immunosuppression after transplantation, it would be necessary to establish a long-lasting immune response prior to organ transplantation, because immunosuppressed patients may fail to produce HPV-specific antibodies and T-cells. Furthermore, no HPV types predominating in nonmelanoma skin cancers have yet been identified. It is probable that a broad range of different HPV types is associated with skin tumors. Consequently, a vaccine should be able to induce a cross-reactive immune response against a number of different HPV types.

**Acknowledgements.** This work has been generously supported by a grant of the Hensel-Stiftung, University of Kiel.

# References


1. Jensen P, Hansen S, Moller B, Leivestad T, Pfeffer P, Geiran O, Fauchald P, Simonsen S (1999) Skin cancer in kidney and heart transplant recipients and different long-term immunosuppressive therapy regimens. J Am Acad Dermatol 40:177–186
2. Bouwes Bavinck JN, Hardie DR, Green A, et al (1996) The risk of skin cancer in renal transplant recipients in Queensland, Australia. A follow-up study. Transplantation 61:715–721
3. Bouwes Bavinck JN, Vermeer BJ, van der Woude FJ, Vandenbroucke JP, Geziena M, Schreuder GMT, et al (1991) Relation between skin cancer and HLA antigens in renal-transplant recipients. N Engl J Med 325:843–848
4. Espana A, Redondo P, Fernandez AL, Zambala M, Herreros J, Llorens R, Quintanilla E (1995) Skin cancer in heart transplant recipients. J Am Acad Dermatol 32:458–465
5. Boyle J, Mackie RM, Briggs JD, Junor BJR, Aitchison TC (1984) Cancer, warts, and sunshine in renal transplant patients. A case-control study. Lancet I:702–704
6. Leigh IM, Buchanan JA, Harwood CA, Cerio R, Storey A (1999) Role of human papillomaviruses in cutaneous and oral manifestations of immunosuppression. J Acquir Immune Defic Syndr 21:S49–S57
7. Gupta AK, Cardella CJ, Habermann HF (1986) Cutaneous malignant neoplasms in patients with renal transplants. Arch Dermatol 122:1288–1293
8. Hardie IR, Strong RW, Hartley LC, Woodruff PW, Clunie GJ (1980) Skin cancer in Caucasian renal allograft recipients living in a subtropical climate. Surgery 87:177–183
9. Penn I, Brunson ME (1996) Malignant melanoma in organ allograft recipients. Transplantation 61:274–278
10. Leveque L, Dalac S, Dompmartin A, Louvet S, Euvrard S, et al (2000) Melanoma in organ transplant patients. Ann Dermatol Venerol 127:160–165
11. Penn I, Brunson ME (1988) Cancers after cyclosporine therapy. Transplant Proc 20:885–892
12. Penn I (1998) Occurrence of cancers in immunosuppressed organ transplant recipients. Clin Transplant 1998:147–158
13. O'Connell BM, Abel EA, Nickoloff BJ, et al (1986) Dermatologic complications following heart transplantation. J Heart Lung Transplant 5:430–436
14. Hojo M, Morimoto T, Maluccio M, Asano T, Morimoto K, Lagman M, Shimbo T, Suthanthiran M (1999) Cyclosporine induces cancer progression by a cell-autonomous mechanism. Nature 397:530–534
15. Stockfleth E, Ulrich C, Meyer T, Arndt R, Christophers E (2001) Skin diseases following organ transplantation-risk factors and new therapeutic approaches. Transplant Proc 33:1848–1853
16. Ong CS, Keogh AM, Kossard S, Macdonald PS, Spratt PM (1999) Skin cancer in Australian heart transplant recipients. J Am Acad Dermatol 40:27–34

17. Majewski S, Jablonska S (1995) Epidermodysplasia verruciformis as a model of human papillomavirus-induced genetic cancer of the skin. Arch Dermatol 131:1312–1318
18. Orth G, Jablonska S, Jarzabek-Chorzelsk M, et al (1979) Characteristics of the lesions and risk of malignant conversion associated with the type of human papillomavirus involved in epidermodysplasia verruciformis. Cancer Res 39:1074–1082
19. Orth G (1987) Epidermodysplasia verruciformis. In: Salzman NP, Howley PM (eds) The Papovaviridae, the papillomaviruses. Plenum, New York, pp 199–235
20. Blessing K, McLaren LM, Benton EC, et al (1989) Histopathology of skin lesions in renal allograft recipients: an assessment of viral features and dysplasia. Histopathology 14:129–139
21. Pfister H, ter Schegget J (1997) Role of HPV in cutaneous premalignant and malignant tumors. Clin Dermatol 15:335–348
22. Berkhout RJ, Tieben LM, Smits HL, et al (1995) Nested PCR approach for detection and typing of epidermodysplasia verruciformis-associated human papillomavirus types in cutaneous cancers from renal transplant recipients. J Clin Microbiol 33:690–695
23. Meyer T, Arndt R, Christophers E, et al (2000) Frequency and spectrum of HPV types detected in cutaneous squamous cell carcinomas depend on the HPV detection system: a comparison of four PCR assays. Dermatology 201:204–211
24. De Villiers EM, Lavergne D, McLaren K, et al (1997) Prevailing papillomavirus types in non-melanoma carcinomas of the skin in renal allograft recipients. Int J Cancer 73:356–361
25. Jackson S, Storey A (2000) E6 proteins from diverse cutaneous HPV types inhibit apoptosis in response to UV damage. Oncogene 27:592–598
26. Purdie KJ, Pennington J, Proby CM, et al (1999) The promotor of a novel human papillomavirus (HPV 77) associated with skin cancer displays UV responsiveness, which is mediated through a consensus p53 binding sequence. EMBO J 18:5359–5369
27. Astori G, Lavergne D, Benton C, et al (1998) Human papillomaviruses are commonly found in normal skin of immunocompetent hosts. J Invest Dermatol 110:752–755
28. Boxman ILA, Berkhout RJM, Mulder LHC, et al (1997) Detection of human papillomavirus DNA in plucked hairs from renal transplant recipients and healthy volunteers. J Invest Dermatol 108:712–715
29. Bens G, Wieland U, Hofmann A, Höpfl R, Pfister H (1998) Detection of a new human papillomavirus sequence in skin lesions of a renal transplant recipient and characterization of the complete genome related to epidermodysplasia verruciformis associated types. J Gen Virol 79:779–787
30. Edwards L, Levine N, Weidner M, Piepkorn M, Smiles K (1986) Effect of intralesional alpha 2-interferon on actinic keratoses. Arch Dermatol 122:779–782
31. Aranay I, Tyring SK, Stanley MA, Tomai MA, Miller RL, Smith MH, McDermott DJ, Slade HB (1999) Enhancement of the innate and cellular immune response in patients with genital warts treated with topical imiquimod cream 5%. Antiviral Res 43:55–63
32. Tyring SK, Arany I, Stanley MA, Tomai MA, Miller RL, Smith MH, McDermott DJ, Slade HB (1998) A randomized, controlled, molecular study of condylomata acuminata clearance during treatment with Imiquimod. J Infect Dis 178:551–555
33. Hengge UR, Esser S, Schultewolter T, Behrendt C, Meyer T, Stockfleth E, Goos M (2000) Self-administered topical 5% imiquimod for the treatment of common warts and molluscum contagiosum. Br J Dermatol 143:1026–1031
34. Stockfleth E, Meyer T, Benninghoff B, et al (2001) Successful treatment of actinic keratosis with imiquimod cream 5%: a report of 6 cases. Br J Dermatol 144:1050–1053
35. Schiller JT (1999) Papillomavirus-like particle vaccines for cervical cancer. Mol Med Today 5:209–215
36. Müller M, Zhou J, Reed TD, Rittmüller C, Burger A, Gabelsberger J, Braspenning J, Gissmann L (1997) Chimeric papillomavirus-like particles. Virology 234:93–111
37. Schäfer K, Müller M, Faath S, Henn A, Osen W, Zentgraf H, Benner A, Gissmann L, Jochmus I (1999) Immune response to human papillomavirus 16 L1E7 chimeric virus-like particles: induction of cytotoxic T-cells and specific tumor protection. Int J Cancer 81:881–888

# New Treatment Modalities for Basal Cell Carcinoma

E. Stockfleth and W. Sterry

## Abstract

Basal cell carcinoma (BCC) is a subtype of nonmelanoma skin cancer (NMSC), a potentially fatal disease linked to overexposure to the sun during childhood. BCC has been associated with UV-induced mutations of the *PTC* and *p53* tumor suppressor genes, and to polymorphisms in the melanocortin-1 receptor and *XPD* genes. Mortality rates due to BCC are low, but its increasing incidence and prolonged morbidity means the disease is costly to treat. Early recognition and effective treatment are therefore important, to reduce the incidence of BCC and lighten the economic burden of its management. This paper reviews current treatments for BCC, including excision and curettage, electrodessication, surgery, cryosurgery, radiotherapy, and treatment with 5-fluorouracil and intralesional/perilesional cytokines. It also deals with two new treatment modalities, photodynamic therapy and imiquimod 5% cream, an immune response modifier that effectively resolves BCC lesions.

## Introduction

The worldwide incidence of nonmelanoma skin cancer (NMSC) is increasing rapidly. Basal cell carcinoma (BCC), which arises from the abnormal growth of epidermal keratinocytes, accounts for the majority of NMSC cases (Salasche 2000). In 1998, approximately 900 000–1 200 000 cases of NMSC were diagnosed in the United States, 80% of which were cases of BCC; this means there has been a 70% increase in disease incidence since 1978 (Salasche 2000; Miller and Weinstock 1994). BCC is a common condition in Australia, where its incidence has increased by 130% since 1985–1995 (Staples et al. 1998). The number of cases reported in Europe has also risen in recent years (Ko et al. 1994; Plesko et al. 2000).

Recent Results in Cancer Research, Vol. 160

BCC tumors occur as superficial, nodular, or infiltrative (morphea- or non-morphea-type) lesions in the dermis, which may bleed, ulcerate, regress or become fibrotic. The clinical presentation varies, making BCC difficult to diagnose (Goldberg 1996), so that the most accurate method of diagnosis is biopsy (Poinsford et al. 1983). Evidence of regression is seen in approximately 50% of tumors (Barnetson and Halliday 1997), but the frequency of complete regression is unknown. BCCs can metastasize, and may be fatal in an estimated 0.1% of cases (Miller and Weinstock 1994); however, long-term morbidity, with disease recurrence after therapy, the ability of lesions to enlarge progressively, and the appearance of multiple lesions in many patients, means that BCC is expensive to treat. High incidence rates have led to concern about the economic burden imposed by BCC management in many countries (Marks et al. 2001).

The main risk factor associated with BCC is overexposure to UV light, and particularly nonoccupational or recreational exposure (Armstrong et al. 1997). This is reflected in the relatively high incidence of BCC lesions on body sites only occasionally exposed to the sun (such as the trunk). There is some evidence suggesting that the onset of BCC may be linked with the level of sun exposure early in life; for example, sunburn in childhood may be an important risk factor (Kricker et al. 1995; Zanetti et al. 1996). The incidence has been shown to increase with age (Levi et al. 1988), suggesting that cumulative exposure to the sun may also affect disease progression. Phenotypic characteristics of individuals at higher risk of developing BCC include fair or red/blond hair and blue–green eyes, i.e., those typically affected are persons with Fitzpatrick skin type 1 (Lear et al. 1997; Marks 1997). Melanocortin-1 receptor (*MC1R*) gene variants strongly associated with this phenotype have been identified as important independent risk factors for NMSC (Bastiaens et al. 2001). There is also strong evidence that early-onset, sporadic BCC can be caused by UV-specific genetic mutations in the *PTC* and *p53* tumor suppressor genes (Zhang et al. 2001). In addition, polymorphisms in the *XPD* gene, which is important for basal transcription and nucleotide excision repair, are associated with an increased risk of disease (Vogel et al. 2001).

High incidence rates in organ transplant patients undergoing therapy with immunosuppressant drugs suggests that the immune response is important in the development of NMSC (Stockfleth et al. 2001b). In a study by Otley et al. (2001), four of six patients who stopped therapy because of allograft failure or onset of unacceptable cutaneous carcinogenesis experienced decelerated development of cutaneous carcinomas and an improvement in skin quality. Cessation of immunosuppression may have led to restoration of the immune response in these patients and therefore to enhanced immune surveillance and destruction of cancerous cells. However, further studies are needed to investigate the mechanism of regression in this patient group.

## Current Treatments

A range of treatments can be applied for the reduction and removal of BCC tumors. The type of treatment chosen may depend on a number of factors, including the patient's age and ability to heal, and the location, size and type of the tumor(s) (Goldberg 1996; Preston and Stern 1992). Cost may also be a factor in the physician's choice, as this can vary very widely depending on the treatment chosen.

## Excision and Curettage

Excision is a common method of removing BCC tumors, and is most appropriate for the treatment of small nodular and superficial BCC lesions (Thissen et al. 1999). However, incomplete excision occurs in approximately 7–14% of cases and can lead to disease recurrence, further surgery and scarring (Griffiths 1999; Schreuder and Powell 1999). Curettage before the excision of BCC lesions helps the surgeon to define the tumor border and can decrease the treatment failure rate by up to 24%. It is particularly effective in improving the treatment of lesions situated in the head and neck region (Chiller at al. 2000). The size of the excision margin removed with the tumor can also affect the success of the procedure. BCC lesions often occur on the head, face and neck; therefore, in order to obtain a cosmetically acceptable result, a minimal amount of surrounding tissue is removed with the lesion. A clinical excision margin of 1–2 mm has been shown to be successful in 95–97% of patients treated (Lalloo and Sood 2000; Niederhagan et al. 2000). Dermatologists have a higher success rate with this method of treatment than otolaryngologists and plastic surgeons, which indicates that the specialty of the physician may affect treatment failure rates (Fleischer et al. 2001).

## Surgery

High-risk morphea-type BCC lesions greater than 1.5 cm in diameter, recurrent lesions, and also those present on the face may be referred for Mohs' micrographic surgery (Goldberg 1996; Lindgren et al. 2000). This method of tissue removal allows the surgeon to examine the tumor borders serially as they are removed, and thus to keep the loss of tissue to a minimum. Rates of success are high, at above 95% (Preston and Stern 1992), and this treatment has the added benefit of lower recurrence rates than other treatment modalities (Thissen et al. 1999). Mohs' surgery allows the surgeon to detect perineural invasion, which is a strong indicator of high-risk tumors (Ratner et al. 2000). However, this method can be expensive owing to extended periods in the operating room and can result in scarring. In addition, some patients will not be eligible for surgery because of poor health or old age.

## Curettage and Electrodessication

A widely used treatment for superficial and nodular BCC lesions less than 1.5 cm in diameter is a combination therapy, with curettage followed by electrodessication. The cure rate is approximately 95%, and the 5-year recurrence rates (1.3–18.8%) are comparable to those achieved with other forms of treatment (Preston and Stern 1992). As physicians need only a sharp curette and an electrodessicator the treatment is widely available, as both are commonly available in any dermatologist's clinic. Curettage can also be combined with freezing to destroy malignant tissue, but this treatment then often leaves a white, irregular scar that can easily be seen (Goldberg 1996).

## Cryosurgery

Cryosurgery using liquid nitrogen delivered through a cryoprobe can also be effective against superficial BCC (Vine 2001). The tissue at the base of the tumor is frozen and then thawed three or four times (to −40 °C to −60 °C) to ensure that the malignant tissue has been destroyed. On average, 5-year recurrence rates are lower after cryosurgery than after curettage and electrodessication (Preston and Stern 1992); however, this treatment is not effective against large, recurrent or aggressive tumors.

## Radiotherapy

Radiotherapy is useful for the management of large or recurrent lesions, particularly in individuals whose age or general health prevents them from undergoing surgery, and also for the treatment of facial lesions for which surgery would have unacceptable cosmetic results (Caccialanza et al. 2001). In a study by Seegenschmiedt et al. (2001) external beam radiotherapy resulted in a 99% remission rate 3 months after the end of therapy. However, treatment is not recommended for patients under the age of 50 years because of less favorable cosmetic results (Thissen et al. 1999; Vine 2001) and a significant risk of secondary malignancy (van Vloten et al. 1987). Recurrence rates of up to 31% have also been reported (Rowe et al. 1989).

## 5-Fluorouracil

5-Fluorouracil (5-FU), a topically applied preparation used for the treatment of BCC, actinic keratosis, and genital warts, inhibits cell growth by interfering with DNA and RNA synthesis. 5-FU therapy combined with curettage (Epstein 1985) or cryosurgery (Tsuji et al. 1993) can be effective in the treatment of BCC, but when 5-FU is used in isolation the treatment failure rates are higher than with other modes of treatment (Epstein 1985). It also induces a high level of irritation at the site of application, which may affect compliance. Injecting 5-FU gel or combining it with phosphatidyl choline (PC), a carrier that aids penetration of the cream through the epidermis (Romagosa et al. 2000), improved efficacy; response rates were comparable to those of surgery (Miller et al. 1997). However, 5-FU is not recommended for use in the American Academy of Dermatology BCC treatment guidelines (Drake et al. 1992).

## Intralesional/Perilesional Cytokine Treatment

T cell cytokines have been used successfully in the treatment of BCCs by several investigators. Intralesional injection of superficial BCCs (sBCCs) with interferon alpha (IFN$\alpha$)-2a or -2b cleared approximately 67% of lesions when used individually (Alpsoy et al. 1996; Chimenti et al. 1995). Efficacy increased to 73.3% when the cytokines were combined. Human natural leukocytic interferon (HNLI) and recombinant IFN$\alpha$-2c have also been successfully combined (Ikic et al. 1991); with this combination 72% of patients were histologically clear of BCC after 6 weeks of treatment. Side effects can include local erythema, pain, swelling and inflammation, and the need for injections given up to three times per week by a trained professional makes this treatment costly and inconvenient. Intralesional interferon is not recommended in US treatment guidelines but is currently being evaluated.

## New Treatment Modalities

### Photodynamic Therapy

Photodynamic therapy (PDT) directly targets and destroys BCC lesions though selective accumulation of $\delta$-aminolevulinic acid (ALA; Soler et al. 2000), photofrin (a dihematoporphyrin derivative; Schweitzer 2001), or metatetrahydroxyphenylchlorine (mTHPC; Baas et al. 2001) in malignant tumor cells. Exposure of cells containing a high concentration of any of these compounds to nonionizing radiation results in cell death. A recent study has shown that PDT is as effective as cryosurgery for the treatment of BCC (Wang et al. 2001). The main side effect of treatment is a sunburn-like reaction characterized by edema and erythema; however, in contrast to the situation after cryotherapy, healing times are short and scarring is minimal. PDT is more effective against sBCC (87% cured) than against nodular BCC lesions (53% cured) (Wang et al. 2001) and is particularly useful for the treatment of disseminated or large BCCs with wide margins and for those in such cosmetically sensitive areas as the face (Haller et al. 2000; Varma et al. 2001). It is also useful for the treatment of multiple lesions in elderly patients who can no longer undergo surgery (Schweitzer 2001). However, 12 months after PDT treatment a relatively high rate of recurrence was detected (25% of treated lesions) compared with that after cryosurgery (15% of treated lesions), so that patients should be monitored for recurrence. Treatment is also associated with severe cutaneous photosensitivity that can last up to 4 weeks (Preston and Stern 1992). PDT has not yet been approved for the treatment of BCC.

## Imiquimod

Imiquimod is the first in a new class of drugs named immune response modifiers (IRM). The compound has been used successfully for the treatment of cutaneous cancers such as actinic keratosis, an early form of squamous cell carcinoma (Stockfleth et al. 2001a), and Bowen's disease or squamous cell carcinoma in situ (Mackenzie-Wood et al. 2001). In a pilot study by Beutner et al. (1999), imiquimod successfully cleared sBCC lesions in 15 of 15 patients who applied the cream at least three times per week. Clearance was confirmed by histological examination. Local inflammatory reactions to treatment were reported, but the majority of side effects were mild to moderate.

A series of phase II trials have confirmed that imiquimod is an effective treatment for sBCC. In an Australian trial, application three times per week for 6 weeks cleared lesions in 70% of patients, and daily application cleared lesions in 88% of patients (Marks et al. 2001). Efficacy was measured in terms of complete histological clearance of the excised post-treatment site. A vehicle-controlled US trial in which patients were treated for 12 weeks yielded similar efficacy rates, with clearance of 87% of lesions after daily application, 81% after treatment five times per week, and 52% after treatment three times per week (Geisse et al. 2001). Both studies showed a dose–response effect. The findings from the US trial also suggested that extending the duration of treatment did not increase the efficacy rate. The final study in this series was conducted in Europe and investigated the effect of occlusion on clearance rates. In this open-label study patients were treated for 6 weeks two or three times per week, both with and without occlusion. The rates for three times per week were comparable to those achieved in the previous studies (76%), and occlusion was shown to cause a moderate increase (to 88%) in clearance (Sterry et al. 2001a). Again, clearance was defined as histological freedom from tumor. Application site reactions in all studies included mild to moderate itching, erythema, discharge and tenderness and were dose dependent; however, the treatment was well tolerated by the majority of patients and cosmetic results were good.

Imiquimod has also been used successfully for the treatment of a patient with basal cell nevus syndrome, a condition that causes the formation of multiple BCCs on the epidermis (Kagy and Amonette 2000). Treatment three times per week for 18 weeks resolved two of three superficial BCC lesions, but the patient reported a strong inflammatory response to treatment. Clearly further studies are needed to assess the optimum treatment regimen for basal cell nevus patients.

Nodular BCC lesions can also be treated successfully with 5% imiquimod cream; daily application cleared lesions in 71 and 76% of patients after 6 and 12 weeks of treatment, respectively (Robinson et al. 2001; Shumack et al. 2001). Local reactions were mostly mild to moderate, and occlusion was shown to improve efficacy (Sterry et al. 2001b).

In preclinical trials, application of imiquimod up-regulated the production of interferon alpha (IFN$\alpha$) and tumor necrosis factor alpha (TNF$\alpha$) in the dermis 1–2 h after application (Stanley 1999). In vitro, imiquimod has also stimulated production of IFN$\alpha$, TNF$\alpha$ and IL12 from monocytes and macrophages, cells that are important for innate and acquired immunity (Wagner et al. 1999). Production of these cytokines suggests that imiquimod may induce a cell-mediated immune response similar to that found in spontaneously regressing BCC lesions (Wong et al. 2000). Imiquimod-induced IFN$\alpha$ can have long-term in vivo antitumor effects (Borden et al. 1991), but it is not yet known whether imiquimod treatment can induce a memory T cell response in BCC patients.

## Conclusions

Many therapies are available for the treatment of BCC. When deciding on the most appropriate therapy for any individual the physician must take into account a range of factors, including the type, size and location of the lesion. As BCCs frequently occur in the head and neck region the cosmetic effects of treatment are often important to the patient. In some areas of high incidence, such as Australia, where the long-term management of BCC has a significant impact on healthcare resources, cost must also be taken into account. Surgery is the most popular and successful treatment for advanced or morphea-type lesions; however, the benefits and success rates of treatments for superficial and nodular BCC vary. Recent studies have shown that imiquimod 5% cream is a safe and effective treatment for both forms of BCC. Further large-scale trials investigating imiquimod for the treatment of superficial and nodular BCC are currently ongoing.

## References


Alpsoy E, Yilmaz E, Basaran E, Yazar S (1996) Comparison of the effects of intralesional interferon alfa-2a, 2b and the combination of 2a and 2b in the treatment of basal cell carcinoma. J Dermatol 23:394–396

Armstrong BK, Kricker A, English DR (1997) Sun exposure and skin cancer. Australas J Dermatol 38:S1–S6

Baas P, Saarnak AE, Oppelaar H, Neering H, Stewart FA (2001) Photodynamic therapy with meta-tetrahydroxyphenylchlorine for basal cell carcinoma: a phase I/II study. Br J Dermatol 145:75–78

Barnetson RStC, Halliday GM (1997) Regression in skin tumours: a common phenomenon. Australas J Dermatol 38:S63–S65

Bastiaens MT, ter Huurne JA, Kielich C, Gruis NA, Westendorp RG, Vermeer BJ, Bavinck JN, The Leiden Skin Cancer Study Team (2001) Melanocortin-1 receptor gene variants determine the risk of non-melanoma skin cancer independently of fair skin and red hair. Am J Hum Genet 68:884–894

Beutner KR, Geisse JK, Helman D, Fox TL, Ginkel A, Owens ML (1999) Therapeutic response of basal cell carcinoma to the immune response modifier imiquimod 5% cream. Am Acad Dermatol 41:1002–1007

Borden EC, Sidky YA, Weeks CE (1991) Mechanisms of anti-tumour action of the interferon inducer R-837. Proc Am Assoc Cancer Res 32:258

Caccialanza M, Piccinno R, Grammatica A (2001) Radiotherapy of recurrent basal and squamous cell skin carcinomas: a study of 249 re-treated carcinomas in 229 patients. Eur J Dermatol 11:25–28

Chiller K, Passaro D, McCalmont T, Vin-Christian K (2000) Efficacy of curettage before excision in clearing surgical margins of non-melanoma skin cancer. Arch Dermatol 136:1327–1332

Chimenti S, Peris K, Di Cristofaro S, Fargnoli MC, Torlone G (1995) Use of recombinant interferon alfa-2b in the treatment of basal cell carcinoma. Dermatology 190:214–217

Drake LA, Ceilley RI, Cornelison RL et al (1992) Guidelines of care for basal cell carcinoma. The American Academy of Dermatology Committee on Guidelines of Care. J Am Acad Dermatol 26:117–120

Epstein E (1985) Fluorouracil paste treatment of thin basal cell carcinomas. Arch Dermatol 121:207–213

Fleischer AB Jr, Feldman SR, Barlow JR, Zheng B, Hahn HB, Chuang TY, Draft KS, Golitz LE, Wu E, Katz AS, Maize JC, Knapp T, Leshin B (2001) The specialty of the treating physician affects the likelihood of tumor-free resection margins for basal cell carcinoma: results from a multi-institutional retrospective study. J Am Acad Dermatol 44:224–230

Geisse JK, Marks R, Owens ML, Andres K, Ginkel AM (2001) Imiquimod 5% cream for 12 weeks treating superficial BCC. 8th world congress on cancers of the skin, Zurich, 18–21 July

Goldberg LH (1996) Basal cell carcinoma. Lancet 347:663–667

Griffiths RW (1999) Audit of histologically incompletely excised basal cell carcinomas: recommendations for management by re-excision. Br J Plast Surg 52:24–28

Haller JC, Cairnduff F, Slack G, Schofield J, Whitehurst C, Tunstall R, Brown SB, Roberts DJ (2000) Routine double treatments of superficial basal cell carcinomas using aminolaevulinic acid-based photodynamic therapy. Br J Dermatol 143:1270–1275

Ikic D, Padovan I, Pipic N, Knezevic M, Djakovic N, Rode B, Kosutic I, Belicza M (1991) Basal cell carcinoma treated with interferon. Int J Dermatol 30:734–737

Kagy MK, Amonette R (2000) The use of imiquimod 5% cream for the treatment of superficial basal cell carcinomas in a basal cell nevus syndrome patient. Dermatol Surg 26:577–579

Ko CB, Walton S, Keczkes K, Bury HP (1994) The emerging epidemic of skin cancer. Br J Dermatol 130:269–272

Kricker A, Armstrong BK, English DR, Heenan PJ (1995) Does intermittent sun exposure cause basal cell carcinoma? A case-control study in Western Australia. Int J Cancer 60:489–494

Lalloo MT, Sood S (2000) Head and neck basal cell carcinoma: treatment using a 2 mm clinical excision margin. Clin Otolaryngol 25:370–373

Lear JT, Tan BB, Smith AG, Bowers W, Jones PW, Heagerty AH, Strange RC, Fryer AA (1997) Risk factors for basal cell carcinoma in the UK: case-control study in 806 patients. J R Soc Med 90:371–374

Levi F, La Vecchia C, Te VC, Mezzanotte G (1988) Descriptive epidemiology of skin cancer in the Swiss Canton of Vaud. Int J Cancer 42:811–816

Lindgren G, Lindblom B, Bratel AT, Molne L, Larko O (2000) Mohs micrographic surgery for basal cell carcinomas on the eyelids and medial canthal area. I. Characteristics of the tumours and details of the procedure. Acta Opthalmol Scand 78:425–429

Mackenzie-Wood A, Kossard S, de Launey J, Wilkinson B, Owens ML (2001) Imiquimod 5% cream in the treatment of Bowen's disease. J Am Acad Dermatol 44:462–470

Marks R (1997) Epidemiology of non-melanoma skin cancer and solar keratoses in Australia: a tale of self-immolation in Elysian fields. Australas J Dermatol 38:S26–S29

Marks R, Gebauer K, Shumack S, Amies M, Bryden J, Fox TL, Owens ML, The Australian Multicenter Trial Group (2001) Imiquimod 5% cream in the treatment of superficial basal cell carcinoma: results of a multicenter 6-week dose-response trial. J Am Acad Dermatol 44:807–813

Miller BH, Shavin JS, Cognetta A, Taylor RJ, Salasche S, Korey A, Orenberg EK (1997) Non-surgical treatment of basal cell carcinomas with intralesional 5-fluorouracil/epinephrine injectable gel. J Am Acad Dermatol 36:72–77

Miller DL, Weinstock MA (1994) Non-melanoma skin cancer in the United States: incidence. J Am Acad Dermatol 30:774–778

Niederhagan B, von Lindern JJ, Berge S, Appel T, Reich RH, Kruger E (2000) Staged operations for basal cell carcinoma of the face. Br J Oral Maxillofac Surg 38:477–479

Otley CC, Coldiron BM, Stasko T, Goldman GD (2001) Decreased skin cancer after cessation of therapy with transplant-associated immunosuppressants. Arch Dermatol 137:459–463

Plesko I, Severi G, Obsitnikova A, Boyle P (2000) Trends in the incidence of non-melanoma skin cancer in Slovakia, 1978–1995. Neoplasma 47:137–142

Poinsford MW, Goodman G, Marks R (1983) The prevalence and accuracy of diagnosis of non-melanocytic skin cancers in Victoria. Australas J Dermatol 24:153–166

Preston DS, Stern RS (1992) Non-melanoma cancers of the skin. N Engl J Med 327:1649–1662

Ratner D, Lowe L, Johnson TM, Fader DJ (2000) Perineural spread of basal cell carcinomas treated with Mohs micrographic surgery. Cancer 88:1606–1613

Robinson JK, Marks R, Owens ML, Andres K, Ginkel AM (2001) Imiquimod 5% cream for 12 weeks treating nodular BCC. 8th world congress on cancers of the skin, Zurich, 18–21 July

Romagosa R, Saap L, Givens M, Salvarrey A, He JL, Hsia SL, Taylor JR (2000) A pilot study to evaluate the treatment of basal cell carcinoma with 5-fluorouracil using phosphatidyl choline as a transepidermal carrier. Dermatol Surg 26:338–340

Rowe DE, Carroll RJ, Day CL (1989) Long-term recurrence rates in previously untreated (primary) basal cell carcinoma: implications for patient follow-up. J Dermatol Surg Oncol 15:315–328

Salasche SJ (2000) Epidemiology of actinic keratoses and squamous cell carcinoma. J Am Acad Dermatol 42:S4–S7

Schreuder F, Powell BW (1999) Incomplete excision of basal cell carcinomas: an audit. Clin Perform Qual Health Care 7:119–120

Schweitzer G (2001) Photofrin-mediated photodynamic therapy for treatment of aggressive head and neck non-melanomatous skin tumours in elderly patients. Laryngoscope 111:1091–1098

Seegenschmiedt MH, Oberste-Beulmann S, Lang E, Lang B, Guntrum F, Olschewski T (2001) Radiotherapy for basal cell carcinoma. Local control and cosmetic outcome. Strahlenther Onkol 177:240–246

Shumack S, Marks R, Amies M, Andres K, Ginkel AM (2001) Imiquimod 5% cream for 6 weeks treating nodular BCC. 8th world congress on cancers of the skin, Zurich, 18–21 July

Soler AM, Warloe T, Tausjo J, Giercksky KE (2000) Photodynamic therapy of residual or recurrent basal cell carcinoma after radiotherapy using topical 5-aminolaevulinic acid or methylester aminolaevulinic acid. Acta Oncol 39:605–609

Stanley MA (1999) Mechanism of action of imiquimod. Papillomavirus Rep 10:23–29

Staples M, Marks R, Giles G (1998) Trends in the incidence of non-melanocytic skin cancer (NMSC) treated in Australia 1985–1995: are primary prevention programs starting to have an effect? Int J Cancer 78:144–148

Sterry W, Bichel J, Andres K, Ginkel AM (2001a) Imiquimod 5% cream for 6 weeks with occlusion treating superficial BCC. 8th world congress on cancers of the skin, Zurich, 18–21 July

Sterry W, Bichel J, Ding L, Ginkel AM (2001b) Imiquimod 5% cream for 6 weeks with occlusion treating nodular BCC. 8th world congress on cancers of the skin, Zurich, 18–21 July

Stockfleth E, Meyer T, Benninghoff B, Christophers E (2001a) Successful treatment of actinic keratosis with imiquimod cream 5%: a report of 6 cases. Br J Dermatol 144:1050–1058

Stockfleth E, Ulrich C, Meyer T, Arndt R, Christophers E (2001b) Skin diseases following organ transplantation–risk factors and new therapeutic approaches. Transplant Proc 33:1848–1853

Thissen MR, Neumann MH, Schouten LJ (1999) A systematic review of treatment modalities for primary basal cell carcinomas. Arch Dermatol 135:1177–1183

Tsuji T, Otake N, Nishimura M (1993) Cryosurgery and topical fluorouracil: a treatment method for widespread basal cell epithelioma in basal cell nevus syndrome. J Dermatol 20:507–513

van Vloten WA, Hermans J, van Daal WA (1987) Radiation-induced skin cancer and radiodermatitis of the head and neck. Cancer 59:411–414

Varma S, Wilson H, Kurwa HA, Gambles B, Charman C, Pearse AD, Taylor D, Anstey AV (2001) Bowen's disease, solar keratoses and superficial basal cell carcinomas treated by photodynamic therapy using a large-field incoherent light source. Br J Dermatol 144:567–574

Vine JE (2001) Treatment alternatives for basal cell and squamous cell carcinoma. NJ Med 98:35–37

Vogel U, Hedayati M, Dybdahl M, Grossman L, Nexo BA (2001) Polymorphisms of the DNA repair gene XPD: correlations with risk of basal cell carcinoma revisited. Carcinogenesis 22:899–904

Wagner TL, Ahonen CL, Couture AM, Gibson SJ, Miller RL, Smith RM et al (1999) Modulation of Th1 and Th2 cytokine production with the immune response modifiers R848 and imiquimod. Cell Immunol 191:10–19

Wang I, Bendsoe N, Klinteberg CA, Enejder AM, Andersson-Engels S, Svanberg S, Svanberg K (2001) Photodynamic therapy vs cryosurgery of basal cell carcinomas: results of a phase III clinical trial. Br J Dermatol 144:832–840

Wong DA, Bishop GA, Lowes MA, Cooke B, Barnetson RStC, Halliday GM (2000) Cytokine profiles in spontaneously regressing basal cell carcinomas. Br J Dermatol 143:91–98

Zanetti R, Rosso S, Martinez C, Navarro C, Schraub S, Sancho-Garnier H, Franceschi S, Gafa L, Perea E, Tormo MJ, Laurent R, Schrameck C, Cristofolini M, Tumino R, Wechsler J (1996) The multicenter south European study 'Helios' I: skin characteristics and sunburns in basal cell and squamous cell carcinomas of the skin. Br J Cancer 73:1440–1446

Zhang H, Ping XL, Lee PK, Wu XL, Yao YJ, Zhang MJ, Silvers DN, Ratner D, Malhotra R, Peacocke M, Tsou HC (2001) Role of PTCH and p53 genes in early-onset basal cell carcinoma. Am J Pathol 158:381–385

# Lymphoma 5

## Pathogenesis
Clinical Presentations
Diagnosis
Therapy

# From Inflammation to Neoplasia:
# New Concepts in the Pathogenesis
# of Cutaneous Lymphomas

Günter Burg, Werner Kempf, Andreas Haeffner, Udo Döbbeling,
Frank O. Nestle, Roland Böni, Marshall Kadin, and Reinhard Dummer

## Abstract

Mycosis fungoides is a clinicopathologic term which describes a neoplasm of
cerebriform T lymphocytes that form plaques and tumors. We further suggest that mycosis fungoides arises in a background of chronic inflammation
or as a response to chronic antigenic stimulation. Subsequently, a series of
mutations results in the stepwise progression from eczematous patches, to
plaques, tumors and eventual hematogenous dissemination. The pathogenetic
process is driven by various, probably individually different, exogenous factors, e.g. environmental foreign antigens, bacterial superantigen, and/or endogenous factors, e.g. autocrine cytokine loops, CD40/CD40L and B7/CD28
interaction.

## Introduction

With respect to the pathogenesis of cutaneous T-cell lymphoma (CTCL) there
are two possibilities: (1) CTCLs are neoplastic diseases from the beginning,
even though definitive criteria for a neoplastic process are missing in early-
stage disease; (2) preneoplastic reactive inflammatory conditions evolve into
neoplasia with reproducible clinicopathologic criteria of malignancy in the
transformed stages. The answer to this question is of special importance to
the taxonomy and epidemiology of subtypes of lymphoproliferative disorders, to their prognosis and therapy, and especially to the individual patient
and his or her physician.

In order to disprove the first and to prove the latter statement, which is fa-
vored by us, it must be shown that parapsoriasis en plaques (PPP) and preneoplastic conditions (PNC) are lacking from the diagnostic criteria of mycosis fungoides (MF) and reflect criteria of reactive inflammatory processes. If
PPP and PNC do not exhibit criteria of MF, but of inflammation, the next

Recent Results in Cancer Research, Vol. 160
© Springer-Verlag Berlin Heidelberg 2002

question to be answered is which event or sequence of events are possibly associated with the transition of reactive inflammatory conditions into neoplasia.

The same problem concerns the discrimination of B pseudolymphoma from cutaneous B-cell lymphoma (CBCL). In many cases of lymphomas of mucosa-associated lymphoid tissue (MALT), there is a history of chronic inflammatory processes like *Helicobacter pylori*-associated chronic gastritis in gastric MALT lymphomas, or of *Borrelia* infection-associated acrodermatitis chronica atrophicans in respective MALT-type cutaneous lymphomas (Braun-Falco et al. 1978; Cerroni et al. 1997; Garbe et al. 1991).

There are many other epidemiologically evidenced and experimentally proven examples that show a switch from preneoplastic "abortive" to neoplastic conditions due to physical irritants such as chronic heat, UV radiation, X-rays, chemical irritants (e.g. tar, cyclic polyphenols), smoking in lung cancer, or viral infection including HTLV in adult T-cell leukemia/lymphoma, EBV in Burkitt's lymphoma, Hodgkin's disease and various cancers, hepatitis B virus in hepatocellular carcinoma, human papilloma virus in genital cancer.

Thus the question is raised as to the pathogenesis of lymphomas arising against the background of viral infection or chronic irritation and inflammation. In this chapter this question is addressed with special reference to CTCL.


## Definitions: Inflammation vs Neoplasia

To discriminate between inflammation and neoplasia it is necessary to define both conditions. Inflammation is a reactive process due to irritative internal or external factors, which regresses spontaneously after cessation of the irritation. Neoplasia, in contrast, is a self-sustaining process with autonomous cell proliferation and the capacity for dissemination.

From a historical point of view in the early descriptions of MF as a neoplastic disease by Alibert (1806), the patient Lukas presented with tumors or elevated plaques, but not with preneoplastic eczematous patches, which would not have prompted a person to see a doctor at that time. From a clinical point of view, neoplasms are locally aggressive or systemic proliferations of cells, exhibiting a tendency to infiltrate beyond normal tissue borders, and to spread by metastasis.

Histo- and cytologically, neoplasms are characterized by atypical morphology. Phenotypically, neoplastic cells may show altered differentiation with loss of surface antigens and/or gain of tumor-associated antigens. Genotypically, clonality of proliferating cells is the hallmark of malignancy –even if insufficient as a single criterion. The cytogenetic fingerprint will define a neoplasm on a molecular basis.

## PPP and PNC: Do They Exhibit the Diagnostic Criteria of MF?

Significant histologic features of the lymphoid neoplasia, designated as MF by Alibert almost 200 years ago, are lacking in the patches seen in PPP. There may be a few epidermotropic cells along the dermal-epidermal junction. There is no significant papillary dermal fibrosis. Significant numbers of dermal blastlike cells are lacking (Santucci et al. 2000; Smoller 1995). These features are compatible with the inflammatory reactions seen in eczema, psoriasis, lichen planus and other inflammatory conditions.

The most important features for the diagnosis of lymphoma are the presence of lymphocytes with extremely convoluted, medium-large ($>7$ µm in diameter) cerebriform nuclei, singly or clustered within the epidermis (Pautrier's microabscesses) and in monomorphic sheets within the dermis. In the epidermis the cells are often surrounded by clear spaces (halos). In a study performed by the International Society for Cutaneous Lymphomas (ISCL), the group of lesions clinically designated as "parapsoriasis" ($n=33$) showed histologic features indistinguishable from those of the control group ($n=33$; eczema, psoriasis and other inflammatory disorders), rather than those of the MF group ($n=33$) (unpublished study of the ISCL on early diagnosis of MF).

Pheno- and genotypically the infiltrate of PPP usually does not show an abnormal antigen profile or loss of differentiation antigens such as CD7 and does not show clonal rearrangement of T-cell antigen receptor genes.

Frequent occurrence of clonal T cells have been demonstrated in the peripheral blood but not in the skin of patients with small plaque parapsoriasis (Muche et al. 1997). From these findings, it was hypothesized that a sufficient cutaneous antitumor response and also an extracutaneous origin of the T-cell clones might explain the failure to detect skin-infiltrating clonal T cells. In four of ten patients with PPP described by Rubegni (2001) and followed over a period ranging from 14 to 36 months, clonal rearrangement of the TCR-g could be detected in skin infiltrates of patients with PPP. One explanation for these apparently contradictory results may be the fact that the follow-up time was not long enough to free allocate the patients studied to the different diagnostic categories in manner free from bias.

In our series of patients registered as PPP at time of first presentation ($n=239$) and followed over periods between 10 and 30 years ($n=31$), only one developed clear-cut MF according to the criteria described above, and genotypically had changed from germline to clonal rearrangement of the TCR-$\gamma$ gene. Rubegini (2001) claims a percentage ranging from 0% to 46% of PPP patients who progress to clear-cut lymphoma. These controversial findings and wide range of figures reflect the lack of clear-cut reproducible criteria in PPP and in preneoplastic conditions which are normally seen in neoplasias.

In conclusion, provided that MF as presented by Alibert in 1806 is considered to be a neoplasm, there is insufficient evidence for a diagnosis of MF in

PPP and premycotic conditions, which both exhibit morphologic, phenotypic and genotypic features of reactive inflammatory processes.

## The Pathogenesis of Cutaneous Lymphomas. When Does MF Start?

MF starts when the criteria normally used to make a diagnosis are fulfilled. These criteria are clinical (progression to plaques or tumors), histo- and cytomorphologic (atypical cells in the context of distinct histologic patterns), phenotypic (loss of differentiation markers or gain of tumor markers) and genotypic (clonal proliferation). The question to be answered is which events or which sequence of events on a molecular level drive lymphocytes from a reactive inflammatory premycotic disorder into a neoplastic process.

There are many phenomena which have been found to be, or not to be, associated with the evolution of CTCL. However the etiology and the exact steps in the pathogenesis of CTCL are not completely understood. Potential pathogenetic factors may be exogenous – environmental foreign antigens, infectious agents – or endogenous – genomic instability, gene mutations, autocrine or paracrine cytokine loops and interactions. A pathogenetic algorithm for MF is presented in Fig. 1.

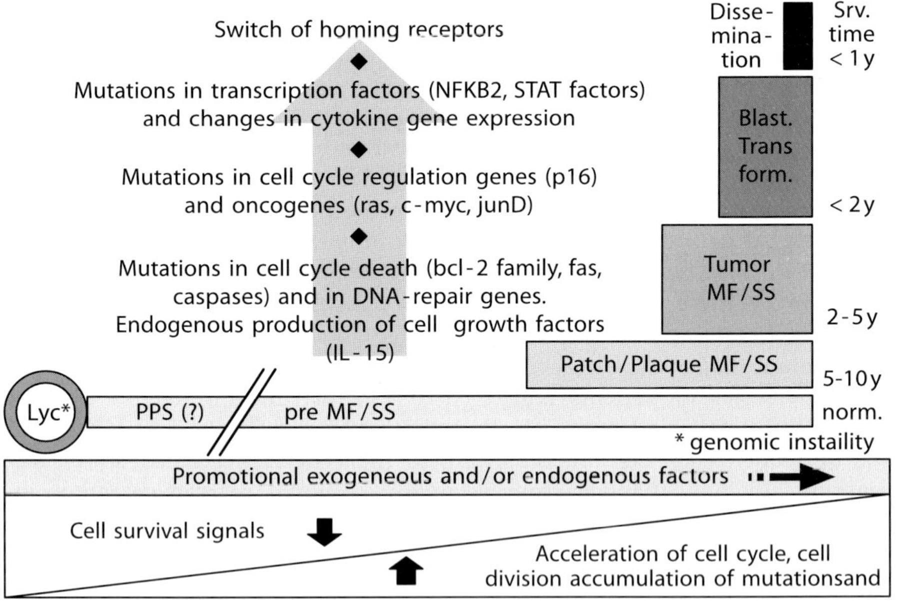


**Fig. 1.** Potential pathogenetic algorithm in MF. Lymphocytes harboring genomic instability due to promotional exogenous or endogenous factors over time accumulate in a background of chronic inflammation a series of mutations, resulting in stepwise progression from eczematous patches, to plaques, tumors and eventual hematogenous dissemination in MF. Breaks in the biologic course are reflected in different survival times, depending on the stage of the disease

*Chromosomal abnormalities* occur regularly in CTCL. Karenko et al. (1997) studied the pattern of chromosomal abnormalities with G-banding and interphase in situ hybridization methods in blood mononuclear cells from 17 patients representing the different phases of CTCL or the premalignant condition, PPP, and from ten control individuals. Numerical aberrations in chromosomes 6, 13, 15, and 17, marker chromosomes, and structural aberrations in chromosomes 3, 9, and 13 were increased in MF compared with healthy controls. These studies indicate that chromosomally abnormal cells can be found in the peripheral blood of both PPP and CTCL patients.

Combined immunophenotyping and karyotyping in peripheral T-cell lymphomas demonstrating different clonal and nonclonal chromosome aberrations in T helper cells (Schlegelberger et al. 1994). In one case of Sézary's syndrome, two or possibly even three different clones as well as nonclonal aberrations were identified within the T (helper/inducer) cell population, providing further evidence that chromosomal instability is a characteristic feature of CTCL.

An association with certain histocompatibility antigens has been described (MacKie et al. 1976).

Reports on the significance of *environmental factors* (Fransway 1988; Schuppli 1976; Shupp 1985) in the pathogenesis of CTCL are contradictory. Patients with chronic skin disease who have long-term exposure to combinations of chemicals, physical agents, and biologic agents, heavy smokers, or patients who have recurrent herpes simplex appear to be prime candidates for developing MF or Sézary syndrome (Fischmann et al. 1979). However, no consistent or biologically plausible differences between patients and controls with respect to types of job held, or to occupational or vacational exposure to chemicals could be demonstrated by others (Teixeira et al. 1994; Whittemoreet al. 1989). MF and PPP have been observed following exposure to plutonium (Zachariae and Sogaard 1990).

In summary, these observations indicate that there is not one specific environmental factor involved in the pathogenesis of CTCL, but that many different irritants in some patients may play an important role in promoting cells with clonal instability to develop into tumor cells.

Turning to *viruses* as pathogenetic factors, Wood et al. found no evidence of HTLV-I proviral integration in lymphoproliferative disorders associated with cutaneous T-cell lymphoma (Boni et al. 1996; Wood et al. 1997). Applying nested PCR with virus-specific primers, Kempf et al. were not able to detect any evidence for the association between lymphomatoid papulosis (Lyp) and Herpes virus types 6, 7 or 8 (Kempf et al. 2001).

Patients with hydroa vacciniforme-like eruptions and malignant potential have been reported from Asia and Mexico, and these patients frequently had an associated latent Epstein-Barr virus (EBV) infection (Iwatsuki et al. 1999). Among T-non-Hodgkin's lymphomas (T-NHL), nasal T-NHL can be regarded as a distinct clinicopathologic entity associated with EBV, which could be derived either from immature T cells or from NK cells (Kanavaros et al. 1995). The EBV genome in lymphoma cells exists in a latently infected form but not in an actively replicating form. There is no prognostic significance for CTCL (Peris et al. 1995).

It has been shown that Sézary cells proliferate in response to *bacterial superantigens* in a manner that is restricted by their VB usage. The addition of interleukin-1 (IL-1) in combination with staphylococcal exfoliating toxin (ExT) has been shown to enhance the stimulative response of VB 2.1-bearing CTCL cells precultured with ExT for 7 days, suggesting that IL-1 may be a cofactor for the stimulation. The study indicated that the superantigen reaction occurs with CTCL cells and implies a possible involvement of bacterial toxins in the pathogenesis of CTCL (Jackow et al. 1997; Tokura et al. 1992).

There is some controversy relating to the immune biology of CTCL with respect to the T helper 1/2 system and their *cytokine profile* (Dummer et al. 1996; Saed et al. 1994; Vowels et al. 1994). The dominance of TH2 cells (Dummer et al. 1996) explains the well-known clinical phenomena seen in most CTCL patients, such as reduced cutaneous delayed-type hypersensitivity reactions, hypereosinophilia, alterations in serum immunoglobulin levels (IgE, IgA), an increased risk of second malignancies and immunologic abnormalities of peripheral blood mononuclear cells (PBMC) such as reduced NK cell activity and decreased mitogen-induced proliferation (Qin et al. 1999).

Cell growth factors such as IL-7 and IL-15 lead to the expression of cell survival genes including NFkB, mcl-1 and bcl-xL (Dobbeling et al. 1998). CTCL cells express constitutive NFkB, c-Myb and STAT-5 (Qin et al. 1999) promoting the transcription of apoptosis inhibitors cIAP2 and bcl-2.

IL-15 is expressed by basal layer keratinocytes and skin dendritic cells. It interacts with the beta chain of the IL-2 receptor, is a potent growth factor for the IL-2-dependent CTCL cell line SeAx, and prolongs the in vitro survival of CTCL cells isolated from Sézary syndrome patients (Dobbeling et al. 1998).

A protein playing an important role in cell cycle regulation is p16. CTCL cell lines (HUT 78, Myla 2059, SeAx) do not express p16 protein and show loss of expression of p16 mRNA, but this is not lost in CTCL peripheral blood cells (Peris et al. 1999). Lymphocytes in CTCL coexpress CD40 and CD40 ligand, leading to autocrine growth stimulation (Storz et al. 2001). The interaction between costimulatory molecules B7 and CD28 (Nickoloff et al. 1994) is another stimulatory factor.

In the evolution from normal to neoplastic lymphocytes, it appears that lymphocytes are driven into activation and reactive cell proliferation by an antigen which may be viral or nonviral, self, altered self, or cross-reactive with other antigens. They may subsequently develop genomic instability ("genotraumatic lymphocytes") (Thestrup and Kaltoft 1994). The risk of occurrence of mutations in the setting of genomic instability increases with each new cell division which usually is limited by controlling mechanisms such as programmed cell death (apoptosis). In CTCL, apoptosis is blocked by increased bcl-2 protein expression (Dummer et al. 1995).

Another mechanism by which cells normally die, is cellular senescence due to excision of telomeres. These repetitive base sequences (TTAGGG) at the end of each chromosome are responsible for the maintenance of chromosomal structure and function. Immortal cells overcome this regulation by reactivation of telomerase activity. Skin-homing T cells and PBMC from CTCL have high telomerase activity and short telomere length. In parapsoriasis and premycotic stages respectively, abnormal telomerase activity characteristic of CTCL may be already present (Wu et al. 1999), as shown also in CTCL cell lines (own unpublished data). The accumulation of mutations evolves in a stepwise sequence, affecting DNA repair genes (Kaltoft et al. 1994) oncogenes, tumor suppressor genes and cell cycle-regulating genes (Garatti et al. 1995; Kanavaros et al. 1994; Marks et al. 1996; Neri et al. 1995; Pezzella et al. 1993; van Haselen et al. 1997), NF-kappa B and signaling factors (Dobbeling et al. 1998; Dummer et al. 2001; Kadin et al. 1994; Neri et al. 1995; Nielsen et al. 1997). Finally, a highly abnormal cell clone evolves which grows independently from external stimuli possibly due to autocrine growth-stimulating factors, e.g. IL-15, IL-7 and IL-2 (Qin et al. 1999), and loss of response to growth inhibitory factors, e.g. transforming growth factor-beta (Kadin et al. 1994).

*Cytogenetic studies* of bone marrow, peripheral blood, and skin tumor cells from a patient with MF at an early stage have shown chromosome abnormalities in 100% of the cells harvested from the cutaneous specimen, whereas the cells of the bone marrow and blood are karyotypically normal. Three related clones, showing increasing cytogenetic complexity, have been found, suggesting a polyphasic evolution of this chronic T lymphoproliferative disease (Barbieri et al. 1986). Recurrent abnormalities of the genes that encode T-cell antigen receptors have not been demonstrated in CTCL (Thangavelu et al. 1997). The region between 1p22 and 1p36 has been identified as a region of the genome that requires detailed analysis to identify the potential gene(s) involved in the process of malignant transformation and/or progression in MF. Unfortunately, cytogenetic studies using modern techniques have not been done so far to identify genetic alterations in skin lesions of premycotic conditions and parapsoriasis, probably due to the small number of dividing cells. Perhaps newer techniques of comparative genomic hybridization or fluorescent in situ hybridization (FISH) could help to detect early mutations.

# References


Alibert JLM (1806) Tableau du pian fongoide. Description des maladies de la peau, observées à l'Hôpital Saint-Louis et exposition des meilleurs méthodes suivies pour leur traitement. Barrois L'Ainé, Paris

Barbieri D, Spanedda R, Castoldi GL (1986) Involvement of chromosomes 12 and 14 in the cutaneous stage of mycosis fungoides: cytogenetic evidence for a multistep pathogenesis of the disease. Cancer Genet Cytogenet 20:287–292

Boni R, Davis-Daneshfar A, Burg G, Fuchs D, Wood GS (1996) No detection of HTLV-I proviral DNA in lesional skin biopsies from Swiss and German patients with cutaneous T-cell lymphoma. Br J Dermatol 134:282–284

Braun-Falco O, Guggenberger K, Burg G, Fateh-Moghadam A (1978) Immunozytom unter dem Bild einer Acrodermatitis chronica atrophicans. Hautarzt 29:644–647

Cerroni L, Zochling N, Putz B, Kerl H (1997) Infection by *Borrelia burgdorferi* and cutaneous B-cell lymphoma. J Cutan Pathol 24:457–461

Dobbeling U, Dummer R, Laine E, Potoczna N, Qin JZ, Burg G (1998) Interleukin-15 is an autocrine/paracrine viability factor for cutaneous T-cell lymphoma cells. Blood 92:252–258

Dummer R, Michie S, Kell D, Gould J, Haeffner A, Smoller B, Warnke R, Wood G (1995) Expression of BCL-2 protein and Ki-67 nuclear proliferation antigen in benign and malignant cutaneous T-cell infiltrates. J Cutan Pathol 22:11–17

Dummer R, Heald PW, Nestle FO, Ludwig E, Laine E, Hemmi S, Burg G (1996) Sezary syndrome T-cell clones display T-helper 2 cytokines and express the accessory factor-1 (interferon-gamma receptor beta-chain). Blood 88:1383–1389

Dummer R, Dobbeling U, Geertsen R, Willers J, Burg G, Pavlovic J (2001) Interferon resistance of cutaneous T-cell lymphoma-derived clonal T-helper 2 cells allows selective viral replication. Blood 97:523–527

Fischmann AB, Bunn PJ Jr, Guccion JG, Matthews MJ, Minna JD (1979) Exposure to chemicals, physical agents, and biologic agents in mycosis fungoides and the Sezary syndrome. Cancer Treat Rep 63:591–596

Fransway AF, Winkelmann RK (1988) Chronic dermatitis evolving to mycosis fungoides: report of four cases and review of the literature. Cutis 41:330–335

Garatti SA, Roscetti E, Trecca D, Fracchiolla NS, Neri A, Berti E (1995) bcl-1, bcl-2, p53, c-myc, and lyt-10 analysis in cutaneous lymphomas. Recent Results Cancer Res 139:249–261

Garbe C, Stein H, Dienemann D, Orfanos CE (1991) *Borrelia burgdorferi*-associated cutaneous B cell lymphoma: clinical and immunohistologic characterization of four cases. J Am Acad Dermatol 24:584–590

Iwatsuki K, Xu Z, Takata M, Iguchi M, Ohtsuka M, Akiba H, Mitsuhashi Y, Takenoshita H, Sugiuchi R, Tagami H, Kaneko F (1999) The association of latent Epstein-Barr virus infection with hydroa vacciniforme. Br J Dermatol 140:715–721

Jackow CM, Cather JC, Hearne V, Asano AT, Musser JM, Duvic M (1997) Association of erythrodermic cutaneous T-cell lymphoma, supcrantigen-positive Staphylococcus aureus, and oligoclonal T-cell receptor V beta gene expansion. Blood 89:32–40

Kadin ME, Cavaille-Coll MW, Gertz R, Massague J, Cheifetz S, George D (1994) Loss of receptors for transforming growth factor beta in human T-cell malignancies. Proc Natl Acad Sci USA 91:6002–6006

Kaltoft K, Hansen BH, Thestrup-Pedersen K (1994) Cytogenetic findings in cell lines from cutaneous T-cell lymphoma. Dermatol Clin 12:295–304

Kanavaros P, Ioannidou D, Tzardi M, Datseris G, Katsantonis J, Delidis G, Tosca A (1994) Mycosis fungoides: expression of C-myc p62 p53, bcl-2 and PCNA proteins and absence of association with Epstein-Barr virus. Pathol Res Pract 190:767–774

Kanavaros P, De Bruin PC, Briere J, Meijer CJ, Gaulard P (1995) Epstein-Barr virus (EBV) in extranodal T-cell non-Hodgkin's lymphomas (T-NHL). Identification of nasal T-NHL as a distinct clinicopathological entity associated with EBV. Leuk Lymphoma 18:27–34

Karenko L, Hyytinen E, Sarna S, Ranki A (1997) Chromosomal abnormalities in cutaneous T-cell lymphoma and in its premalignant conditions as detected by G-banding and interphase cytogenetic methods. J Invest Dermatol 108:22–29

Kempf W, Kadin ME, Kutzner H, Lord CL, Burg G, Letvin NL, Koralnik IJ (2001) Lymphomatoid papulosis and human herpesviruses – a PCR-based evaluation for the presence of human herpesvirus 6, 7 and 8 related herpesviruses. J Cutan Pathol 28:29–33

MacKie R, Dick HM, de Sousa MB (1976) HLA and mycosis fungoides (letter). Lancet 1:1179

Marks DI, Vonderheid EC, Kurz BW, Bigler RD, Sinha K, Morgan DA, Sukman A, Nowell PC, Haines DS (1996) Analysis of p53 and mdm-2 expression in 18 patients with Sezary syndrome. Br J Haematol 92:890–899

Muche JM, Lukowsky A, Asadullah K, Gellrich S, Sterry W (1997) Demonstration of frequent occurrence of clonal T cells in the peripheral blood of patients with primary cutaneous T-cell lymphoma. Blood 90:1636–1642

Neri A, Fracchiolla NS, Roscetti E, Garatti S, Trecca D, Boletini A, Perletti L, Baldini L, Maiolo AT, Berti E (1995) Molecular analysis of cutaneous B- and T-cell lymphomas. Blood 86:3160–3172

Nickoloff BJ, Nestle FO, Zheng XG, Turka LA (1994) T lymphocytes in skin lesions of psoriasis and mycosis fungoides express B7-1: a ligand for CD28. Blood 83:2580–2586

Nielsen M, Kaltoft K, Nordahl M, Ropke C, Geisler C, Mustelin T, Dobson P, Svejgaard A, Odum N (1997) Constitutive activation of a slowly migrating isoform of Stat3 in mycosis fungoides: tyrphostin AG490 inhibits Stat3 activation and growth of mycosis fungoides tumor cell lines. Proc Natl Acad Sci USA 94:6764–6769

Peris K, Niedermeyer H, Chimenti S, Radaskiewicz T, Kerl H, Hoefler H (1995) Detection of Epstein-Barr virus in cutaneous and lymph nodal anaplastic large cell lymphomas (Ki-1+). Br J Dermatol 133:542–546

Peris K, Stanta G, Fargnoli MC, Bonin S, Felli A, Amantea A, Chimenti S (1999) Reduced expression of CDKN2a/P16INK4a in mycosis fungoides. Arch Dermatol Res 291:207–211

Pezzella F, Morrison H, Jones M, Gatter KC, Lane D, Harris AL, Mason DY (1993) Immunohistochemical detection of p53 and bcl-2 proteins in non-Hodgkin's lymphoma. Histopathology 22:39–44

Qin JZ, Dummer R, Burg G, Dobbeling U (1999) Constitutive and interleukin-7/interleukin-15 stimulated DNA binding of Myc, Jun, and novel Myc-like proteins in cutaneous T-cell lymphoma cells. Blood 93:260–267

Rubegni P, De Aloe G, Di Renzo M, Pompella G, Pasqui AL, Auteri A, Andreassi L, Fimiani M (2001) Cytokine production profile of peripheral blood mononuclear cells in patients with large-plaque parapsoriasis. Arch Dermatol 137:966–967

Saed G, Fivenson DP, Naidu Y, Nickoloff BJ (1994) Mycosis fungoides exhibits a Th1-type cell-mediated cytokine profile whereas Sezary syndrome expresses a Th2-type profile. J Invest Dermatol 103:29–33

Santucci M, Biggeri A, Feller AC, Massi D, Burg G (2000) Efficacy of histologic criteria for diagnosing early mycosis fungoides: an EORTC Cutaneous Lymphoma Study Group investigation. Am J Surg Pathol 24:40–50

Schlegelberger B, Weber-Matthiesen K, Sterry W, Bartels H, Sonnen R, Maschmeyer G, Feller AC, Grote W (1994) Combined immunophenotyping and karyotyping in peripheral T cell lymphomas demonstrating different clonal and nonclonal chromosome aberrations in T helper cells. Leuk Lymphoma 15:113–125

Schuppli R (1976) Is mycosis fungoides an "immunoma"? Dermatologica 153:1–6

Shupp DL, Winkelmann RK (1985) Patch tests in Sezary syndrome and mycosis fungoides. Contact Dermatitis 13:180–185

Smoller BR, Bishop K, Glusac E, Kim YH, Hendrickson M (1995) Reassessment of histologic parameters in the diagnosis of mycosis fungoides. Am J Surg Pathol 19:1423–1430

Storz M, Zepter K, Kamarashev J, Dummer R, Burg G, Haffner AC (2001) Coexpression of CD40 and CD40 ligand in cutaneous T-cell lymphoma (mycosis fungoides). Cancer Res 61:452–454

Teixeira F, Ortiz-Plata A, Cortes-Franco R, Dominguez-Soto L (1994) Do environmental factors play any role in the pathogenesis of mycosis fungoides and Sezary syndrome? Int J Dermatol 33:770–772

Thangavelu M, Finn WG, Yelavarthi KK, Roenigk HH Jr, Samuelson E, Peterson L, Kuzel TM, Rosen ST (1997) Recurring structural chromosome abnormalities in peripheral blood lymphocytes of patients with mycosis fungoides/Sezary syndrome. Blood 89:3371–3377

Thestrup-Pedersen K, Kaltoft K (1994) Genotraumatic T cells and cutaneous T-cell lymphoma. A causal relationship? Arch Dermatol Res 287:97–101

Tokura Y, Heald PW, Yan SL, Edelson RL (1992) Stimulation of cutaneous T-cell lymphoma cells with superantigenic staphylococcal toxins. J Invest Dermatol 98:33–37

van Haselen CW, Vermeer MH, Toonstra J, van der Putte SC, Mulder PG, van Vloten WA, Willemze R (1997) p53 and bcl-2 expression do not correlate with prognosis in primary cutaneous large T-cell lymphomas. J Cutan Pathol 24:462–467

Vowels BR, Lessin SR, Cassin M, Jaworsky C, Benoit B, Wolfe JT, Rook AH (1994) Th2 cytokine mRNA expression in skin in cutaneous T-cell lymphoma. J Invest Dermatol 103: 669–673

Whittemore AS, Holly EA, Lee IM, Abel EA, Adams RM, Nickoloff BJ, Bley L, Peters JM, Gibney C (1989) Mycosis fungoides in relation to environmental exposures and immune response: a case-control study. J Natl Cancer Inst 81:1560–1567

Wood GS, Schaffer JM, Boni R, Dummer R, Burg G, Takeshita M, Kikuchi M (1997) No evidence of HTLV-I proviral integration in lymphoproliferative disorders associated with cutaneous T-cell lymphoma. Am J Pathol 150:667–673

Wu K, Lund M, Bang K, Thestrup-Pedersen K (1999) Telomerase activity and telomere length in lymphocytes from patients with cutaneous T-cell lymphoma. Cancer 86:1056–1063

Zachariae H, Sogaard H (1990) Plutonium-induced mycosis fungoides and parapsoriasis en plaques – a new entity? Curr Probl Dermatol 19:81–89

# Lymphoma 5

Pathogenesis
**Clinical Presentations**
Diagnosis
Therapy

# Cutaneous Lymphomas and Pseudolymphomas: Newly Described Entities

Dmitry V. Kazakov, Günter Burg, Reinhard Dummer, and Werner Kempf

## Abstract

This chapter summarizes some recently described cutaneous lymphomas and pseudolymphomas with regard to their clinicopathological presentation, biological behavior and classification place. Among cutaneous lymphomas, the group of cytotoxic lymphomas, angioimmunoblastic T-cell lymphoma, intravascular lymphoma, hydroa-like lymphoma, marginal zone lymphoma, spindle-cell B-cell lymphoma, and B-cell lymphoma with a dermatomal distribution are presented. In the context of pseudolymphomas, cutaneous follicular lymphoid hyperplasia with monotypic plasma cells, pleomorphic reactions in molluscum contagiosum, and CD30$^+$ reactions to parapoxvirus are discussed.

## Introduction

The diagnosis of cutaneous lymphoma (CL) remains a challenge for pathologists and clinicians (Kempf et al. 1999). More than 30 types of malignant lymphoid neoplasms may involve the skin. These either arise primarily in the skin or occur as secondary involvement due to progression of nodal lymphomas or other extracutaneous lymphomas or leukemia. The introduction of modern diagnostic tools has allowed the identification of a variety of lymphoproliferative entities with distinct clinical, morphological and immunological features. These entities have been included in recently developed classifications of lymphoid tissue neoplasms such as the Revised European-American Lymphoma (REAL) classification (Harris et al. 1994), the WHO classification (Harris et al. 1999; Jaffe et al. 2000), and the European Organization for Research and Treatment of Cancer (EORTC) classification (Willemze et al. 1997). However, some other entities or rare subtypes remain beyond the scope of these classifications. The aim of this chapter is to summarize some of the recently described lymphoproliferative disorders and discuss clinicopathological features, biological behavior, and nosological classification.

Recent Results in Cancer Research, Vol. 160
© Springer-Verlag Berlin Heidelberg 2002

## T-cell Lymphomas

One of the largest groups of CL that has undergone a considerable revision in the last few years is cytotoxic lymphomas of the skin. These are heterogeneous entities derived from lymphoid cells expressing cytotoxic proteins such as TIA-I, granzyme A and B, and perforin. Cytologically these cells often contain azurophilic granules in their cytoplasm (Giemsa staining). Cells with such properties are NK cells, NK-like T cells, and a small proportion of $\alpha\beta^+$T cells and $\gamma\delta^+$T cells, which can give rise to a corresponding lymphoma.

## CD8$^+$ Epidermotropic T-cell Lymphoma

CD8$^+$ epidermotropic T-cell lymphoma is characterized clinically by lesions that are either necrotic nodules or patches and plaques similar to those seen in mycosis fungoides (MF). Some cases are identical clinicopathologically to previously described pagetoid reticulosis. Histological features include pagetoid infiltration of the basal layer by small convoluted lymphocytes, a band-like infiltrate and prominent edema in the dermis (see Fig. 1). Extravasated erythrocytes can be seen. The tumor cells have the phenotype of CD2$^-$, CD3$^+$, CD4$^-$, CD5$^-$, CD8$^+$ lymphocytes and express other cytotoxic proteins (TIA-I, perforin, granzyme B). TCR genes are clonally rearranged in the majority of cases. The disease demonstrates a rapid fatal progression notwithstanding aggressive treatment. However, in some cases an indolent course can be observed. Expression of CD7 antigen is associated with a more favor-

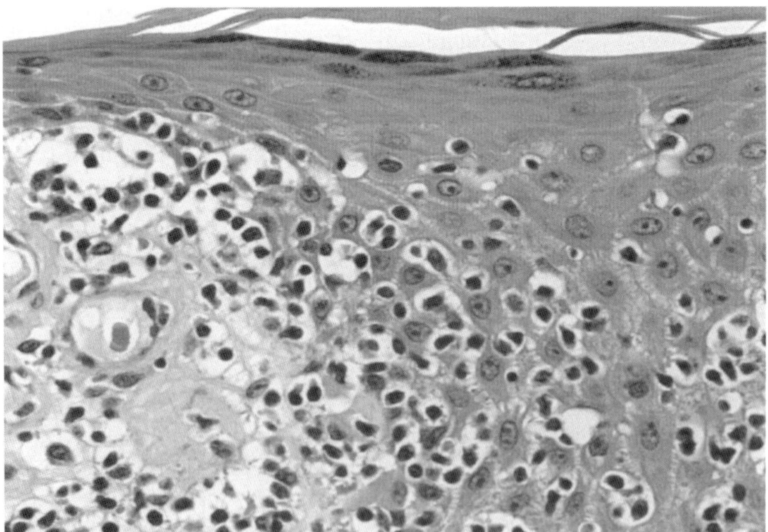

**Fig. 1.** CD8$^+$ epidermotropic T-cell lymphoma. Infiltration of the epidermis by atypical lymphocytes in a pagetoid pattern

able prognosis while CD8$^+$, CD7$^-$ lymphomas run a very aggressive course (Agnarsson et al. 1990; Berti et al. 1999; Dummer et al. 2002).

## NK Lymphomas

NK lymphomas are a group of lymphoproliferative disorders derived from natural killer (NK) cells or their precursors that express NK cell-associated markers (CD56, CD57, CD16). At least three distinctive types of this disease have been identified: (1) pure NK lymphoma, (2) NK/T-cell lymphoma, (3) blastic (blastoid) NK-lymphoma. All these entities are systemic disorders and can affect the upper aerodigestive tract, skin, central nervous system, bone marrow, spleen, testis, and muscles. All the conditions run a very aggressive course usually resulting in the patient's death within 1 year. Primary CLs of this type are encountered extremely rarely. Systemic tumors are usually associated with Epstein Barr virus (EBV) infection (Jaffe 1996).

PURE NK LYMPHOMA. Pure NK lymphoma is derived from cells that immunologically and genetically correspond to true NK cells, that is they lack expression of CD3 antigen on their surface and show no TCR gene rearrangement. Skin lesions are rapidly growing, ulcerated nodules, plaques or tumors that may sometimes have a bruise-like appearance. Histologically, there is an intradermal proliferation of small to large pleomorphic lymphoid cells with cytoplasmic azurophilic granules (usually in larger cells on Giemsa staining). The tumor cells stain positive for one or more NK markers (CD16, CD56, CD57). Typically, they are negative for surface CD3 but sometimes demonstrate a cytoplasmic positivity using polyclonal antibodies against CD3-$\varepsilon$. In addition, they can show positivity for other T-cell antigens (especially for CD2) and cytotoxic proteins (TIA-I, perforin, granzyme B) (Dummer et al. 1996; Jaffe 1996).

T/NK LYMPHOMA. T/NK lymphoma is derived from neoplastic counterparts of so-called NK-like T-cells that are characterized by the expression of CD3 molecule on their surface and usually show rearrangement of their TCR. The disease is characterized by the development of infiltrative erythematous plaques or large, rapidly growing tumors or demarcated, swollen, bruise-like areas. Histologically, the tumor population is a mixture of small lymphocytes with round or cleaved nuclei and medium-sized to large lymphoid cells. The latter demonstrate azurophilic granules in the cytoplasm. Atypical lymphocytes tend to infiltrate and destroy vessel walls with a resultant zonal necrosis (angiocentric and angiodestructive pattern). The typical phenotype of the neoplastic cells is CD2$^+$, sCD3$^+$, CD16$^+$, CD56$^+$, CD57$^{+/-}$. Genotyping reveals monoclonal rearrangement of TCR genes in the majority of the cases (Jaffe 1996).

Blastic (Blastoid) NK Lymphoma. Blastic NK lymphoma is a malignant systemic lymphoproliferative disease derived from precursors of NK cells. Sometimes skin involvement is the first manifestation of the condition. Skin lesions are multiple indurated plaques or ulcerated tumors located on the face, trunk or lower extremities. In some cases the lesions have a bruise-like appearance. Histologically, the disease is characterized by the proliferation of medium-sized cells with irregularly folded delicate nuclear membranes, fine chromatin and inconspicuous nucleoli. The tumor cells are positive for CD56 and TdT. TCR genes are in a germline configuration. EBV is not detected (Jaffe 1996; Ginarte et al. 2000).

## Subcutaneous Panniculitic T-cell Lymphoma

Subcutaneous panniculitic T-cell lymphoma is an aggressive T-cell lymphoma arising in the subcutaneous tissue. Clinical features include multiple or solitary tumors or nodules located mainly on the limbs. Less frequently, the trunk or head is involved. When located on the lower extremities, the lesions are apt to simulate reactive inflammatory panniculitis such as acute erythema nodosum. General symptoms include fever, weight loss and malaise. Histologically, the disease corresponds to the pattern of a lobular panniculitis with a dense, focal or diffuse infiltrate in the subcutis. The infiltrate consists of small, medium-sized or large pleomorphic cells and macrophages engulfing neoplastic cells and nuclear fragments. Rimming of the tumor cells around lipocytes is a typical but not pathognomonic finding. Erythrophagocytosis can be found. The lower dermis displays perivascular aggregates of neoplastic cells. The tumor cells demonstrate a suppressor cell (CD3$^+$, CD4$^-$, CD8$^+$, TIA-1$^+$, CD56$^-$), a helper cell (CD3$^+$, CD4$^+$, CD8$^-$, TIA-1$^-$, CD56$^-$) or sometimes a NK cell (CD56$^+$) phenotype.

Apart from cases with TCR$\beta$ gene rearrangement, $\gamma/\delta^+$ variants of the disease have been described. The latter are probably better categorized as $\gamma/\delta^+$-cell CLs with fat tissue involvement. The median survival of patients after diagnosis is approximately 2 years. Patients with a CD3$^+$, CD4$^+$, CD8$^-$, CD56$^-$, TCR$\alpha/\beta^+$ phenotype have a more favorable prognosis than those with the CD3$^+$, CD4$^-$, CD8$^-$, CD56$^{+/-}$, TCR$\gamma/\delta^+$ variant (Wang et al. 1996; Salhany et al. 1998).

## $\gamma/\delta^+$ T-cell Lymphoma

$\gamma/\delta^+$ T-cell lymphoma is a malignant lymphoproliferative disease derived from T lymphocytes bearing $\gamma/\delta$ heterodimer of T-cell receptor on their surface. These cells comprise an immunologically distinct lymphocyte population. The classification of tumors with the $\gamma/\delta$ configuration of TCR is still unclear. These neoplasms are sometimes encountered among NK lymphomas and subcutaneous panniculitic T-cell lymphomas. More often, $\gamma/\delta^+$ T-cell lymphoma manifests itself as plaques and/or tumors situated mainly on the limbs. Histologically, an epidermotropic infiltrate of cerebriform lymphocytes or a diffuse dermal infiltrate constituted of medium-sized pleomorphic lymphocytes is observed. In some instances, the histological picture is similar to that seen in subcutaneous panniculitic lymphoma.

The typical phenotype of the tumor cells is $CD3^+$, $CD4^-/CD8^-$, $TIA-I^+$, perforin$^+$, granzyme $B^+$. The immunological hallmark of the disease is a positive staining for TCR$\delta$ and negative staining for TCR$\alpha/\beta$ ($\beta$F1$^-$) on frozen sections. Cases with TCR$\gamma^+/J_H^+$ rearrangement have been described. The disease runs a very aggressive course. Precise survival data are not available due to the small number of cases reported. In the majority of the cases death occurs between 15 and 29 months after diagnosis notwithstanding aggressive treatment modalities (Burg et al. 1991; Heald et al. 1992; Harris et al. 1994; Toro et al. 2000).


## Angioimmunoblastic T-cell Lymphoma

Angioimmunoblastic T-cell lymphoma (AITCL, previously called angioimmunoblastic lymphadenopathy with dysproteinemia) is a systemic malignant lymphoproliferative disorder characterized by a clonal growth of atypical lymphoid cells accompanied by the proliferation of postcapillary venules and dermal dendritic cells (Jaffe et al. 2000). The disease is characterized by fever, weight loss, night sweats, lymphadenopathy, hepato- and splenomegaly. Peripheral blood shows anemia, leukocytosis, and polyclonal hypergammaglobulinemia. Skin involvement occurs as maculopapular, urticarial or purpura-like lesions with a predilection for the trunk.

The histological patterns of skin involvement have been summarized (Martel et al. 2000). These authors identified four types of pathological presentation of AITCL in the skin. The first one is characterized by nonspecific scant perivascular infiltrates composed of eosinophils and lymphocytes without atypia accompanied by hyperplasia of capillaries. In the second, more specific, pattern perivascular infiltrates composed of pleomorphic lymphocytes with large reniform nuclei are found. Vascular hyperplasia is also present. The third pattern is typified by dense infiltrates of pleomorphic cells in combination with vascular hyperplasia. The fourth pattern corresponds to that of a vasculitis with no nuclear atypia of infiltrating lymphoid cells.

The tumor cells express the phenotype of mature T-helper cells ($CD3^+$, $CD4^+$, $CD8^{+/-}$). Staining for factor XIIIa reveals increased numbers of dermal dendritic cells in the infiltrate. Study of the TCR$\gamma$ gene with PCR-based techniques allows the identification of the same clone in the skin, lymph nodes, and peripheral blood. The disease runs an aggressive course with a mortality rate ranging from 50% to 70% and a median survival ranging from 11 to 30 months (Martel et al. 2000).

## Intravascular (Angiotropic) Lymphoma

Intravascular lymphoma (IVL) is a malignant lymphoproliferative disease characterized by the growth of neoplastic lymphocytes within blood vessels. Previously, those cases were regarded as malignant angioendotheliomatosis. The introduction of immunohistochemistry allowed the distinction of at least two subtypes of this lymphoma, namely *intravascular large B-cell lymphoma* and *intravascular T-cell lymphoma.*

Primary cutaneous IVL are rarely encountered. More commonly, IVL manifests itself as a systemic disease with secondary specific cutaneous involvement. Neurological symptoms are the first manifestation of the disease in 70% of patients. The skin lesions are plaques or deep-seated subcutaneous nodules situated on the lower extremities or trunk. Some patients present with a clinical picture resembling that of panniculitis. In addition, patients presenting clinically with generalized telangiectasia, diffuse black discoloration of 50% of the body surface, pitting edema, and palpable purpura have been described. Pathology reveals an increased number of dermal vessels with the lumina filled with atypical lymphoid cells. In addition, one may find so-called "glomeruloid" structures that result from vascular occlusion and ensuing recanalization. The intraluminar lymphoid cells express leukocyte common antigen (LCA) as well as pan-B-cell antigens or pan-T antigens depending on the immunological type of the tumor. Antibodies for endothelial markers (factor VIII, CD31) allow the intravascular locations of the neoplastic infiltrate to be confirmed. Specific genetic abnormalities have not been described so far. Most cases demonstrate monoclonal $J_H$ or TCR gene rearrangement. The disease usually runs an aggressive course with an estimated 5-year survival of approximately 50%. However, spontaneous regression of skin lesions can occur on rare occasions (Chang et al. 1998).

## Mycosis Fungoides

MF is the most common type of CL. Apart from the classic clinical presentation, the disease may occur as poikiloderma, solitary, pustular, bullous, verrucous, ichthyosiform, and hypo- and hyperpigmented forms. It has recently been accepted that MF could have another atypical clinicopathological presentation. At least a proportion of so-called *persistent pigmented purpuric dermatitis* have features consistent with MF. Patients with this condition present clinically with persistent pigmented purpuric lesions. Histologically, there is usually a lichenoid infiltrate composed of small cerebriform lymphocytes and siderophages. Epidermal changes are variable but the presence of lining-up of lymphoid cells is typical. These cells share many properties with those of MF including a near absence of cytopathic effects on adjacent keratinocytes and limited ability to induce spongiosis. Some of the cells are CD8$^+$ but most are CD4$^+$. Clonal rearrangement can be demonstrated in a subset of cases. Follow-up is crucial to distinguish between benign pigmented purpuric dermatoses and MF (Toro et al. 1997).

## Hydroa-Like Lymphoma

Several cases of so-called hydroa-like lymphoma have been documented in the past few years (Magano et al. 1999). Most of the affected patients are children from Asia and Latin America. Clinically, the condition shows similarity to hydroa vacciniforme and is typified by vesiculopapular eruptions on the face, trunk and limbs. Necrotic areas, edema, and scars can be found. Histologically, dense infiltrates composed of large pleomorphic lymphocytes, histiocytes and eosinophils are present in the dermis and subcutis. An angiocentric and angiodestructive growth pattern with resultant necrosis can be seen in some cases. The atypical lymphocytes express pan-T-cell antigens and up to 40% of them are CD30$^+$. PCR reveals the presence of EBV DNA sequences in most cases. The disease is fatal in many cases. The patients die as a result of involvement of internal organs and the central nervous system. The atypical lymphocytes are also found in autopsy specimens in various organs (Iwatsuki et al. 1999; Magano et al. 1999). Further observations are warranted to clarify the exact character of this peculiar condition.

## B-cell Lymphomas

### Marginal Zone B-cell Lymphoma

Marginal zone B-cell lymphoma is a low-grade malignant lymphoproliferative disease derived from cells resembling those seen in the marginal zone of a lymph node. The skin lesions are nodules, plaques or tumors situated predominantly on the upper limbs and trunk. Histological features include nodular or diffuse infiltrates with the characteristic "inverse pattern", typified by a darker center constituted of small lymphocytes, and a surrounding brighter zone of centrocyte-like cells. In addition, germinal centers of typical appearance may be present. In some cases infiltration of the germinal centers by neoplastic cells of the marginal zone – so-called follicular colonization – is seen. The cellular population in the interfollicular areas is composed of small lymphocytes, plasma cells, lymphoplasmacytoid cells, monocytoid B cells, and occasional blasts. The plasma cells tend to be collected in small aggregations at the periphery of the infiltrate. The centrocyte-like cells have a CD19$^+$, CD20$^+$, CD22$^+$, CD79a$^+$, CD5$^-$, CD10$^-$, CD23$^-$ immunophenotype. Monotypic expression of immunoglobulin light chains is found in 40–65% of cases. The tumor often shows clonal rearrangement of $J_H$ genes. No specific cytogenetic abnormality is described. The disease has an indolent course with an estimated 5-year survival of approximately 100% (Cerroni et al. 1997).

## Spindle-Cell B-cell Lymphoma

In 2000, Cerroni and colleagues described five patients with spindle-cell B-cell lymphoma. Three women and two men presented clinically with large tumors, plaques or nodules that histologically showed a diffuse dense proliferation of elongated and spindle-shaped cells resembling those of dermatofibrosarcoma protuberans in the dermis and/or subcutis. A storiform or fascicular growth pattern was seen in some areas, representing up to 50% of the infiltration. Typical appearing centroblasts and centrocytes were located at the periphery of the infiltrate. In addition, large bizarre cells and spermatozoalike cells were observed. The spindle cells possessed B-cell phenotype ($CD20^+$, $CD79a^+$, $CD3^-$, $CD5^-$, $CD43^-$, $CD45RO^-$). At least two patients met the criteria for primary cutaneous B-cell lymphoma. Staging revealed disseminated involvement of bones in one patient. The clinical course of this particular morphological subtype of B-cell lymphoma remains to be clarified (Cerroni et al. 2000).

Another unusual clinico-pathological presentation of *B-cell lymphoma with a dermatomal distribution* was reported by Marzano et al. (1999). They described a 61-year-old woman presenting clinically with multiple erythematous papules and nodules and large ulcerated plaques located on her back and abdomen arranged in a dermatomal distribution. Histologically, the disease was categorized as B-cell lymphoma of follicular center cell according to the EORTC scheme. No systemic involvement was detected at the initial presentation after complete staging. However, approximately 6 months later the patient developed axillary lymph node involvement demanding administration of chemotherapy (Marzano et al. 1999).

## Pseudolymphomas

In addition to true lymphomas, several pseudolymphomatous lesions with unusual clinicopathological features have recently been described. Among the group of B-cell pseudolymphomas, so-called *cutaneous follicular lymphoid hyperplasia with monotypic plasma cells* was reported by Schmid et al. in 1995. The authors described 18 patients with various clinical presentations (solitary or multiple plaques located on the trunk, limbs and face), but unique histological features. These included diffuse dermal or subcutaneous infiltrates with prominent follicular pattern growth and rims of plasma cells with monotypic Ig kappa or lambda expression at the border of florid germinal centers. In the majority of the patients the number of plasma cells did not exceed 5% of the total cellular infiltrate, whereas in one-third of the patients plasma cells accounted for up to 50% of the infiltration. Other pathological features included an increased number of postcapillary venules in interfollicular areas similar to those seen in the paracortex, and a mixture of macrophages, eosinophils, and immunoblasts in the infiltrate. In 8 of 13 specimens available for clonality studies clonal Ig heavy chain rearrangement was detected. Of the 18 patients, 16 were followed up (median duration of follow up 33 months) to find persistent disease in one and local recurrences in three others (Schmid et al. 1995).

Among the group of T-cell pseudolymphomas, pronounced pleomorphic lymphoid reactions have been reported in *molluscum contagiosum* (MC). Clinically, these lesions do not differ from ordinary MC, but histologically there is a florid infiltrate surrounding a cavity with molluscum bodies. The infiltrate is composed of small to large pleomorphic cells expressing CD3 and CD8. Up to 30% of the lymphocytic population express CD30. The mitotic rate is high. However, clonal TCR rearrangement could not be demonstrated. The reasons for these changes in lymphocytes have been suggested to be a lymphoblastic transformation in response to the MC virus (Guitart and Hurt 1999).

Besides the MC virus, an infection with *parapoxvirus* can be added to the spectrum of cutaneous CD30$^+$ benign lymphoproliferations. Rose and coauthors described three members of one family who developed multiple erythematous nodules and plaques on the dorsal aspects of both hands accompanied in one patient by axillary lymphadenopathy. Biopsy showed in all cases a dense miscellaneous dermal infiltrate composed of lymphocytes, eosinophils, and plasma cells as well as large pale-staining lymphoid cells with a pleomorphic nucleus and prominent nucleoli. Immunohistochemically, the majority of cells expressed CD3 and CD4 antigens, with very few cells expressing CD8. In addition, abundant CD30$^+$ cells both arranged in small clusters and scattered throughout the infiltrate were found. The proliferative index was up to 70%. Molecular analysis for TCR gene rearrangement revealed a polyclonal nature of the infiltrate in all three cases. Parapoxvirus particles were demonstrated in epidermal keratinocytes in two of the patients by electron microscopy (Rose et al. 1999).

In summary, various new variants and diseases of primary CLs have been described recently. Since the number of reported cases is small there is a need for multicenter studies to clarify clinico-pathological and prognostic features of these cases. Therefore, the referral of patients with unusual forms of CL to specialists is recommended.

# References

Agnarsson BA, Vonderheid EC, Kadin ME (1990) Cutaneous T cell lymphoma with suppressor/cytotoxic (CD8) phenotype: identification of rapidly progressive and chronic subtypes. J Am Acad Dermatol 22:569–577

Berti E, Tomasini D, Vermeer MH, Meijer CJ, Alessi E, Willemze R (1999) Primary cutaneous CD8-positive epidermotropic cytotoxic T cell lymphomas. A distinct clinicopathological entity with an aggressive clinical behavior. Am J Pathol 155:483–492

Burg G, Dummer R, Wilhelm M, Nestle F, Ott MM, Feller A, Hefner H, Lanz U, Schwinn A, Wiede J (1991) A subcutaneous delta-positive T-cell lymphoma that produces interferon gamma. N Engl J Med 325:1078–1081

Cerroni L, Signoretti S, Höfler G, Annessi G, Pütz B, Lackinger E, Metze D, Giannetti A, Kerl H (1997) Primary cutaneous marginal zone B-cell lymphoma: a recently described entity of low-grade malignant cutaneous B-cell lymphoma. Am J Surg Pathol 21:1307–1315

Cerroni L, El-Shabrawi-Caelen L, Fink-Puches R, LeBoit PE, Kerl H (2000) Cutaneous spindle-cell B-cell lymphoma. A morphological variant of cutaneous large B-cell lymphoma. Am J Dermatopathol 22:299–304

Chang A, Zic JA, Boyd AS (1998) Intravascular large cell lymphoma: a patient with asymptomatic purpuric patches and a chronic clinical course. J Am Acad Dermatol 39:318–321

Dummer R, Potoczna N, Haeffner A, Zimmermann DR, Gilardi S, Burg G (1996) A primary non-T, non-B CD4+ CD56+ lymphoma. Arch Dermatol 132:550–553

Dummer R, Kamarashev J, Kempf W, Häffner A, Hess-Schmid M, Burg G (2002) Junctional CD8+ cutaneous lymphoma with non-aggressive clinical behavior, a CD8+ variant of mycosis fungoides? Arch Dermatol (in press)

Ginarte M, Abalde MT, Peteiro C, Fraga M, Alonso M, Toribio J (2000) Blastoid NK cell leukemia/lymphoma with cutaneous involvement. Dermatology 201:268–271

Guitart J, Hurt MA (1999) Pleomorphic T-cell infiltrate associated with molluscum contagiosum. Am J Dermatopathol 21:178–180

Harris NL, Jaffe ES, Stein H, Banks PM, Chan JK, Cleary ML, Delsol G, DeWolf Peeters C, Falini B, Gatter KC (1994) A revised European-American classification of lymphoid neoplasms: a proposal from the International Lymphoma Study Group. Blood 84:1361–1392

Harris NL, Jaffe ES, Diebold J, Flandrin G, Muller-Hermelink HK, Vardiman J, Lister TA, Bloomfield CD (1999) The World Health Organization classification of neoplastic diseases of the hematopoietic and lymphoid tissues. Report of the Clinical Advisory Committee Meeting, Airlie House, Virginia, November 1997. Ann Oncol 10:1419–1432

Heald P, Buckley P, Gilliam A, Perez M, Knobler R, Kacinski B, Edelson R (1992) Correlations of unique clinical, immunotypic, and histological findings in cutaneous gamma/delta T-cell lymphoma. J Am Acad Dermatol 26:865–870

Iwatsuki K, Xu Z, Takata M, Iguchi M, Ohtsuka M, Akiba H, Mitsuhashi Y, Takenoshita H, Sugiuchi R, Tagami H, Kaneko F (1999) The association of latent Epstein-Barr virus infection with hydroa vacciniforme. Br J Dermatol 140:715–721

Jaffe ES (1996) Classification of natural killer (NK) cell and NK-like T-cell malignancies. Blood 87:1207–1210

Jaffe ES, Sander CA, Flaig MJ (2000) Cutaneous lymphomas: a proposal for a unified approach to classification using the R.E.A.L./WHO Classification. Ann Oncol 11:17–21

Kempf W, Dummer R, Burg G (1999) Approach to lymphoproliferative infiltrates of the skin. The difficult lesions. Am J Clin Pathol 111:S84–S93

Magana M, Sangueza P, Gil-Beristain J, Sanchez-Sosa S, Salgado A, Ramon G, Sangueza OP (1999) Angiocentric cutaneous T-cell lymphoma of childhood (hydroa-like lymphoma): a distinctive type of cutaneous T-cell lymphoma. J Am Acad Dermatol 38:574–579

Martel P, Laroche L, Courville P, Larroche C, Wechsler J, Lenormand B, Deflau MH, Bodemer C, Bagot M, Joly P (2000) Cutaneous involvement in patients with angioimmunoblastic lymphadenopathy with dysproteinemia. A clinical, immunohistological, and molecular analysis. Arch Dermatol 136:881–886

Marzano AV, Berti E, Alessi E (1999) Primary cutaneous B-cell lymphoma with a dermatomal distribution. J Am Acad Dermatol 41:884–886

Rose C, Starostik P, Broecker EB (1999) Infection with parapoxvirus induces CD30-positive cutaneous infiltrates in humans. J Cutan Pathol 26:520–522

Salhany KE, Macon WR, Choi JK, Elenitsas R, Lessin SR, Felgar RE, Wilson DM, Przyblski GK, Lister J, Wasik MA, Swerdlow SH (1998) Subcutaneous panniculitis-like T-cell lymphoma: clinicopathologic, immunophenotypic, and genotypic analysis of alpha/beta and gamma/delta subtypes. Am J Surg Pathol 22:881–893

Schmid U, Eckert F, Griesser H, Steinke C, Cogliatti SB, Kaudewitz P, Lennert K (1995) Cutaneous follicular lymphoid hyperplasia with monotypic plasma cells. Am J Surg Pathol 19:12–20

Toro JR, Sander CA, LeBoit PE (1997) Persistent pigmented purpuric dermatitis and mycosis fungoides: stimulant, precursor, or both? Am J Dermatopathol 19:108–118

Toro JR, Beaty M, Sorbara L, Turner ML, White J, Kingma DW, Raffeld M, Jaffe ES (2000) Gamma delta T-cell lymphoma of the skin: a clinical, microscopic, and molecular study. Arch Dermatol 136:1024–1032

Wang CY, Su WP, Kurtin PJ (1996) Subcutaneous panniculitic T-cell lymphoma. Int J Dermatol 35:1–8

Willemze R, Kerl H, Sterry W, Berti E, Cerroni L, Chimenti S, Diaz Peréz JL, Geerts ML, Goos M, Knobler R, Ralfkiaer E, Santucci M, Smith N, Wechsler J, van Vloten WA, Meijer CJ (1997) EORTC classification for primary cutaneous lymphomas: a proposal from the Cutaneous Lymphoma Study Group of the European Organization for Research and Treatment of Cancer. Blood 90:354–371

# Clinical Aspects and Pathology of Primary Cutaneous B-Cell Lymphomas

H. Kerl, R. Fink-Puches, and L. Cerroni

## Abstract

Primary cutaneous B-cell lymphomas (pCBCL) occur more frequently than generally believed. The most important subtypes are: marginal zone B-cell lymphoma/immunocytoma, follicle center-cell lymphoma and large B-cell lymphoma of the leg. A correct diagnosis can be rendered only in the context of knowledge of the clinical findings. Progress in terms of classification and biology is associated with the application of modern techniques including immunohistology and laser beam microdissection followed by molecular analysis. Future definitions of pCBCL will be based on their molecular abnormalities and their etiology and pathogenesis. Awareness of the special clinical behavior of pCBCL should prevent unnecessarily aggressive treatment.

Patients with cutaneous lymphomas can be divided into those with primary and those with secondary cutaneous lymphoma. Those with primary cutaneous lymphomas reveal cutaneous disease alone with no evidence of extracutaneous manifestations over a period of at least 6 months when a complete staging examination has been performed. Patients with secondary cutaneous lymphomas show extracutaneous disease and subsequent development of skin lesions.

Primary cutaneous B-cell lymphomas (pCBCL) are defined as malignant B-cell proliferations with a specific homing pattern to the skin. pCBCL occur far more frequently than generally believed. It is extremely important to emphasize that pCBCL differ significantly from their nodal counterparts in showing characteristic clinical, histopathologic, immunophenotypic and molecular features. A correct diagnosis can be rendered only in the context of knowledge of the clinical findings (Kerl and Cerroni 1996; Burg et al. 1997). Progress in diagnosis in terms of lymphoma biology is associated with the application of modern methods. In particular the new technique of laser beam microdissection of lymphocytes followed by PCR analysis allows precise correlation of morphologic features with molecular results.

Recent Results in Cancer Research, Vol. 160
© Springer-Verlag Berlin Heidelberg 2002

In this chapter we discuss the most common types of pCBCL, namely cutaneous marginal zone B-cell lymphoma/immunocytoma, cutaneous follicle center-cell lymphoma and large B-cell lymphoma of the leg. Awareness of their special prognostic aspects should prevent unnecessarily aggressive treatment.

## Classification of Primary Cutaneous B-cell Lymphomas

Classifications of lymphomas have always been controversial. The European Organization for Research and Treatment of Cancer (EORTC) Cutaneous Lymphoma Project Group proposed a new classification for primary cutaneous lymphomas in 1997 (Willemze et al. 1997). The classification is based on well-defined clinicopathologic entities with emphasis on clinical features, including prognosis. The new approach also considers immunohistologic and genetic criteria. This EORTC classification has been the subject of criticism and debate. It was suggested to classify primary cutaneous lymphomas according to the recently proposed WHO-classification (Harris et al. 2000). The criticism was not very helpful because a significantly better model for classification of cutaneous lymphomas has not yet been formulated. The EORTC classification allows a more precise categorization of patients with cutaneous lymphomas than the WHO classification, especially for pCBCL.

Table 1 compares equivalent categories in the EORTC and WHO classifications for the most frequent pCBCL. One problem concerns primary cutaneous follicle center-cell lymphomas (Cerroni and Kerl 2001) because many cases are characterized histologically by a diffuse growth pattern with predominance of medium to large centrocytes and centroblasts. These lymphomas would probably be classified among the diffuse large B-cell lymphomas in the WHO classification.

Concepts about lymphomas continuously evolve. Therefore, it is difficult to establish an internationally accepted classification scheme. We also recognize, of course, that the EORTC classification for primary cutaneous lymphomas can also only be seen as a transitional concept. Looking towards the future, cutaneous malignant lymphomas will soon be defined in relation to their molecular abnormalities (Alizadeh et al. 2000) and their etiology and pathogenesis. This information will encourage further progress and the development of better therapies.

**Table 1.** Comparison of the EORTC classification for primary cutaneous B-cell lymphomas with the WHO classification for B-cell neoplasms

| EORTC classification | WHO classification |
| --- | --- |
| Primary cutaneous marginal zone B-cell lymphoma/ immunocytoma | Extranodal marginal zone B-cell lymphoma of MALT type |
| Primary cutaneous follicle center-cell lymphoma | Follicular lymphoma |
| Primary cutaneous large B-cell lymphoma of the leg | Diffuse large B-cell lymphoma |

## Marginal Zone B-cell Lymphoma

Marginal zone B-cell lymphoma (MZL) has been recognized as a distinct variant of a pCBCL (Bailey et al. 1996; Baldassano et al. 1999; Cerroni et al. 1997a). It is closely related to immunocytoma and MALT lymphomas. The term SALT (skin-associated lymphoid tissue) lymphoma has also been used for these tumors (Santucci et al. 1991). Clinically, there are solitary or clustered erythematous patches, papules, nodules, or plaques located on the upper extremities or trunk. Generalized lesions can be observed in a minority of patients. The prognosis is excellent despite frequent recurrences. In a recent study of 62 patients with primary cutaneous marginal zone B-cell lymphoma/immunocytoma a 5-year survival of 98% was found.

Histology is characterized by dense nodular, diffuse or patchy perivascular/periadnexal infiltrates throughout the entire dermis and subcutaneous fat. At scanning power, a characteristic pattern can be observed: dark areas composed of small lymphocytes (lymphoid nodules) are surrounded by and contrast with pale areas containing medium-sized cells with indented nuclei and abundant pale cytoplasm (marginal zone cells, centrocyte-like cells). Reactive (polytypic) germinal centers are a frequent finding; lymphoplasmacytoid cells, plasma cells, blasts, and eosinophils are also present.

Immunohistology shows a monotypic intracytoplasmic expression of immunoglobulins in about 70% of cases. Neoplastic cells are positive for B-cell-associated markers (CD20, CD79a) and display negativity for CD5, CD10 and bcl-6. A typical intracytoplasmic granular reactivity for the monocytoid B-cell-associated antibody KiM1p is frequently found. Molecular analysis reveals rearrangement of $J_H$ genes in about two-thirds of the cases. Table 2 shows the important features of primary cutaneous MZL.

There is ongoing controversy concerning the question as to whether primary cutaneous MZL and immunocytoma are the same disease (Kerl and Cerroni 2000). It is clear that MZL is closely related to immunocytoma (LeBoit et al. 1994; Rijlaarsdam et al. 1993). However, there are morphologic differences between MZL and immunocytoma. Clinically, immunocytomas usually appear as solitary or clustered bluish-red or reddish-brown plaques, or dome-shaped tumors with a smooth surface. Predilection sites are the lower extremities. The prognosis is excellent. The histopathologic features are characterized by dense nodular or diffuse infiltrates within the entire dermis extending into the subcutis. The pattern of growth and the infiltrates

**Table 2.** Primary cutaneous marginal zone B-cell lymphoma

| |
| --- |
| Young adults; upper extremities, trunk; prognosis excellent |
| Nodules of reactive B lymphocytes surrounded by neoplastic marginal zone cells; sheets of plasma cells; reactive follicles |
| CD20$^+$, cIg$^+$, CD5$^-$, CD10$^-$, bcl-6$^-$ |
| Ig genes rearranged |

look monomorphous and differ from the "marginal zone pattern" of cutaneous MZL. Cytomorphologically a predominance of small lymphocytes and lymphoplasmacytoid cells is found. A diagnostic clue is PAS-positive intranuclear inclusions (Dutcher bodies) which are sometimes observed. *Borrelia burgdorferi* probably plays a role in the pathogenesis of this lymphoma (Cerroni et al. 1997b; Goodland et al. 2000). Immunocytomas can arise in areas affected by acrodermatitis chronica atrophicans or in association with erythema chronicum migrans.

## Follicle Center-Cell Lymphoma

Primary cutaneous follicle center-cell lymphoma (FCL) is a neoplasm of B lymphocytes of the germinal center, characterized by the neoplastic proliferation of centrocytes and centroblasts confined to the skin. The exact incidence of this type of pCBCL is a matter of discussion. Some authors believe that it represents a common type of CBCL, whereas others maintain that true FCLs of the skin are very rare. In our opinion, it represents a relatively common subtype of pCBCL.

To this group belong most of the patients diagnosed in the past as "reticulohistiocytoma of the dorsum" or "Crosti's lymphoma", typically located on the back. The prognosis for patients with cutaneous FCL is favorable (5-year survival 94% in 60 patients). Clinically solitary or grouped reddish-brown to reddish-blue papules, plaques or tumors surrounded by erythematous patches can be seen. Preferential locations are the head (scalp, forehead) and the back. Recurrences are observed in about 50% of patients, but dissemination to internal organs is rare.

Histopathologically, FCL is usually characterized by a diffuse growth pattern. A typical follicular pattern with proliferation of neoplastic centrocytes and centroblasts is, however, observed in a distinct proportion of patients with FCL as demonstrated by laser beam microdissection followed by PCR analysis of $J_H$ gene rearrangement (Cerroni et al. 2000) (Fig. 1). Within the neoplastic infiltrate of centrocytes and centroblasts a variable number of immunoblasts, small lymphocytes, histiocytes, and in some cases eosinophils and plasma cells can be admixed.

The tumor cells express monotypic surface Ig and B cell-associated antigens (CD20, CD79a), reveal CD21 (DRC, dendritic reticulum cells) positivity and are CD5 negative, whereas variable results are found for CD10(+/–) and bcl-6(+/–) depending on the histopathologic pattern. Staining for bcl-2 protein is frequently negative, which is a major difference from nodal FCL. Aberrant positivity for MT2 (CD45RA) can be seen in neoplastic follicles in about 20% of FCLs of the skin. Clonal rearrangement of $J_H$ genes can be demonstrated in a majority of cases. The interchromosomal 14;18 translocation typically observed in nodal follicular lymphomas is usually not found in primary cutaneous FCL.

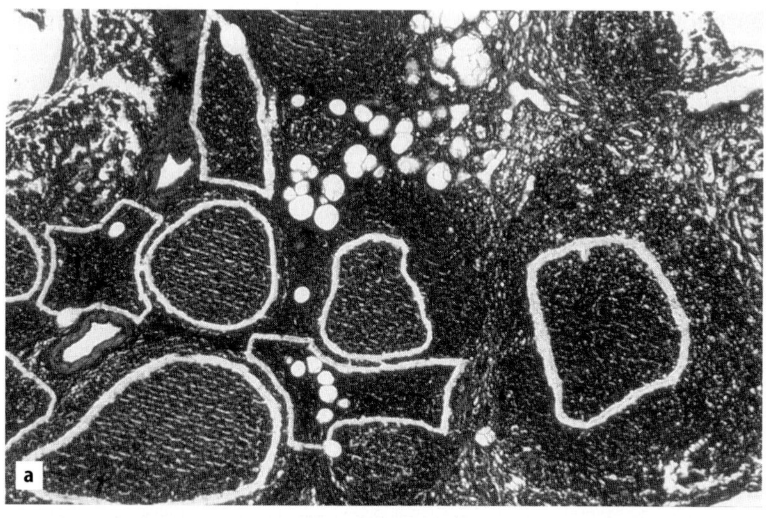

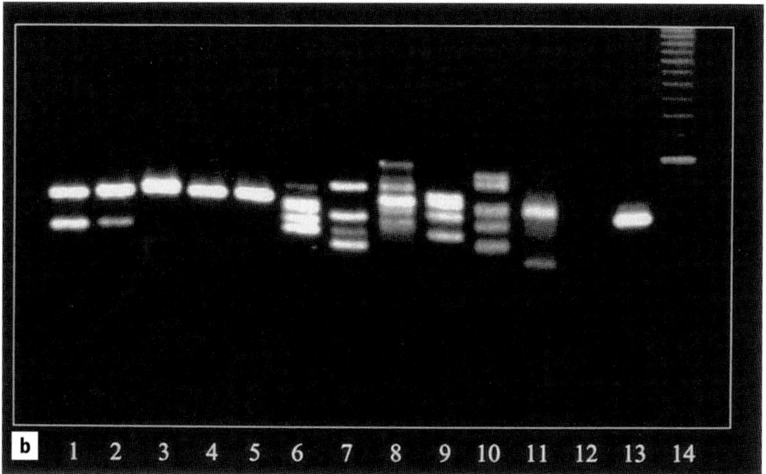


**Fig. 1a,b.** Primary cutaneous follicle center-cell lymphoma. **a** Preparation of follicle center cells and inter-follicular cells by laser beam for computerized microdissection. **b** Example of a monoclonal pattern of J$_H$ gene rearrangement of cells within the follicles after laser beam microdissection (*lanes 1–5* five different follicles; *lanes 6–11* six different interfollicular areas; *lane 12* negative control, no DNA; *lane 13* positive control, cutaneous B-cell lymphoma; *lane 14* molecular ladder)

**Table 3.** Primary cutaneous follicle center-cell lymphoma

| |
|---|
| Middle-aged patients; head, trunk; prognosis excellent |
| Diffuse/follicular pattern; centrocytes, centroblasts |
| CD20$^+$, CD10$^{+/-}$, bcl-6$^{+/-}$, bcl-2$^{-/+}$, DRC$^+$ |
| Ig genes rearranged |

Synthesis of morphologic, immunohistochemical and molecular data suggests that FCLs originating in the lymph nodes and the skin, though characterized by a similar morphologic pattern, have different pathogenetic mechanisms. Table 3 summarizes the important features of primary cutaneous FCL.

## Large B-cell Lymphoma of the Leg

Primary cutaneous large B-cell lymphomas (LBCL) are neoplasms of B lymphocytes consisting predominantly of large cells with features of centroblasts, large centrocytes, and immunoblasts (Vermeer et al. 1996; Lair et al. 2000; Wechsler and Bagot 2000). Clinically, reddish-brown to bluish-red solitary or grouped tumors and plaques which are located most frequently on the lower legs can be observed. Tumors with similar morphologic features can arise also on body areas other than the lower extremities. Ulceration is not uncommon. Older females are frequently affected. The prognosis is more unfavorable than in other types of pCBCL, with a 5-year survival rate of approximately 60% (number of patients in our study 23).

Histology is characterized by dense, diffuse infiltrates of large cells in the entire dermis and subcutis. Infiltration of the epidermis simulating a T-cell lymphoma can sometimes be observed. Cytomorphologically neoplastic cells resemble either immunoblasts or centroblasts. Mitotic figures are frequent. Often an exact classification is not possible. It has been proposed that most cases of LBCL represent large-cell lymphomas originating from the lymphocytes of the germinal center.

Immunohistology reveals monotypic surface immunoglobulins and/or cytoplasmic immunoglobulin. Neoplastic cells are CD20$^+$ and bcl-2$^+$. Molecular analysis shows rearrangement of $J_H$ genes in most cases. The t(14;18) is not present.

LBCL must be differentiated from anaplastic large-cell lymphoma and from non-lymphoid tumors such as metastases among others. The clinicopathologic pattern, together with immunohistochemical and molecular features of the tumors, allows the correct classification in most cases. In Table 4 the important features of LBCL (of the leg) are summarized.

**Table 4.** Large B-cell lymphoma of the leg

| |
|---|
| Elderly patients; 5-year survival approximately 60% |
| Centroblasts, immunoblasts |
| CD20$^+$, bcl-2$^+$, CD10$^{-/+}$, bcl-6$^{+/-}$ |
| Ig genes rearranged |

## References

Alizadeh AA, Eisen MB, Davis RE, et al (2000) Distinct types of diffuse large B-cell lymphoma identified by gene expression profiling. Nature 403:503–511

Bailey EM, Ferry JA, Harris NL, et al (1996) Marginal zone lymphoma (low-grade B-cell lymphoma of mucosa-associated lymphoid tissue type) of skin and subcutaneous tissue. A study of 15 patients. Am J Surg Pathol 20:1011–1023

Baldassano MF, Bailey EM, Ferry JA, et al (1999) Cutaneous lymphoid hyperplasia and cutaneous marginal zone lymphoma. Comparison of morphologic and immunophenotypic features. Am J Surg Pathol 23:88–96

Burg G, Kempf W, Haeffner AC, et al (1997) Cutaneous lymphomas. Curr Probl Dermatol 9:137–204

Cerroni L, Kerl H (2001) Primary cutaneous follicular lymphoma. Arch Dermatol 137:489–490

Cerroni L, Signoretti S, Hoefler G, et al (1997a) Primary cutaneous marginal zone B-cell lymphoma: a recently described entity of low-grade malignant cutaneous B-cell lymphoma. Am J Surg Pathol 21:1307–1315

Cerroni L, Zoechling N, Puetz B, Kerl H (1997b) Infection by *Borrelia burgdorferi* and cutaneous B-cell lymphoma. J Cutan Pathol 24:457–461

Cerroni L, Arzberger E, Puetz B, et al (2000) Primary cutaneous follicle center cell lymphoma with follicular growth pattern. Blood 95:3922–3928

Goodlad JR, Davidson MM, Hollowood K, et al (2000) Primary cutaneous B-cell lymphoma and *Borrelia burgdorferi* infection in patients from the highlands of Scotland. Am J Surg Pathol 24:1279–1285

Harris NL, Jaffe ES, Diebold J, et al (2000) The World Health Organization classification of neoplastic diseases of the haematopoietic and lymphoid tissues: report of the Clinical Advisory Committee Meeting, Airlie House, Virginia, November, 1997. Histopathology 36:69–89

Kerl H, Cerroni L (1996) The morphologic spectrum of cutaneous B-cell lymphomas. Arch Dermatol 132:1376–1377

Kerl H, Cerroni L (2000) Controversies in cutaneous lymphomas. Semin Cutan Med Surg 19:157–160

Lair G, Parant E, Tessier MH, et al (2000) Primary cutaneous B-cell lymphomas of the lower limbs: a study of integrin expression in 11 cases. Acta Derm Venereol 80:367–369

LeBoit PE, McNutt NS, Reed JA, et al (1994) Primary cutaneous immunocytoma. A B-cell lymphoma that can easily be mistaken for cutaneous lymphoid hyperplasia. Am J Surg Pathol 18:969–978

Rijlaarsdam JU, van der Putte SCJ, Berti E, et al (1993) Cutaneous immunocytomas: a clinicopathologic study of 26 cases. Histopathology 23:117–125

Santucci M, Pimpinelli N, Arganini L (1991) Primary cutaneous B-cell lymphoma: a unique type of low-grade lymphoma. Cancer 67:2311–2326

Vermeer MH, Geelen FAMJ, van Haselen CW, et al (1996) Primary cutaneous large B-cell lymphomas of the legs. A distinct type of cutaneous B-cell lymphoma with an intermediate prognosis. Arch Dermatol 132:1304–1308

Wechsler J, Bagot M (2000) Primary cutaneous large B-cell lymphoma. Semin Cutan Med Surg 19:130–132

Willemze R, Kerl H, Sterry W, et al (1997) EORTC classification for primary cutaneous lymphomas: a proposal from the Cutaneous Lymphoma Study Group of the European Organization for Research and Treatment of Cancer. Blood 90:354–371

# Lymphoma 5

**Pathogenesis**
**Clinical Presentations**
## Diagnosis
**Therapy**

# Modern Diagnosis of Cutaneous Lymphoma

B. Giannotti and N. Pimpinelli

## Abstract

The issue of primary cutaneous lymphoma (CL) has been greatly influenced by the increasing knowledge about lymphoid cell biology, the widespread use of sensitive and specific immunological and molecular markers, and the careful correlation among clinical, histological and immunomolecular features. This latter is the key element of the classification of CL proposed by the EORTC Cutaneous Lymphoma Study Group in 1997, which categorizes distinct clinicopathological entities with prognostic and therapeutic relevance. With few exceptions, no reliable diagnosis and subtyping of CL can be made without the aid of immunohistochemistry and/or molecular analysis. On the other hand, the acritical use of immunological and molecular markers can be misleading if not combined properly with a correct clinical and histological evaluation. For this reason, a step-by-step diagnosis and staging protocol is exceedingly important. Finally, great caution should be used in the interpretation of lymphoid cell infiltrates of the skin which show a monoclonal rearrangement in the absence of reliable clinical and/or pathological evidence of neoplasia.

The first prerequisite for a correct diagnosis and classification of cutaneous lymphoma (CL) is its definition, i.e. non-Hodgkin's lymphoma primarily presenting in the skin, without any evidence of extracutaneous disease at presentation [1, 2].

The issue of a "modern" diagnosis of CL has been – and is – greatly influenced by the increasing knowledge about lymphoid cell biology, the widespread use of sensitive and specific immunohistochemical and molecular techniques, and the proper correlation among clinical, histological and immunomolecular features. This latter is the key element of the classification of CL proposed by the EORTC Cutaneous Lymphoma Study Group in 1997 (Table 1) [2], which categorizes distinct clinicopathological entities with prognostic and therapeutic relevance.

Recent Results in Cancer Research, Vol. 160
© Springer-Verlag Berlin Heidelberg 2002

**Table 1.** EORTC classification for primary cutaneous lymphomas (Willemze R. et al. (1997) Blood 90:354–371)

| T cell lymphoma | | B cell lymphoma | |
|---|---|---|---|
| Indolent | MF | Indolent | Follicle center-cell lymphoma |
| | MF + follicular mucinosis | | Immunocytoma (marginal zone BCL) |
| | Pagetoid reticulosis | | |
| | Lymphomatoid papulosis | Intermediate | Large-cell lymphoma of the leg |
| | CD30$^+$ large-cell lymphoma | | |
| Aggressive | CD30$^-$ large-cell lymphoma | | |
| | Sézary syndrome | | |
| Provisional | Granulomatous slack skin | Provisional | Intravascular lymphoma |
| | Pleomorphic small/medium sized | | Plasmacytoma |
| | Subcutaneous panniculitis-like | | |

**Table 2.** Diagnosis of cutaneous lymphoma

| Level 1 | Evaluation by experienced dermatologist |
|---|---|
| | Histology (EE, PAS, Giemsa) |
| | Immunohistochemistry (embedded tissue) |
| | – typing of the infiltrate (CD3, CD4, CD8, CD20, CD79a) |
| | – cIg light chain monoclonality (CBCL) |
| | – prognostically relevant antigen expression (CD30, TIA-1, CD56) |
| Level 2 | Immunohistochemistry (embedded and/or frozen tissue) |
| | – sIg light chain monoclonality (CBCL) |
| | – subtyping CBCL (CD5, CD10) |
| | – aberrant phenotype (CTCL) |
| | – proliferation markers (MIB-1, Ki-67) |
| | – specific oncogene-related protein expression (bcl-2) |
| Level 3 | Molecular analysis (Southern blot, PCR) |
| | – clonal rearrangement (TCR, Ig heavy chain) |
| | – specific oncogene expression (bcl-1/2/6, c-myc, etc) |

Generally speaking, no reliable (early) diagnosis and subtyping of CL can be made without the aid of immunohistochemistry and/or molecular analysis. The only current exception in this regard is mycosis fungoides (MF), the most well known and widely recognized subtype of CL, whose diagnosis – and even early diagnosis – is based on histomorphological features as the gold standard [3]. Therefore, we would propose the use of different levels of diagnostic accuracy, in which the clinical and histological features are combined with basic (Table 2, level 1) and/or more sensitive immunohistochemistry (Table 2, level 2) and/or molecular analysis (Table 2, level 3). Concerning prognostically relevant markers, it is important to emphasize that their expression is relevant when specific clinicopathological conditions do occur [1, 2, 4]. For example, CD30 antigen expression means a favorable prognosis when found at presentation and associated with specific clinical features (localized infiltrative lesions, often with partial spontaneous regression, in CD30$^+$ large-cell CTCL; crops of

**Table 3.** Staging of cutaneous lymphoma

| Level 1 | Blood chemistry<br>– hemogram, immunoelectrophoresis, LHD, $\beta$-2-microglobulin, ferritin, quantitative Ig<br>Biopsy of clinically suspicious nodes<br>– histology, immunochemistry<br>Chest radiography<br>CT scan (PET scan)<br>Bone marrow biopsy facult. in MF stage I-II and CBCL (low-grade) |
|---|---|
| Level 2 | Peripheral blood lymphocyte typing<br>– possible TCR V$\beta$ clone analysis<br>Molecular analysis<br>– histology of suspicious nodes, peripheral blood |

papulonodular lesions with ulceronecrotic evolution and with complete spontaneous regression in lymphomatoid papulosis). In contrast, CD30 expression has no prognostic relevance when found in tumor-stage MF, associated with blastic transformation. In this latter case, the prognosis, which overall is poor, is not influenced at all by CD30 expression.

Concerning TIA-1 antigen expression, a cytotoxic functional marker, it is crucial to identify newly recognized, specific clinicopathological subtypes of CTCL with an overall bad prognosis, i.e. subcutaneous panniculitis-like CTCL [5] and aggressive, epidermotropic cytotoxic CTCL [6]. Nevertheless, it has to be clearly stressed that no prognostic importance is linked to TIA-1 expression in other conditions, e.g. CD30$^+$ CTCL [7]. Finally, great caution should be used in the interpretation of lymphoid cell monoclonality in the skin and/or peripheral blood in the absence of a reliable clinical and/or pathological evidence of neoplasia.

Once a "modern" diagnosis is made, performing adequate staging procedures (Table 3) is mandatory for a correct final classification of the case and a proper scheduling of treatment [1, 2].

# References


1. Pimpinelli N, Santucci M, Giannotti B (1993) Cutaneous lymphomas: a clinically relevant classification. Int J Dermatol 32:695–700
2. Willemze R, Kerl H, Sterry W, et al (1997) EORTC classification for primary cutaneous lymphomas: a proposal from the cutaneous lymphoma study group of the European Organization for Research and Treatment of Cancer. Blood 90:354–371
3. Santucci M, Biggeri A, Feller AC, et al (2000) Efficacy of histologic criteria for diagnosing early mycosis fungoides: an EORTC Cutaneous Lymphoma Study Group investigation. Am J Surg Pathol 24:40–50
4. Willemze R, Mejier CJLM (1998) Classification of cutaneous lymphomas: crosstalk between pathologist and clinician. Curr Diagn Pathol 5:23–33
5. Gonzales CL, Medeiros LJ, Braziel RM, Jaffe ES (1991) T-cell lymphoma involving the subcutaneous tissue. A clinicopathologic entity commonly associated with hemophagocytic syndrome. Am J Surg Pathol 15:17–27

6. Berti E, Tommasini D, Vermeer MH, et al (1999) Primary cutaneous CD8-positive epidermotropic cytotoxic T-cell lymphomas. A distinct clinicopathologic entity with an aggressive clinical behavior. Am J Pathol 155:483–492
7. Kummer JA, Vermeer MH, Dukers D, et al (1997) Most primary cutaneous CD30-positive lymphoproliferative disorders have a CD4-positive cytotoxic T-cell phenotype. J Invest Dermatol 109:636–640

# Lymphoma  5

Pathogenesis
Clinical Presentations
Diagnosis
**Therapy**

# Treatment of Cutaneous T Cell Lymphoma: 2001

Eric C. Vonderheid

## Abstract

The neoplastic cells of mycosis fungoides (MF) and Sézary syndrome are recognized to be clonal expansions of "memory" T cells that home into the upper dermis and epidermis via the interplay of adhesion molecules and chemokines, and this may account for the marked effectiveness and even curative potential of various skin-directed therapies utilized to treat clinically early disease. However, because neoplastic T cells freely circulate and are detectable in extracutaneous tissues by PCR prior to other methods, effective long-term control of more advanced MF and Sézary syndrome, i.e. reduction of tumor burden and decreased risk of transformation into aggressive lymphoma, often requires long-term administration of a therapy with systemic activity in addition to skin-directed therapies. Therapies with immunomodulatory activities, e.g. interferon alfa, bexarotene or extracorporeal photochemotherapy (ECP), are probably superior to traditional cytotoxic drugs in this regard although the response rates are relatively low. Selected patients with advanced or biologically aggressive CTCL should be considered for an allogeneic stem cell transplantation regimen to induce a graft-versus-tumor response. New and emerging treatments include immunotoxins such as denileukin diftitox that selectively target neoplastic T cells, potent immunomodulatory cytokines such as rIL-12 to enhance innate antitumor immune mechanisms, novel immunotherapeutic approaches that use dendritic cells loaded with tumor-associated antigens or vaccination using synthetic peptides or DNA plasmids that express the variable region of the T cell receptor beta chain, and possibly gene and protein transduction therapy to correct intracellular defects in neoplastic T cells. Overall the future of therapy for CTCL seems quite optimistic.

Recent Results in Cancer Research, Vol. 160
© Springer-Verlag Berlin Heidelberg 2002

## Introduction

Cutaneous T cell lymphoma (CTCL) is a form of extranodal non-Hodgkin's lymphoma with initial manifestations arising in the skin. The major clinical subsets of CTCL are mycosis fungoides (MF) and Sézary syndrome. These entities are characterized by a clonal proliferation of neoplastic T cells with highly infolded "cerebriform" nuclei (Sézary cells) and a surface immunophenotype of previously activated or "memory" T cells, most often of the CD4$^+$ T helper subset (Kim and Hoppe 1999). In addition, expression of homing receptors such as the cutaneous lymphocyte antigen and chemokine receptors such as CXCR by the neoplastic cells appear to mediate cell trafficking into the upper dermis and epidermis (Rook and Heald 1995; Tensen et al. 1998). As such, CTCL may be regarded as a malignant lymphoma of skin-associated lymphoid tissue (SALT).

Current evidence also indicates that neoplastic T cells, like their normal counterparts, readily circulate among the skin, regional lymph nodes and blood, a phenomenon that accounts for the multifocal skin involvement of most patients at presentation and the high frequency (40–60%) of T cell clones detected in the peripheral blood by sensitive molecular genetic techniques based on the polymerase chain reaction (PCR). However, because T cell clones in the blood are often different from the T cell clones in skin lesions, it appears that T cell clones in the blood of many patients may actually represent an expanded normal T cell population rather than circulating neoplastic T cells (Delfau-Larue et al. 2000). Moreover, the prognostic significance of T cell clonality in the blood of patients with clinically early MF is uncertain at this time (Fraser-Andrews et al. 2000; Muche et al. 2000). Additional studies are needed to clarify this issue.

The localization of neoplastic T cells in the skin and other tissue compartments in CTCL does not occur randomly due to the effect of adhesion molecules and chemokines (Rook and Heald 1995; Tensen et al. 1998). In clinically early MF, lesions tend to develop initially on areas not habitually exposed to the sun (at least in patients with light skin color), thereby implying a direct inhibitory effect of ultraviolet radiation on neoplastic T cells and/or an indirect effect via keratinocytes or other epidermal cells. In early patch or plaque lesions, neoplastic T cells localize within the epidermis (epidermotropism), particularly along the basal layer and about Langerhans cells, as demonstrated by split skin preparations, immunohistochemistry using V$\beta$ antibodies, and most recently by the laser microdissection technique (Gellrich et al. 2000). The associated dermal infiltrate of early lesions is thus composed mostly of normal cells, and it is thought that CD8$^+$ T suppressor cells in the infiltrate mediate an antitumor immune response against the disease (Hoppe et al. 1995). With disease progression and the development of thicker plaques and tumor nodules in the skin, neoplastic T cells become apparent within the dermal infiltrate in increasing numbers, sometimes with loss of epidermotropism.

These observations concerning the biology of CTCL have several important therapeutic implications. Firstly, phototherapy or chemotherapeutic agents delivered solely to the skin are quite effective in promoting complete responses (CR) of lesions in clinically early disease while the neoplastic cells are located in the epidermis and upper dermis. Conversely, such topical treatments alone often prove to be inadequate with thicker plaques/nodules or infiltrates localized around hair follicles presumably because malignant cells extend more deeply into the dermis. Secondly, the fact that neoplastic T cells readily circulate has lead to considerable pessimism about the curative potential of skin-directed therapies. However, the strong homing of cells into the skin may explain the 30–50% sustained CR rates and probable cures even in patients with multiple skin lesions. Thirdly, treatments that reduce malignant cells in one tissue compartment often reduce the tumor burden in another compartment. For example, repetitive leukapheresis to remove the circulating neoplastic T cells of Sézary syndrome can also clear the skin and lymph nodes. The author has documented several instances of disappearance of T cell clones in the blood of patients treated only with topical therapy. Finally, strategies to enhance antitumor immune responses can be fruitful, e.g. extracorporeal photochemotherapy (ECP), administration of immunomodulating cytokines such as IL-2 and IL-12, and vaccines.

## Approach to the Management of CTCL

The goals of treatment of patients with CTCL are to relieve the signs and symptoms of disease, and to provide effective long-term control by minimizing tumor burden and thereby discouraging further tumor progression and/ or transformation into a more aggressive lymphoma. The possibility that intensive topical therapy can achieve sustained complete remissions without the need for maintenance therapy (probable cures) in 30–50% of patients with clinically early CTCL must also be considered as a goal of treatment when appropriate.

An estimate of the curative potential of therapy can be derived from relapse-free survival curves in patients who achieve a CR from treatment and then are monitored for recurrent disease off treatment. A horizontal plateau in the curve after the passage of time provides both an estimate of the cure rate and the minimum time that patients need to be followed before relapses become quite unlikely. This type of analysis is easiest to obtain when treatments are administered over a short interval of time, such as occurs with total skin electron beam (TSEB) or a course of systemic chemotherapy. Similar analyses could also be performed with photochemotherapy (PUVA) and topically applied chemotherapy, but at most centers these treatments are given chronically to maintain the CR, probably because cure is not judged to be a likely end point.

At present TSEB provides the clearest example of the curative potential of a skin-directed therapy in CTCL (Jones et al. 1995). Experience indicates that relapses rarely occur beyond 8–10 years after treatment and therefore the 10-year freedom-from-relapse (FFR) rate provides a reasonable estimate of the cure rate. For patients treated with TSEB at Stanford University, the 10-year FFR rate is 52% for stage Ia, 14% for stage Ib, 16% for stage IIa, and 7% for stage III. The experience at the Hamilton Regional Cancer Center is similar, although the follow-up intervals are shorter, with 33%, 11%, and 11% FFR for stages Ia, Ib, and IIa, respectively. Long-term sustained CRs exceeding 10 years also have been reported in patients who are treated with topical mechlorethamine (HN2), carmustine (BCNU), and PUVA. Thus, it appears that a significant proportion of patients with patch/plaque phase MF (T1/T2 skin rating) and some patients with non-Sézary erythrodermic CTCL (T4 rating) will achieve cure from various treatments administered solely to the skin.

The most important indicator of prognosis for patients with CTCL is derived from the stage of disease as well as the age and general health status of the patient. Another important, but less well-characterized prognostic factor may be the pace of disease progression. The staging classification system in widespread use today is based on the tumor-node-blood-metastasis (TNBM) format that was developed at a workshop sponsored by the National Cancer Institute in 1978, and subsequently modified by Sausville and coworkers in 1988. T rating reflects the status of skin involvement by CTCL: T1 and T2 refers to patch or plaque phase disease involving less than or more than 10% of the skin surface, respectively; T3 refers to presence of one or more tumors; and T4 refers to generalized erythroderma. However, T rating does not provide detailed information about the depth of infiltration by tumor cells (lesion thickness) and exact location of skin involvement, particularly regions that are often difficult to treat, e.g., palms and soles, eyelids, scalp, etc. Moreover, the current staging system does not take into account histopathologic findings of prognostic importance such as evidence of host resistance ($CD8^+$ cells in the dermal infiltrate) and transformation into aggressive large-cell lymphoma.

Histologic involvement of lymph nodes or visceral organs signifies a relatively poor prognosis for patients with CTCL regardless of the status of the skin, and these patients are classified as having stage IV disease (de Coninck et al. 2001). However, the prognosis of patients with histologically involved lymph nodes (N3 rating) also depends on the morphology of the infiltrating tumor cells: nodes involved with small "cerebriform" cells have a more favorable outlook than other patterns (Vonderheid et al. 1992). Finally, the use of Sézary cell counts exceeding 20% of the lymphocytes as a criterion for blood involvement (B1 rating) has not been found to retain independent significance in a multivariate analysis with T rating and other measures of tumor burden (Sausville et al. 1988). Recently, in its consensus report on erythrodermic CTCL, the International Society for Cutaneous Lymphoma proposed hematologic criteria for "leukemic" blood involvement in CTCL (B2 rating) and recommended that patients with these findings be considered to be at stage IV (Vonderheid et al. 2002).

## Importance of Complete Responses

Several studies have shown that patients who achieve a CR from treatment have a better prognosis than those who do not, and that a CR retains significance as a prognostic factor in multivariate models that include stage of disease (van Doorn et al. 2000). However, no study has addressed whether the survival of patients who achieve a CR is superior to patients who achieve a partial response (PR) to treatment. In addition, the issue of whether local therapy directed solely to involved areas provides similar long-term results compared to therapy directed to both lesional and uninvolved skin has never been formally studied in a clinical trial. However, it is well known that the cutaneous manifestations of early MF are often clinically subtle or unapparent, and that such lesions often become "unmasked" when treatment such as topical HN2 chemotherapy or PUVA are administered to most of the skin surface. This phenomenon seems to be analogous to the effect of topically applied 5-fluorouracil on photodamaged skin.

If the goal of treatment is to induce a sustained CR and hopefully cure in clinically early MF, then it would seem desirable to deliver topical treatment to as much of the skin surface as possible in order not to miss areas of subtle involvement. For these reasons, the author generally recommends that skin-directed treatments be administered to both involved and uninvolved skin areas for most patients with CTCL with the intention of inducing a CR (and hopefully cure in early MF). The major exceptions are patients with only one lesion (unilesional MF) or perhaps two lesions in which local treatment alone may be curative, and patients of advanced age or poor general health where the impact of the CTCL on survival is likely not to be important and palliative treatment is acceptable.

## Treatment Options

A number of therapeutic modalities have activity in CTCL. The treatments that are frequently utilized for skin manifestations (skin-directed therapy) include surgical excision of solitary lesions, high potency topical corticosteroids, and bexarotene gel which are administered only to lesional skin, while ultraviolet phototherapy, PUVA, topical chemotherapy with HN2 or BCNU, and radiation therapy may be administered also to clinically uninvolved skin if desired. Treatments that may be given for systemic effects include relatively well-tolerated agents that dermatologists often utilize and more intensive treatments that are usually administered by medical oncologists at least in the United States. The first group (those used by dermatologists) includes systemic corticosteroids, bexarotene (Targretin), interferon alfa or gamma, methotrexate, ECP or an alkylating drug such as chlorambucil (Leukeran), and the second group (those administered by oncologists) includes denileukin diftitox (Ontak), pentostatin (Nupent) or another purine nucleoside analog, and multidrug regimens. For selected patients with advanced CTCL, high-dose chemotherapy supported by stem cell or bone marrow transplantation has also been utilized.

The selection of which external therapy or combination of therapies should be utilized to achieve a CR is best individualized to the particular patient's situation. A composite experience with the common skin-directed therapies is shown in Table 1. To avoid misleading conclusions, the reader is cautioned not to use the average response rates given in the Table 1 to draw conclusions about the relative efficacy among the various treatments because of differences that exist among patients selected for each treatment, e.g., although the average CR rate for patients with patch/plaque MF who are treated with PUVA and TSEB appears to be comparable, it is likely that most patients who receive total skin electron beam have relatively more advanced disease than patients selected for PUVA.

The effectiveness of conventional ultraviolet phototherapy (broad-band UVB or heliotherapy) is limited to patients with patch phase disease with CR rates of about 70% (higher CR rates in patients with fair complexions, lower CR rates in patients with dark complexions). Long-term disease-free intervals off treatment occurred in 23% of patients in one series (Resnik and Vonderheid 1993). The CR rates reported for PUVA monotherapy are about 80% (range 58–100%). As with UVB phototherapy, skin complexion probably influences response rates but to a lesser degree, and patients with plaque phase disease respond better to treatment. CRs are more difficult to achieve in patients with widespread skin involvement because lesions may persist in skin areas that are shielded from ultraviolet exposure. Topical chemotherapy with HN2 or BCNU has the advantage of not requiring a specialized facility for treatment and the entire skin surface can be treated if desired. The reported CR rate with topical HN2 is about 65% (range 37–82%) and depends on the formulation of the drug utilized for treatment (lower CR rate with anhydrous ointment, higher CR rate with aqueous solution) and whether treatment is given locally or to the entire skin surface. The CR rate achieved with topical

**Table 1.** Composite experience with external therapies used in patch and plaque phase mycosis fungoides (*UV-B* broad-band ultraviolet phototherapy, *PUVA* oral methoxsalen photochemotherapy, *HN2* mechlorethamine, *BCNU* carmustine, *TSEB* total skin electron beam)

| Modality | No. of series[a] | No. of patients | Complete remission | |
|---|---|---|---|---|
| | | | Number | % (range) |
| UV-B[b] | 3 | 205 | 139 | 68 (32–75) |
| PUVA | 9 | 312 | 245 | 79 (58–100) |
| Topical HN2 | 7 | 697 | 440 | 63 (37–82) |
| Topical BCNU | 1 | 109 | 72 | 66 |
| TSEB | 8 | 701 | 552 | 79 (46–100) |

[a] Ten or more cases in series
[b] Mostly patch phase

BCNU is similar to that with topical HN2 although this result was derived from only one series. Thicker plaques or nodules or lesions involving the scalp, palms or soles may not respond adequately to topical HN2 whereas such lesions may respond to topical BCNU or PUVA presumably because these agents penetrate more deeply into the dermis.

Long-term CRs after treatment is discontinued (probable cures) have been observed for both topical HN2 and BCNU, but such a result is not yet established for PUVA. Total skin electron beam (TSEB) is regarded as the most effective external therapy with reported CR rates of about 80% (range 46–100%) for patch/plaque phase MF. The advantage of radiation therapy is that thicker, more infiltrated lesions respond more completely than to other topical therapies. However, no significant beneficial effect on overall survival has been shown for patients treated with TSEB compared to those treated with topical HN2 chemotherapy.

Thus, for most patients with clinically early MF, the author's practice is to treat patients initially with either PUVA or topical HN2 chemotherapy to as much of the skin surface as possible in an attempt to induce a CR (and possible cure), and to utilize TSEB as a primary treatment for patients with widespread involvement with thick plaques and/or nodules.

The probability that a CR attained from a skin-directed therapy will be durable is related to the extent of skin surface involvement in patients without overt extracutaneous involvement (stage I to III). For example, patients with unilesional MF are more likely to remain clear after local field radiation than patients with two or three lesions (Wilson et al. 1998), and patients with less than 10% involvement of the skin surface with patch/plaque phase MF (T1 skin rating) are less apt to experience recurrence of disease following topical chemotherapy, PUVA, or TSEB than patients with more extensive involvement. Patients with non-Sézary erythrodermic CTCL (T4 skin rating) also have a high rate of disease recurrence after a CR is achieved, similar to patients with extensive plaque phase disease.

For patients whose disease recurs off treatment, intermittent or sustained therapy will be required for disease control and consideration should be given to agents and treatment regimens that minimize the potential for adverse side effects related to chronic treatment such as the induction of other skin cancers. For example, conventional UVB might be preferred over topical chemotherapy or PUVA for long-term control of patch phase MF in patients with persistent or recurrent disease despite initial treatment with curative intent. There appears to be no difference between topical HN2 chemotherapy and PUVA in terms of long-term side effects as both treatments given chronically increase the incidence of basal and squamous cell carcinomas. Treatment delivered to involved skin areas only may be preferred in this situation.

## A Stratified Approach to Treatment

Based on the above considerations, the author's approach is to administer skin-directed therapies with "curative intent" initially to patients with patch/ plaque MF or non-Sézary erythrodermic CTCL with biologically non-aggressive disease and overt disease manifestations limited to the skin because a substantial proportion of these patients achieve a sustained CR without the need for chronic maintenance therapy. The selection of a skin-directed therapy is typically made between topical HN2 chemotherapy and PUVA because both treatments can be administered to most or all of the skin surface (involved and uninvolved) and both provide high CR rates without undue toxicity. Ultraviolet phototherapy is not preferred for initial treatment because of the lower potential to induce a sustained CR, and TSEB usually is reserved for patients with numerous thick plaques and is often combined with an adjunct therapy (see below). In the author's experience, successful therapy with topical HN2 chemotherapy or PUVA, i.e., long-term control or in some instances cure, occurs in most patients with disease at stage Ia (T1N0), many with stage Ib or IIa (T2N0, T1–2N1) disease and occasional patients with stage III (T4N0–1) disease.

For many patients with extensive or advanced skin involvement, a skin-directed therapy alone would in most instances be inadequate to keep the disease under long-term control and supplemental local or adjuvant systemic therapy is often beneficial. Many of these patients have relatively thick plaques or tumors or involvement of problematic areas such as the face, scalp, genitals, palms or soles. In addition, patients who have evidence of a dominant T-cell clone in the skin and blood (presumably circulating malignant T cells) should be considered as candidates for combined topical and adjuvant systemic therapy in the author's opinion. In terms of staging, such patients tend to have disease at Ib or IIa (T2N0–1), IIb (T3N0–1), or III (T4N0–1). Localized administration of BCNU solution or radiation may be useful to clear any individual resistant lesion in patients treated with topical HN2 chemotherapy or PUVA. For patients with multiple persistent lesions despite treatment with topical HN2 chemotherapy or PUVA, consideration should be given to adding a relatively well-tolerated systemic drug that can be utilized for prolonged intervals such as interferon alfa, bexarotene, methotrexate or ECP to the regimen in an effort to improve the response. For example, interferon alfa may be utilized to enhance the clearing potential of PUVA. An alternative approach is to administer low-dose TSEB to promote clearing of skin lesions, then resume topical HN2 chemotherapy or PUVA along with adjuvant systemic therapy. A similar treatment strategy, i.e., administration of a well-tolerated agent that has systemic effects combined with a skin-directed therapy, is also sometimes successful for patients with overt lymph node or blood involvement such as Sézary syndrome, provided that the disease is not behaving in a biologically aggressive fashion.

For patients who have highly aggressive intracutaneous disease at stage IIb (T3N0–1) and most patients with overt involvement of lymph nodes, blood or visceral organs at stage IV (T2–4N3M0–1 or T2–4N0–1B2M0–1), long-term control is unlikely and treatment is typically given with palliative intent. If transformation to large-cell lymphoma has occurred, intensive treatment with multiagent systemic drugs or total body photon radiation is usually required for initial control and remissions are seldom long-lasting. Stem cell or bone marrow transplantation regimens should be considered for relatively young and healthy patients. Topical HN2 chemotherapy, PUVA or TSEB can be combined with intensive systemic treatment to promote the clearing of skin lesions.

## New and Emerging Treatments

Recent reports on small numbers of patients indicate that narrow-band UVB (312 nm) and UVA1 (340–400 nm) are better tolerated and at least equally effective as conventional broad-band UVB ultraviolet phototherapy or PUVA in clinically early MF (Clark et al 2000; Zane et al. 2001). As with PUVA, the probable mechanism of action of ultraviolet radiation is through the induction of apoptosis by neoplastic T cells. The fact that UVA1 ultraviolet radiation penetrates more deeply into the dermis than the other wavelengths of ultraviolet radiation makes this ultraviolet source of particular interest for treatment of CTCL.

Photodynamic therapy with photosensitizers other than 8-methoxypsoralen is another emerging treatment approach for CTCL. Activity has been demonstrated for topically applied 5-aminolevulinic acid although treatment is somewhat painful (Wolf et al. 1994). Hypericin, a photodynamic compound derived from the plant St. John's Wort and activated by either UVA or visible radiation, is another drug that might be useful in this regard (Fox et al. 1998).

The future systemic therapy of CTCL will likely reflect the development of cytotoxic drugs that selectively target malignant T cells relative to their normal counterparts, biologic approaches that enhance antitumor immunologic responses, and perhaps gene and protein transduction therapies that correct intracellular defects in malignant T cells. Immunotoxins, which satisfy Paul Ehrlich's concept of a "magic bullet" for cancer treatment, selectively kill tumor cells by binding to cell surface markers expressed primarily by malignant cells and a number of such agents have been introduced recently for treatment of other lymphomas. Denileukin diftitox, a diphtheria immunotoxin that binds to the a-chain of the interleukin-2 receptor (Tac or CD25), is the first immunotoxin to become available for treatment of CTCL (Olsen et al. 2001). Other agents that are under investigation include anti-Tac(Fv)-PE38 and RFT5-SMPT-dgA which are anti-CD25 immunotoxins linked to *Pseudomonas* endotoxin and ricin A-chain respectively, and a humanized anti-CD25 antibody that is radiolabeled with yttrium-90.

Immunomodulatory cytokines or other drugs that augment innate antitumor mechanisms and restore the imbalance that exists between $T_H1$ and $T_H2$ cell function in advanced CTCL is another promising approach that is under investigation. Both interferon alfa and gamma are utilized successfully for the treatment of CTCL, and preliminary experience with recombinant interleukin-2 and recombinant interleukin-12 (rIL-12) likewise shows promise (Baccard et al 1997; Rook et al. 1999). The antitumor activity of rIL-12 seems to be mediated through induction of antitumor $CD8^+$ cytotoxic T-cell responses (Rook et al. 1999). Antitumor cellular therapy using T cells primed to react against tumor-specific antigens or dendritic cells that are loaded with tumor-specific antigens is an area of great potential in CTCL because of laboratory evidence that neoplastic T cells express tumor-associated antigens (Berger et al. 1998). Indeed the major mechanism underlying the activity of photopheresis in CTCL is thought to involve the processing of tumor cell antigens present on ECP-induced apoptotic neoplastic T cells that have been ingested by ECP-induced dendritic cells.

Other immunotherapeutic approaches include vaccination of patients with synthetic peptides based on genes encoding these tumor-associated antigens or DNA plasmids that express the variable region of the T-cell receptor beta chain. Another novel approach that might be utilized in advanced CTCL is allogeneic hematopoietic stem cell transplantation to confer a graft-versus-tumor effect against neoplastic T cells (Burt et al. 2000). The risk of severe graft-versus-host disease might be minimized by use of donor cells modified to contain a "suicide" gene such as herpes simplex thymidine kinase, which makes the donor cells susceptible to killing by ganciclovir (Link et al. 2000). Alternatively ECP might be used in such patients to suppress graft-versus-host reactions.

## References


Baccard M, Marolleau JP, Rybojad M (1997) Middle-term evolution of patients with advanced cutaneous T-cell lymphoma treated with high-dose recombinant interleukin-2. Arch Dermatol 133:656

Berger CL, Longley J, Imaeda S, Christensen I, Heald P, Edelson RL (1998) Tumor-specific peptides in cutaneous T-cell lymphoma: association with class I major histocompatibility complex and possible derivation from the clonotypic T-cell receptor. Int J Cancer 76:304–311

Burt RK, Guitart J, Traynor A, Link C, Rosen S, Pandolfino T, Kuzel TM (2000) Allogeneic hematopoietic stem cell transplantation for advanced mycosis fungoides: evidence of a graft-versus-tumor effect. Bone Marrow Transplant 25:111–113

Clark C, Dawe RS, Evans AT, Lowe G, Ferguson J (2000) Narrowband TL-01 phototherapy for patch-stage mycosis fungoides. Arch Dermatol 136:748–752

de Coninck EC, Kim YH, Varghese A, Hoppe RT (2001) Clinical characteristics and outcome of patients with extracutaneous mycosis fungoides. J Clin Oncol 19:779–784

Delfau-Larue M-H, Laroche L, Wechsler J, Lepage E, Lahet C, Asso-Bonnet M, Bagot M, Farcet J-P (2000) Diagnostic value of dominant T-cell clones in peripheral blood in 363 patients presenting consecutively with a clinical suspicion of cutaneous lymphoma. Blood 96:2987–2992

Fox FE, Niu Z, Tobia A, Rook AH (1998) Photoactivated hypericin is an anti-proliferative agent that induces a high rate of apoptotic death of normal, transformed, and malignant T lymphocytes: implications for the treatment of cutaneous lymphoproliferative and inflammatory disorders. J Invest Dermatol 111:327–332

Fraser-Andrews EA, Woolford AJ, Russell-Jones R, Seed PT, Whittaker SJ (2000) Detection of a peripheral blood T cell clone is an independent prognostic marker in mycosis fungoides. J Invest Dermatol 114:117–121

Gellrich S, Lukowsky A, Schilling T, Rutz S, Muche JM, Jahn S, Audring H, Sterry W (2000) Microanatomical compartments of clonal and reactive T cells in mycosis fungoides: molecular demonstration by single cell polymerase chain reaction of T cell receptor gene rearrangements. J Invest Dermatol 115:620–624

Hoppe RT, Medeiros J, Warnke RA, Wood GS (1995) CD8-positive tumor-infiltrating lymphocytes influence the long-term survival of patients with mycosis fungoides. J Am Acad Dermatol 32:448–453

Jones GW, Hoppe RT, Glatstein E (1995) Electron beam treatment for cutaneous T-cell lymphoma. Hematol Oncol Clin North Am 9:1057–1076

Kim YH, Hoppe RT (1999) Mycosis fungoides and the Sézary syndrome. Semin Oncol 26:276–289

Link CJ, Seregina T, Traynor A, Burt RK (2000) Cellular suicide therapy of malignant disease. Stem Cells 18:220–226

Muche J, Lukowsky A, Ahnhudt C, Gellrich S, Sterry W (2000) Peripheral blood T cell clonality in mycosis fungoides: an independent prognostic marker? J Invest Dermatol 115:504–505

Olsen E, Duvic M, Frankel A, Kim Y, Martin A, Vonderheid E, Jegasothy B, Wood G, Gordon M, Heald P, Oseroff A, Pinter-Brown L, Bowen G, Kuzel T, Fivenson D, Foss F, Glode M, Molina A, Knobler E, Stewart S, Cooper K, Stevens S, Craig F, Reuben J, Bacha P, Nichols J (2001) Pivotal phase III trial of two dose levels of denileukin diftitox for the treatment of cutaneous T-cell lymphoma. J Clin Oncol 19:367–388

Resnik KS, Vonderheid EC (1993) Home ultraviolet phototherapy of early mycosis fungoides: long-term follow-up observations. J Am Acad Dermatol 29:73–77

Rook AH, Heald P (1995) The immunopathogenesis of cutaneous T-cell lymphoma. Hematol Oncol Clin North Am 9:997–1010

Rook AH, Wood GS, Yoo EK, Elenitsas R, Kao DMF, Sherman ML, Witmer WK, Rockwell KA, Shane RB, Lessin SR, Vonderheid EC (1999) Interleukin-12 therapy of cutaneous T-cell lymphoma induces lesion regression and cytotoxic T-cell responses. Blood 94:902–908

Sausville EA, Eddy JL, Makuch RW, Fischmann AB, Schechter GP, Matthews M, Glatstein E, Ihde DC, Kaye F, Veach SR, Phelps R, O'Connor T, Trepel JB, Cotelingam JD, Gazdar AF, Minna JD, Bunn PA Jr (1988) Histopathologic staging at initial diagnosis of mycosis fungoides and the Sézary syndrome: definition of three distinctive prognostic groups. Ann Intern Med 109:372–382

Tensen CP, Vermeer MH, van der Stoop PM, van Beek P, Scheper RJ, Boorsma DM, Willemze R (1998) Epidermal interferon-gamma inducible protein-10 (IP-10) and monokine induced by gamma-interferon (Mig) but not IL-8 mRNA expression is associated with epidermotropism in cutaneous T cell lymphomas. J Invest Dermatol 111:222–226

van Doorn R, Van Haselen CW, van Voorst Vader PC, Geerts M-L, Heule F, de Rie M, Steijlen PM, Dekker SK, van Vloten WA, Willemze R (2000) Mycosis fungoides: disease evolution and prognosis in 309 Dutch patients. Arch Dermatol 136:504–510

Vonderheid EC, Diamond LW, Lai SM, Au F, Dellavecchia M (1992) Lymph node histopathologic findings in cutaneous T-cell lymphoma. Am J Clin Pathol 97:121–129

Vonderheid EC, Bernengo MG, Burg G, Duvic M, Heald P, Laroche L, Olsen E, Pittelkow M, Russell-Jones R, Takigawa M, Willemze R (2002) Update on erythrodermic cutaneous T cell lymphoma: report of the International Society for Cutaneous Lymphomas. J Am Acad Dermatol 46:95–106

Wilson LD, Kacinski BM, Jones GW (1998) Local superficial radiotherapy in the management of minimal stage Ia cutaneous T-cell lymphoma (mycosis fungoides). Int J Radiat Oncol Biol Phys 40:109–115

Wolf P, Fink-Puches R, Cerroni L, Kerl H (1994) Photodynamic therapy for mycosis fungoides after topical photosensitization with 5-aminolevulinic acid. J Am Acad Dermatol 31:678–680

Zane C, Leali C, Airò P, De Panfilis G, Pinton PC (2001) "High-dose" UVA1 therapy of widespread plaque-type, nodular, and erythrodermic mycosis fungoides. J Am Acad Dermatol 44:629–633

# New Biologic Agents for the Treatment of Cutaneous T-Cell Lymphoma

Carmela C. Vittorio, Jacqueline M. Junkins-Hopkins, Karen S. McGinnis, Michael Shapiro, Maria Wysocka, Mohamed H. Zaki, Lars E. French, and Alain H. Rook

## Abstract

Cutaneous T-cell lymphoma (CTCL) is typically a skin-infiltrating malignancy of clonally derived CD4$^+$ T lymphocytes. Because the host antitumor response appears to play an important role in disease control, systemic therapeutic agents are used in such a manner as to preserve the integrity of the host antitumor response while selectively targeting the malignant cells. The new biologic response-modifying treatment options currently used to treat CTCL are reviewed.

## Introduction

Cutaneous T-cell lymphoma (CTCL) is typically a lymphoproliferative disorder of clonally derived skin-infiltrating malignant CD4$^+$ T lymphocytes [1]. Diagnosis of the disease in its early stages is often difficult as both the clinical presentation and the histology may not be conclusive. Most patients initially present with erythematous, scaling patches or plaques involving less than 20% of the skin surface. Ultimately, lesions may progress to tumors, and blood and visceral organ involvement may occur. Patients may also develop erythroderma or tumors de novo. The leukemic form of the disease, Sézary syndrome, is characterized by circulating atypical lymphocytes with convoluted nuclei referred to as Sézary cells. T-cell receptor gene rearrangement studies utilizing polymerase chain reaction amplification of reverse-transcribed isolated RNA from peripheral blood mononuclear cells may show circulating clonal T cells even at very early stages of the disease. Peripheral blood involvement at any stage of skin disease signifies a poorer prognosis.

The prognosis is based on stage of the disease at the time of diagnosis. Patients who present with less than 10% skin involvement with patches (stage 1A), if treated, have the same survival as age-matched controls [2]. Patients with erythroderma have 5-year survivals of approximately 40% [1].

Recent Results in Cancer Research, Vol. 160<br>© Springer-Verlag Berlin Heidelberg 2002

Among erythrodermic patients, over 70% of patients have evidence of malignant T cells within the peripheral blood.

## Therapy of Early CTCL

Among patients with limited patch- or plaque-stage disease who receive treatment, progression to serious systemic disease occurs in only 10%. Moreover, the cell-mediated immune response is typically normal. Thus, the majority of these patients can be treated effectively with skin-directed therapies [3, 4]. Such therapies include topical steroids, topical mechlorethamine, topical carmustine, psoralen plus ultraviolet A light (PUVA), and notably, a new effective topical retinoid, bexarotene (discussed below). A significant percentage of patients who use these modalities achieve long-lasting remissions of their disease [5]. Given that a large percentage of the malignant clonal T cells are located within the skin, the host antitumor response most likely mediates an effect outside the skin that presumably eradicates microscopic foci of malignant cells at extracutaneous sites, thus contributing to the success of skin-directed therapy at this stage. Combinations of potent chemotherapeutic drugs are not recommended as they do not appear to cure patients with early disease. Moreover, survival of patients with advanced disease is not prolonged by chemotherapy [6].

## Decline in the Immune Response in Advanced CTCL

In advanced CTCL, especially in patients with Sézary syndrome, there is a decline in the cell-mediated immune response [7]. The production of cytokines necessary for the activation and differentiation of cell-mediated immunity such as interferon gamma (IFN$\gamma$) and interleukin-2 (IL-2), which are produced by T-helper type 1(Th1) cells and IL-12, produced principally by monocyte/macrophages and dendritic cells, becomes depressed with advancing disease. The production of immunosuppressive cytokines, such as IL-4 and IL-10, by malignant T cells directly contributes to the depressed cell-mediated immunity [3, 8]. IL-4 and IL-10 are produced by T-helper type 2 (Th-2) cells and both suppress the production and antagonize the effects of IFN$\gamma$ and IL-2 from Th1 cells [9]. IL-10 negatively regulates the production of IL-12 which regulates the development of cytotoxic T-cell responses [10]. The increased tumor cell burden in advanced CTCL coupled with the associated imbalance between Th1 and Th2 cytokines leads to a profound defect in cell-mediated immunity. Newer treatment strategies with biologic response modifiers, used both singly and particularly in combination, target the tumor cell burden and augment the immune response to the disease.

## Bexarotene

Bexarotene (Targretin) capsules were approved in 1999 by the US Food and Drug Administration for the treatment of all stages of CTCL. Bexarotene is the first of a new class of drugs that bind to the retinoid X receptor (RXR). The antiproliferative and immune potentiating effects of retinoids have long been recognized. Previously available retinoids exerted their effect by binding to the retinoic acid receptors resulting in regulation of cell growth and differentiation. RXR-specific retinoids are thought to regulate apoptosis, or programmed cell death, which may be defective in CTCL [11].

Clinical trials involved patients with both refractory early-stage and refractory advanced disease. The optimum dose of bexarotene which achieved either complete response (complete resolution of all measurable disease) or partial response ($\geq$50% improvement in disease symptoms) for four or more study weeks was 300 mg/m$^2$/day. In patients with refractory or persistent early-stage CTCL the overall response rate was 54%. The overall response rate in patients with refractory or persistent advanced-stage CTCL was 45% at this dosage [12]. Responses have been observed among patients with extensive tumor-stage disease that has been associated with large-cell transformation.

Since the side effects seem to be dose-related, lower doses can be used initially and increased as needed. Nevertheless, efficacy does appear to be dose-related. In our institution, patients are generally started at 150 mg/day, and increased if necessary based on the clinical response. Many of our patients are on combination biologic therapy which appears to permit lowering the dosage of bexarotene necessary to achieve the desired clinical response. Every 3–4 months CD4$^+$ T-cell counts can be followed in Sézary patients by flow cytometry.

The most common adverse events that occur with oral bexarotene are dose-dependent hypertriglyceridemia, hypercholesterolemia, and hypothyroidism. Acute pancreatitis has also been reported. Other side effects include elevated liver enzymes, headache and leukopenia. Bexarotene decreases serum thyrotropin and free thyroxine, thus causing a central hypothyroidism. The degree of suppression is greater in patients treated with higher doses of bexarotene and in those with a history of treatment with interferon alpha (IFN$a$) [13]. Patients have both low TSH and low T4 levels. Treatment is with levothyroxine and should be based upon serum free T4 levels. Laboratory abnormalities normalize with discontinuation of bexarotene.

Marked hypertriglyceridemia can occur within days of beginning treatment with bexarotene. Therefore biweekly monitoring should be done until the patient is stabilized on fenofibrate, atorvastatin, or both. Gemfibrozil must not be used as it worsens hypertriglyceridemia by increasing the serum concentration of bexarotene. We currently recommend initiation of fenofibrate at a dose of 134 mg daily concurrent with initiation of bexarotene therapy.

Bexarotene in a topical 1% gel formulation has also recently been approved. It is indicated for the treatment of stage IA and IB CTCL. An overall response rate of 59% has been reported with twice daily application in patients with early-stage CTCL. Adverse events were restricted to the application site and consisted of irritation, redness, scaling, pruritus and burning pain of usually mild to moderate degree [12]. The gel should be started on an every-other-day basis and gradually increased to twice daily in an effort to minimize irritation.

It is important to stress that both bexarotene capsules and gel are rated as pregnancy category X.


## DAB389-Interleukin-2

DAB389-IL-2 (Ontak) is a recombinant cytotoxic fusion protein that targets the IL-2 receptor on T cells. The molecule combines the receptor binding domain of IL-2 with diphtheria toxin. Once bound to the IL-2 receptor, it is taken up by endocytosis, the diphtheria toxin portion is cleaved and protein synthesis is inhibited [14]. The clinical trials for this agent selected patients with refractory disease and the presence of the CD25 IL-2 receptor on T cells. Patients with advanced stage IIB disease showed a 38% response rate with improvement in quality of life [15].

The drug is administered intravenously for five consecutive days repeated every 3 weeks. Recommended doses are 9 µg/kg per day or 18 µg/kg per day administered over 1 h. Response rates and adverse effects are slightly, but not significantly more frequent at the higher dose. Patients with advanced tumor-stage disease will respond to this therapeutic agent. Symptoms with the infusion are similar to those seen with IFN and IL-2 administration, specifically fever, chills, nausea and a capillary leak syndrome seen about 10 days after treatment. A small percentage of patients have experienced a hypersensitivity reaction associated with acute back pain and hypotension. These adverse effects may be diminished by the pre- and posttreatment infusion of saline and by the use of 4 mg dexamethasone administered twice daily during periods of drug treatment and for several days after its conclusion.


## Recombinant Interferon Alpha

Because Th1 cytokines support antitumor immunity and induce cytotoxic T cells, newer therapeutic strategies have focused on the use of these cytokines to boost the host cell-mediated response to malignant cells. IFNα has been the most frequently used. A significant clinical response is achieved in 50–80% of patients [16, 17]. It is administered subcutaneously, intramuscularly, or intralesionally to plaques and tumors. Although the ideal dose and frequency of administration are not defined, at our institution IFNα is initiated at low doses of between 1 and 1.5 MU subcutaneously three times weekly. Over several weeks the dose is slowly escalated to 3–5 MU three to four times weekly. Symptoms such as chills, fever, headache, myalgia, loose stools, and fatigue are minimized by using a protocol of slow dose escalation. Dosing of IFN prior to bedtime with acetaminophen also minimizes the 'flu-like symptoms.

Induction of an initial clinical response requires 2–5 months of continuous therapy. A maximal response typically requires longer periods of treatment. Maintenance therapy is suggested for any significantly responding patient or for any patient with advanced disease (multiple tumors or erythroderma) as the risk of clinical relapse is high. More frequent administration and higher dose regimens may be employed before abandoning therapy [18].

Recent reports have suggested that IFN$\alpha$ in combination with retinoids yield additional benefits over either treatment alone [19, 20]. Bexarotene orally, in combination with IFN$\alpha$, has been used in our institution and has shown promising results and is well tolerated. We recently treated a patient with skin-restricted, multifocal, persistent CD30$^+$ large T-cell lymphoma with bexarotene and IFN$\alpha$. All the skin lesions regressed and remission was induced after 6 months of treatment. For patients with tumors radiation therapy is initially used. This is followed by long-term IFN$\alpha$ and bexarotene to prevent relapse. IFN$\alpha$ can also be used in combination with topical chemotherapy and PUVA [21]. Sézary syndrome patients treated with extracorporeal photopheresis (ECP) and IFN$\alpha$ appear to derive additional benefit over those treated with either agent alone [22].

The effects of IFN$\alpha$ and other biologic response modifiers on the behavior of malignant cells has been assessed in vitro. IFN$\alpha$ inhibits the proliferative capacity of malignant T cells in response to growth-stimulatory factors such as IL-2, IL-7, and IL-4 [23]. IFN$\alpha$ also inhibits the increased production of IL-4 and IL-5 by malignant T cells [24]. In effect, IFN$\alpha$ has the ability to reverse the immunosuppressive effect of IL-4 and the eosinophilopoietic effect of IL-5. IFN$\alpha$ may also enhance other antitumor immune responses such as cell-mediated cytotoxicity [25].


## Recombinant Interferon Gamma

Experience with IFN$\gamma$ has been much more limited than with IFN$\alpha$. IFN$\gamma$ has been shown to inhibit Th2 cytokine production by malignant T lymphocytes [3]. In one study of 16 CTCL patients, most of whom had advanced disease and had failed one or more treatment modalities, five patients showed significant partial responses with a median duration of response of 10 months. The patients were treated with the maximal tolerated dose of 0.5 mg/m$^2$ [26]. The side effects are similar to those of IFN$\alpha$. For patients who have developed treatment resistance to IFN$\alpha$, possibly due to the development of neutralizing antibodies, IFN$\gamma$ may offer an alternative adjunctive treatment modality. Clearly, more data is needed regarding the potential benefit of this agent for different stages of CTCL.

## Recombinant Interleukin-12

The rationale for the use of IL-12 in CTCL is based on its ability to induce the production of IFNγ by T cells and natural killer cells, and to stimulate cytotoxic T-cell activity [8]. IL-12 also decreases IL-4 production by malignant T cells in vitro [27]. Patients with advanced CTCL have a marked defect in IL-12 production which may be a result of increased production of IL-10 by malignant T cells [8]. In a phase I dose-escalation trial, IL-12 exhibited marked activity when administered intralesionally or subcutaneously with the disappearance of injected tumors or plaques [28]. Subcutaneous dosing resulted in complete responses in two of five plaque patients and partial responses in two of five plaque, and one of two Sézary syndrome patients, for an overall response rate of 56% (five of nine) [28]. In a more recent phase II trial responses were seen in 10 of 23 patients [29]. Future clinical trials combining IL-12 with other immune augmentary cytokines are in the planning stage.

## Extracorporeal Photopheresis

ECP is a leukapheresis-based procedure in which approximately $10^{10}$ 8-methoxypsoralen-treated peripheral blood mononuclear cells are exposed to 1–2 J of ultraviolet A light. The light-exposed cells are returned to the patient. This entire procedure is carried out on two consecutive days every 3 to 5 weeks. The light-activated psoralen has been demonstrated to cause apoptotic death of the treated cells [30]. It is hypothesized that tumor antigens are released during apoptosis, followed by processing by antigen-presenting cells. This leads to the development of a systemic antitumor response due to the induction of anticlonotypic immunity directed against pathogenic clones of T lymphocytes [31].

Our experience with carefully studied patients screened for the presence of peripheral blood involvement with a dominant malignant T-cell population (by T-cell receptor gene rearrangement PCR, by thin section detection of Sézary cells in buffy coats, or by flow cytometry for elevated numbers of $CD4^+/CD7^-$ cells) shows that CTCL patients who lack evidence of peripheral blood disease are much less likely to respond to ECP than patients with leukemic involvement. The ideal candidates for ECP are those with modest to low numbers of circulating atypical cells with a reasonably intact immune response characterized by normal or near-normal numbers of circulating $CD8^+$ and $CD56^+$ cells [22]. Patients who have been immunosuppressed by prior chemotherapy and patients with markedly elevated white blood counts with large numbers of malignant peripheral blood cells usually do not respond to photopheresis as a single treatment agent. For these patients IFNα and bexarotene are added. Topical chemotherapy, PUVA, topical steroids, and electron beam radiation can be used in addition to these modalities. A recent study has demonstrated that for erythrodermic CTCL patients, ECP given concurrently or shortly following total skin electron beam significantly improves progression-free survival compared with total skin electron beam without ECP [32].

## Conclusion

Advanced forms of CTCL are optimally treated with a combination of immune enhancing biologic response modifiers. Skin tumor burden can also be diminished by using topical therapy, phototherapy, and electron beam radiation [33–35]. Biologic response modifiers in combination with photopheresis are used for those with the leukemic phase of the disease. Among the majority of advanced stage patients so treated, immune response augmentation appears to prolong survival [36].

## References


1. Diamandidou E, Cohen PR, Kurzrock R (1996) Mycosis fungoides and Sézary syndrome. Blood 88:2385–2409
2. Kim YH, Chow S, Varghese A, et al (1999) Clinical characteristics and long-term outcome of patients with generalized patch or plaque (T2) mycosis fungoides. Arch Dermatol 135:26–32
3. Vowels BR, Cassin M, Vonderheid E, et al (1992) Aberrant cytokine production by Sézary syndrome patients: cytokine secretion pattern resembles murine Th2 cells. J Invest Dermatol 99:90–94
4. Kin YH, Jensen RA, Watanabe GL, et al (1996) Clinical stage IA (limited patch and plaque) mycosis fungoides. A long-term outcome analysis. Arch Dermatol 132:1309–1313
5. Vonderheid EC, Tan ET, Kantor AF, et al (1989) Long term efficacy, curative potential, and carcinogenicity of topical mechlorethamine chemotherapy in cutaneous T-cell lymphoma. J Am Acad Dermatol 20:416–428
6. Kaye FJ, Bunn PA Jr, Steinberg SM, et al (1989) A randomized trial comparing combination electron-beam radiation and chemotherapy with topical therapy in the initial treatment of mycosis fungoides. N Engl J Med 321:1784–1790
7. Rook AH, Lessin SR, Jaworsky C, et al (1993) Immunopathogenesis of cutaneous T-cell lymphoma: abnormal cytokine production by Sézary T-cells. Arch Dermatol 129:486–489
8. Rook AH, Kubin M, Cassin M, et al (1995) Interleukin 12 reverses cytokine and immune abnormalities in Sézary syndrome. J Immunol 154:1491–1498
9. Peleman R, Wu J, Rargeas C, et al (1989) Recombinant interleukin 4 suppresses the production of interferon gamma by human mononuclear cells. J Exp Med 170:1751–1756
10. D'Andrea A, Aste-Amea M, Valiante NM, et al (1993) Interleukin-10 inhibits human lymphocyte IFN-$\gamma$ production by suppressing natural killer stimulatory factor/interleukin-12 synthesis in accessory cells. J Exp Med 178:1041–1048
11. Boehm MF, Heyman RA, Nagpal S (1997) A new generation of retinoid drugs for the treatment of dermatological disease. Emerging Drugs 2:287–303
12. Lowe MN, Plosker GL (2000) Bexarotene. Am J Clin Dermatol 1:245–250
13. Sherman S, Gopal J, Haugen BR, et al (1999) Central hypothyroidism associated with retinoid X receptor-selective ligands. N Engl J Med 340:1075–1079
14. Nichols J, Foss F, Kuzel TM, et al (1997) Interleukin-2 fusion protein: an investigational therapy for interleukin-2 receptor expressing malignancies. Eur J Cancer 33:S34–S36
15. Duvic M, Cather JC, Maize J, et al (1998) DAB389IL-2 diphtheria fusion toxin reduces clinical responses in tumor stage cutaneous T-cell lymphoma. Am J Hematol 58:78–90
16. Olsen EA, Bunn PA (1995) Interferon in the treatment of cutaneous T-cell lymphoma. Hematol Clin North Am 9:1089–1107

17. Olsen EA, Rosen ST, Vollmer RT, et al (1989) Interferon alpha 2a in the treatment of cutaneous T-cell lymphoma. J Am Acad Dermatol 20:395–407

18. Rook AH, Yoo EK, Grossman DJ, et al (1998) Use of biological response modifiers in the treatment of cutaneous T-cell lymphoma. Curr Opin Oncol 10:170–174

19. Knobler RM, Radaszkiewicz T (1991) Treatment of cutaneous T-cell lymphoma with a combination of low-dose interferon alfa 2b and retinoids. J Am Acad Dermatol 24:247–252

20. Dreno B, Celorier P, Litroux P (1993) Roferon-A in combination with Tegason in cutaneous T-cell lymphomas. Acta Haematol 89 [Suppl 1]:28–32

21. Kuzel TM, Gilyon K, Springer E, et al (1990) Interferon alfa-2a combined with phototherapy in the treatment of cutaneous T-cell lymphoma. J Natl Cancer Inst 82:203–207

22. Gottlieb SL, Wolfe JT, Fox FE, et al (1996) Treatment of cutaneous T-cell lymphoma with extracorporeal photopheresis monotherapy and with recombinant interferon alfa. J Am Acad Dermatol 35:946–957

23. Fox FE, Niu Z, Lessin S, et al (1997) Cytokine regulation of the growth of clonal malignant T-cells from patients with Sézary syndrome (abstract). J Invest Dermatol 108:552

24. Gottlieb SL, Fox FE, Cassin M, et al (1995) Interleukin 5 expression by peripheral blood mononuclear cells in Sézary syndrome correlates with peripheral eosinophilia and is suppressed by interferon alfa (abstract). J Invest Dermatol 104:683

25. Platsoucas CD, Fox FE, Oleszak E, et al (1989) Regulation of natural killer cytotoxicity by recombinant alpha interferons: augmentation by IFN-alpha 7, an interferon similar to IFN-alpha. J Anticancer Res 9:849–858

26. Kaplan EH, Rosen ST, Norris DB, et al (1990) Phase II study of recombinant human interferong for treatment of cutaneous T-cell lymphoma. J Natl Cancer Inst 82:208–212

27. Fox FE, Kubin M, Cassin M, et al (1999) Retinoids synergize with interleukin-12 to augment IFN-gamma and interleukin-12 production by human peripheral blood mononuclear cells. J Interferon Cytokine Res 19:407–415

28. Rook AH, Wood GS, Yoo EK, et al (1999) Interleukin-12 Therapy of cutaneous T-cell lymphoma induces lesion regression and cytotoxic T-cell responses. Blood 94:902–908

29. Rook AH, Foss F, Wood G, et al (2000) A phase 2 open-label study reveals that recombinant human interleukin-12 (rhIL-12) is efficacious in patients with early stage cutaneous T-cell lymphoma (CTCL) (abstract). J Invest Dermatol 114:880

30. Yoo EK, Rook AH, Elenitsas R, et al (1996) Apoptosis induction by ultraviolet A and photochemotherapy in cutaneous T-cell lymphoma: relevance to mechanism of therapeutic action. J Invest Dermatol 107:235–242

31. Rook AH, Suchin KR, Kao DMF, et al (1999) Photopheresis: clinical applications and mechanisms of action. J Invest Dermatol Symp Proc 4:85–89

32. Wilson LD, Jones GW, Kim D, et al (2000) Experience with total skin electron beam therapy in combination with extracorporeal photopheresis in the management of patients with erythrodermic (T4) mycosis fungoides. J Am Acad Dermatol 43:54–60

33. Kuzel TM, Roenigk HH, Samuelson E, et al (1995) Effectiveness of interferon alfa-2a combined with phototherapy for mycosis fungoides and the Sézary syndrome. J Clin Oncol 13:257–263

34. Ramsey DL, Meller JA, Zackheim HS (1995) Topical treatment of early cutaneous T-cell lymphoma. Hematol Oncol Clin North Am 9:1031–1056

35. Clark C, Dawe RS, Evans AT, et al (2000) Narrowband TL-01 phototherapy for patch-stage mycosis fungoides. Arch Dermatol 136:748–752

36. Suchin KR, DeNardo B, Macey W, et al (2000) Treatment of cutaneous T-cell lymphoma with combined immunomodulatory therapy: a 15-year experience at a single institution. Pacific Dermatologic Association; 13–17 Sept 2000; Victoria, British Columbia

# Mesenchymal Tumors   **6**

# Etiology and Pathogenesis of Kaposi's Sarcoma

Brian J. Nickoloff and Kimberly E. Foreman

## Abstract

*Objective:* To provide an overview of the role for HHV-8 as the causative agent responsible for Kaposi's sarcoma, the molecular cross-talk between HHV-8 and HIV-1, and the ability of specific cytokines to influence the pathophysiology of this malignancy. *Patients:* Normal human skin grafts were studied using a SCID mouse xenograft model system in which engrafted skin was injected intradermally with HHV-8 and/or HIV-1, and the subsequent induction of clinical, histologic, and viral titer changes were assessed in serial fashion. *Results:* Following intradermal injection of HHV-8 into engrafted normal human skin, cutaneous lesions resembling Kaposi's sarcoma were created in numerous different grafts. These lesions were characterized by routine light microscopy as well as by immunophenotypic and molecular virological assessments. As several grafts injected with HHV-8 failed to develop Kaposi's sarcoma, we sought to determine whether another cofactor was required and this led us to uncover the ability of HHV-8 and HIV-1 to reciprocally influence each other using both in vitro and in vivo studies. Given the importance of various cytokines, the influence of scatter factor and IFN-$\gamma$ in the pathophysiology of Kaposi's sarcoma was also evaluated. *Conclusion:* Based on these in vivo studies using SCID mice engrafted with human skin and injected with HHV-8, we conclude that HHV-8 is the etiologic agent in Kaposi's sarcoma, and that HIV-1 and HHV-8 can influence each other involving both direct and indirect cross-talk mechanisms.

## Introduction

Kaposi's sarcoma (KS) is a multifocal neoplasm of likely vascular origin characterized by spindle-shaped tumor cells, angiogenesis, extravasated erythrocytes, edema and a mononuclear cell infiltrate. Originally described in the late 1800s by Moritz Kaposi, KS was considered a relatively benign disease occur-

Recent Results in Cancer Research, Vol. 160
© Springer-Verlag Berlin Heidelberg 2002

ring predominantly in elderly men of Mediterranean and Eastern European origin (classic KS). Patients typically present with discrete reddish-brown to brown-violet plaques, which over time can develop into tumor nodules. While the lesions can be disfiguring and cause considerable pain, classic KS is seldom life-threatening. However, three other forms of KS have since been described. Post-transplantation (iatrogenic) KS arises in allograft recipients receiving immunosuppressive therapy, endemic (African) KS occurs mainly in children and young adults in subequatorial Africa, and AIDS-related (epidemic) KS occurs in HIV-infected individuals. Both African and AIDS-KS are more aggressive forms of the disease, which commonly involve visceral and lymphatic organs and have a poor prognosis. Unlike conventional malignancies, rather than being formed by cloned expansion of a transformed cell, KS lesions appear to develop as hyperplastic tissue reactions mediated by local production of cytokines and growth factor (Gallo 1998 a).

Recognition of cutaneous KS lesions in otherwise healthy homosexual males was one of the first signs of the impending AIDS epidemic (Friedman-Kien et al. 1981). As the epidemic spread, KS emerged as the most common neoplasm in these patients affecting up to 20% of HIV-1-positive individuals. The disease is particularly aggressive in the context of HIV-1 infection with approximately 12% of AIDS-KS patients dying due to complications related to KS and the remaining patients suffering significant morbidity. Since the introduction of highly active antiretroviral therapy (HAART), the incidence of KS has declined dramatically (up to a 70% reduction in KS among HIV-positive individuals has been reported) (Jacobson et al. 1999). However, KS still remains the most common neoplasm in these patients, and with HAART failure occurring in over 50% of treated patients, KS continues to be a significant healthcare problem (Bower et al. 1999; Deeks et al. 1999).

The pathogenesis of KS is complex and currently unclear. The exact blend and interrelationships between HIV-1, human herpesvirus 8 (HHV-8), cytokines, and growth factors responsible for producing KS lesions remain to be defined at the molecular level (Ganem 1995). However, the discovery of HHV-8 from KS lesions in 1994 by Chang, Moore and co-workers marked a turning point in our understanding of this disease (Chang et al. 1994). The etiologic agent of KS has now been identified, and studies are currently focused on how this virus actually causes KS. In this chapter the roles of HHV-8 (the etiologic agent of KS), HIV-1 (an important potential cofactor in AIDS-KS) and cytokines in the development of this disease are reviewed with a focus on various model systems, particularly animal models, for studying KS pathogenesis.

## HHV-8: The Etiologic Agent of KS

HHV-8, which is also known as KS-associated herpesvirus (KSHV), is a member of the $\gamma$2-herpesvirus family and is most closely related to Epstein-Barr virus (EBV) and herpesvirus saimiri (HVS). HHV-8 shares a number of features typical of herpesviruses including a large, double stranded DNA genome, replication within the nucleus, and the ability to establish persistent infection within its natural host cell. HHV-8 is stably maintained as an episome in latently infected cells during which time only a small subset of viral genes are expressed (Sarid et al. 1998). During reactivation, the viral genome replicates, progeny virions are produced, and the host cell is ultimately destroyed. It is of interest that HHV-8 does not appear to be ubiquitous. While most herpesviruses have infected a large proportion of the population (EBV and CMV have infected over 95% and 75% of adults, respectively), seroepidemiologic data indicates only a small percentage of normal blood donors (between 3% and 25% in the USA) have been infected with HHV-8 (Gao et al. 1996).

Strong evidence supports the conclusion that HHV-8 is necessary for the development of KS. First, HHV-8 DNA has been detected in virtually all KS lesions including all four epidemiologic forms of KS as well as in all stages of the disease. In contrast, HHV-8 is rarely found in other tumors, with the notable exception of two lymphoproliferative disorders, primary effusion lymphoma (PEL), and a subset of multicentric Castleman's disease (MCD). HHV-8 infects the spindle-shaped tumor cells within the lesions, and nearly all the tumor cells in late-stage lesions are latently infected. Second, serologic studies have found that a majority of KS patients (80–100%) have specific antibodies to HHV-8 antigens. Seropositivity rates, while low in normal donors, are dramatically increased in populations at risk for developing KS, such as HIV-positive homosexual males. Finally, seropositivity or detection of the HHV-8 genome DNA in peripheral blood predicts future development of KS. Whitby et al. found that 54.5% of HIV-1-positive patients without KS went on to develop the disease if HHV-8 was detectable in their peripheral blood mononuclear cells (PBMCs) compared with 9% of those who showed no evidence of HHV-8 infection (Whitby et al. 1995). While these findings individually do not establish causation, taken together they indicate that HHV-8 is the etiologic agent of KS.

It is, however, currently unclear how HHV-8 causes KS. Two scenarios could be considered based on our current knowledge: (1) HHV-8 might play a critical role in creating the necessary microenvironment for lesion development through autocrine/paracrine mechanisms; or (2) HHV-8 might directly transform cells. These scenarios are not necessarily mutually exclusive. It has been postulated that KS begins as a hyperplastic proliferation mediated by growth factors and angiogenic factors, which, under certain conditions, becomes a true malignancy as the disease progresses (Gallo 1998a). Recently, Cesarman and colleagues have demonstrated that infection of cultured endothelial cells with HHV-8 results in cellular transformation, as determined by long-term proliferation and cell survival (Flore et al. 1998). However, only 1–6% of the cells in culture were infected with HHV-8, indicating that paracrine mechanisms were responsible for extending survival of the uninfected cells (Flore et al. 1998).

The HHV-8 genome encodes for more than 85 open reading frames (ORFs) including over 70 conserved genes with sequence similarity to other herpesviruses (many of which encode for replication-associated enzymes and proteins) and approximately 15 additional genes (designated K1 to K15) which appear to be unique to this virus. Many of these genes encode for homologs of cellular proteins and candidate transforming genes, which may play a role in KS pathogenesis. It is of particular interest that HHV-8 encodes genes that inhibit apoptosis (vBcl-2 and vFLIP), promote cell cycle dysregulation (v-cyclin, LANA), and function as cytokines/chemokines (vIL-6, vMIP-1, -II and -III). In addition, HHV-8-encoded proteins (including vMIPs and vGPCR) have been shown to induce angiogenesis either directly or through induction of VEGF secretion, which may promote the neovascularization characteristic of KS lesions (Bais et al. 1998). For interested readers, several excellent review articles have detailed descriptions of these genes and their individual functions (Katano and Sata 2000; Sarid et al. 1999; Schulz 1998).

Although these viral genes/proteins have the potential to alter normal cellular functions contributing to the initiation or progression of KS, many studies are currently focused on determining whether they are expressed in HHV-8-related tumors and how their expression is regulated. Preliminary evidence indicates that there may be important differences in HHV-8 gene regulation in KS, PEL, and MCD. For example, vIL-6 is constitutively expressed at low levels in PEL cell lines, and has been detected in both PEL and MCD biopsies at both the mRNA and protein level; however, there is no evidence of vIL-6 expression in KS lesions (Parravicini et al. 2000). These studies indicate that viral protein expression can be differentially regulated in vivo, in vitro and in different cell types, and that information gained on viral gene expression from PEL cell lines in vitro may not accurately reflect expression in KS, PEL or MCD lesions in vivo (Parravicini et al. 2000). Furthermore, localization studies have demonstrated that a majority of KS cells are latently infected with HHV-8 with only a small proportion of tumor cells undergoing lytic cycle replication (Staskus et al. 1997). Therefore, viral proteins expressed during either the latent or lytic cycle may be important in the paracrine stimulation of the cells within the tumor while only proteins produced during latency are likely to be responsible for cellular transformation.

## HIV-1 and AIDS-KS

Current evidence suggests HHV-8 infection is necessary, but not sufficient, for the development of KS. Indeed, HHV-8 infection alone cannot explain the different clinical forms of KS, the aggressive nature of AIDS-KS or the prevalence of the disease in men. Additional cofactors, such as hormones, genetic predisposition, and/or coinfection with other infectious agents, appear to be necessary for disease development. While HIV-1 infection is clearly not required for KS development, HIV-1 is thought to play an important role in the pathogenesis of AIDS-KS, particularly in explaining the unusually aggressive behavior of this form of the disease. Studies have shown that KS tumor cells themselves are not infected with HIV-1. Therefore, HIV-1 does not appear to play a direct oncogenic role in AIDS-KS. However, it is currently unclear what role HIV-1 plays in KS, and whether HIV simply induces immunosuppression or plays a more direct part in the pathogenesis of this disease is still debated.

Current evidence indicates that immunosuppression alone is unlikely to explain the role of HIV-1 in AIDS-KS. First, there is an overwhelming prevalence of KS in AIDS patients compared with other immunosuppressed patient populations (Beral et al. 1990). Second, KS occurs at all CD4 counts including CD4 levels that are not associated with increased opportunistic infections (Ahmed et al. 2001). Finally, there is an overwhelming association of KS in patients infected with HIV-1, but not in those with HIV-2 (Ariyoshi et al. 1998). Therefore, many investigators have proposed that HIV-1 plays a more direct role in AIDS-KS, and have hypothesized that this role involves cytokines produced in response to HIV-1 infection and production of the HIV-1 Tat protein (Gallo 1998b).

It is well recognized that cytokines are essential to the growth and proliferation of KS tumor cells, and investigators have shown that a variety of cytokines are important in the pathogenesis of KS – including hepatocyte growth factor/scatter factor (HGF/SF), oncostatin M (OSM), IL-1$\beta$, TNF-$\alpha$, IFN-$\gamma$, transforming growth factor $\beta$ (TGF-$\beta$), granulocyte-macrophage colony-stimulating factor (GM-CSF), IL-6, bFGF and platelet-derived growth factor (PDGF) (Polverini and Nickoloff 1995; Ensoli and Sirianni 1998). These cytokines are produced by both autocrine and paracrine mechanisms within the KS lesion to create the necessary microenvironment for tumor initiation and progression.

While it is difficult to determine the exact source of particular cytokines within the KS lesions, clues can be gathered from studying isolated KS cells and HIV-1-infected T cells, monocyte/macrophages and dendritic cells in vitro. KS cells in culture have been shown to produce and release biologically active cytokines, such as bFGF, IL-1$\beta$, PDGF, GM-CSF and IL-6. These cytokines not only act as autocrine growth factors, but also stimulate the proliferation of normal endothelial cells and induce angiogenesis. However, studies performed on isolated KS tumor cells may tell only part of the story as KS cells grown in culture are not infected with HHV-8 (except during early passages) (Foreman et al. 1997). It is currently unknown what effect, if any, HHV-8 infection has on cytokine production and secretion by these cells in vivo. HIV-1-infected cells, including T cells, monocyte/macrophages and dendritic cells, have been shown to secrete inflammatory cytokines such as TNF-$\alpha$ and IL-1$\beta$, and HIV-1-infected patients have been shown to have higher circulating levels of IL-1, IL-3, IL-4, IFN-$\gamma$, TNF-$\alpha$, TNF-$\beta$, TGF-$\beta$ and OSM, probably as a result of chronic viral infection and stimulation of the immune system (Alonso et al. 1997).

While cytokines are clearly important to the growth and proliferation of KS tumor cells, they may also play an important role in induction of HHV-8 replication. A cytokine-driven increase in HHV-8 could be important in increasing the local HHV-8 viral load and explaining the aggressive nature of AIDS-related KS. Studies in our laboratory have recently shown that soluble factors produced by, or in response to, HIV-1-infected T cells induce HHV-8 replication and the production of progeny virions (Mercader et al. 2000). These studies have identified OSM, HGF/SF and IFN-$\gamma$, but not IL-6, IL-2 and TNF-$\alpha$, as cytokines that induce HHV-8 replication. Similar studies by other groups also identified IFN-$\gamma$ as a cytokine that induces HHV-8 replication, but found no effect by TNF-$\alpha$, IL-1, IL-2, IL-6, GM-CSF or bFGF (Blackbourn et al. 2000; Chang et al. 2000; Monini et al. 1999).

In addition to cytokines, HIV-1 Tat protein may play an important role in the pathogenesis of AIDS-KS. Tat is an 86 amino acid protein whose primary function is to increase the processivity of RNA polymerase II and to increase transcription initiation (Gaynor 1995). While HIV-1-infected cells produce Tat intracellularly to facilitate HIV replication, these cells also release soluble Tat protein (Ensoli et al. 1993). Tat can enter neighboring cells through a receptor-independent mechanism, and may directly interact with cellular genes to alter their expression. For example, Tat protein has been shown to increase expression of the TNF-$\beta$ gene, but not the genes encoding for IL-1 and IL-6 in in vitro studies (Buonaguro et al. 1994). Soluble Tat can also bind to both $\alpha_v\beta_3$ and $\alpha_5\beta_1$ integrins. Integrins are receptors for extracellular matrix proteins that are critical to endothelial cell adhesion, migration and invasion. Tat competes with natural integrin ligands to bind to $\alpha_v\beta_3$ and $\alpha_5\beta_1$ through a highly conserved Arg-Gly-Asp (RGD) sequence in the carboxy terminus, and this interaction may function to induce intracellular signals that ultimately lead to changes in gene expression (Barillari et al. 1993).

Studies have demonstrated a variety of biologic activities associated with Tat protein, which may be important in KS pathogenesis. For example, Tat protein has been shown to activate cells (particularly normal endothelial cells and KS tumor cells) resulting in cytokine production, adhesion molecule expression and increased growth, proliferation and migration (Ensoli et al. 1990, 1993; Hofman et al. 1993). Tat protein has also been shown to have angiogenic properties. Recent studies have shown that Tat binds to and activates the tyrosine kinase receptor FLK-1/KDR, a known receptor for VEGF (Albini et al. 1996; Ganju et al. 1998). As KDR is expressed in KS, this may provide a mechanism by which Tat induces angiogenesis in this disease (Skobe et al. 1999). In addition, Tat may play a role in KS pathogenesis by inducing HHV-8 replication (Harrington et al. 1997). Recent studies by Huang et al indicate that coexpression of Tat protein in HHV-8-infected PEL cell lines results in increased expression of HHV-8 ORF25 mRNA (major capsid protein) suggesting that Tat protein may induce reactivation of this virus (Huang et al. 2001).

## Reciprocal Interactions Between HIV and HHV-8

As the studies mentioned above indicate that HIV-1 may alter HHV-8 replication, investigators have begun to evaluate the effect of HHV-8 on HIV-1 replication. Previous studies have demonstrated that coinfection with herpesviruses can modulate HIV-1 replication. This can occur either through a direct interaction between the viruses infecting the same cell or through stimulation by cellular factors produced in response to the herpesvirus infection (Griffiths 1995). This modulation can be either an enhancement of HIV replication (for example, CMV has been shown to transactivate the HIV-1 LTR) or an inhibition (for example, HHV-7 has been shown to compete with HIV for binding to the CD4 receptor). Studies in our laboratories have recently demonstrated that coculture of HIV-1-infected T cells with HHV-8-infected PEL cell lines results in a significant increase in HIV replication as determined by p24 ELISA and reverse transcriptase assays (Mercader et al. 2001). This result was confirmed using an in vivo model system (see below). Injection of purified HHV-8- and HIV-1-infected T cells into human skin transplanted on an immunodeficient mouse resulted in enhanced HIV-1 replication compared to control animals injected with PBS as a control. Studies by Huang et al. (2001) have also demonstrated induction of HIV-1 replication in the presence of HHV-8. They fused an HIV-1-infected cell with an HHV-8-infected cell to create a cell that was infected with both viruses. Although coinfection of cells has not been demonstrated in vivo, these studies show that the ORF45 gene product is able to act synergistically with Tat to activate the HIV-1 LTR (Huang et al. 2001).

## Models for the Pathogenesis of KS

An ongoing problem in the study of KS has been the lack of an appropriate in vivo model system to study the disease. Isolated KS tumor cells have provided invaluable information regarding KS, but studies have consistently shown that HHV-8 is lost from the culture after a few passages (Foreman et al. 1997). When injected into the skin of nude mice, these cells cause transient, angiogenic lesions of mouse origin which resemble early KS (Salahuddin et al. 1988). Similar lesions can be induced by injecting nude mouse skin with conditioned medium from KS cells, bFGF or HIV-1 Tat protein (Ensoli et al. 1994; Nakamura et al. 1992). To date, only a few immortalized KS tumor cell lines have been described, including the SLK and KSY-1 cell lines (Herndier et al. 1994; Lunardi-Iskandar et al. 1995). These cells, which are not infected with HHV-8, readily produce tumors in nude mice (Lunardi-Iskandar et al. 1995). Although these models lack HHV-8 infection, they are well-characterized, reproducible models, which can be used to study various aspects of KS including novel therapeutic approaches, which do not directly target HHV-8 replication.

Recent studies involving HHV-8 have also attempted to demonstrate production of either KS or lymphoproliferative diseases following expression of HHV-8-encoded proteins or infection with the virus. Yang et al. have recently demonstrated that transgenic mice expressing HHV-8 vGPCR transgene under control of the CD2 promoter in NK and T cells develop multicentric erythematous lesions which are histologically similar to KS (Yang et al. 2000). As this model does not contain HHV-8 and very few of the cells within the lesions express vGPCR, the model underscores the importance of paracrine mechanisms in the development of vascular proliferation. In contrast, Dittmer et al. have recently reported HHV-8 infection of CD19[+] B cells in severe combined immunodeficient (SCID) mice implanted with human fetal thymus and liver grafts (Dittmer et al. 1999). HHV-8 infection was limited to the implant, and the animals did not develop KS-like lesions. However, the authors used this model to demonstrate that ganciclovir interferes with both establishment and maintenance of HHV-8 infection in CD19[+] B cells. These findings confirm and extend earlier studies looking at antiviral agents in experiments using PEL cell lines.

Returning to the ORF74 of HHV-8 (i.e. GPCR), it should be noted that it has the highest homology to human CXC chemokine receptor (CXCR) 2 (Cesarman et al. 1996). When this gene is overexpressed in NIH 3T3 cells, upon injection into nude mice, highly vascular tumors develop (Arvantakis et al. 1997; Bais et al. 1998; Schwarz and Murphy 2001). Constitutive signaling by HHV-8 vGPCR induces VEGF production and the transcription factor AP-1 (Arvantakis et al. 1997; Bais et al. 1998; Schwarz and Murphy 2001). While VEGF by itself cannot induce KS, several other proinflammatory cytokines, chemokines and growth factors are produced such as IL-1$\beta$, TNF-$\alpha$, IL-6, IL-8, MCP-1, and bFGF (Schwarz and Murphy 2001). Taken together, these results support a view of KS in which an infectious disease is converted into a hyperplastic tissue response created by locally produced cytokines and growth factors that act in a paracrine and autocrine fashion (Kirshner et al. 1999).

Recently, we have developed a new model for KS using human skin engrafted on SCID mice. This well-characterized system involves transplantation of normal human skin onto SCID mice, resulting in a graft with retention of clinical, histologic, and immunologic characteristics that are remarkably similar to pretransplanted skin (Nickoloff et al. 1995). Injection of this normal human skin with HHV-8 results in a thickened, erythematous lesion after 16–18 weeks, which are not found in control mice injected with heat-killed HHV 8 preparations (Foreman et al. 2001). These lesions are consistent with KS including the presence of angiogenesis, spindle-shaped cells with morphologic and phenotypic characteristics similar to KS tumor cells in vivo (Foreman et al. 2001). In addition, the spindle-shaped cells can be isolated from the lesion, grown in culture and are latently infected with HHV-8 as demonstrated by immunohistochemical staining for ORF73, RT-PCR and Southern blot analysis (Foreman et al. 2001). It is of interest that only 60% of animals injected with KS-derived HHV-8 develop lesions. It is currently unclear whether the lack of consistent lesion development is due to genetic differences related to the human skin donor, to differences in individual mice, or to the absence of an additional cofactor that is necessary to induce KS-like lesions reproducibly. Ongoing studies are focused on determining what factors are necessary to produce KS-like lesions consistently in this model. While still in development, this new model may complement and extend previous KS models for the study of disease pathogenesis as well as evaluation of new therapeutic agents.

## Summary

During the past decade, considerable progress has been made in advancing our understanding of the etiology and pathophysiology of this enigmatic disease. Despite a greater appreciation of the etiologic role HHV-8 and HIV-1 play in KS, and elucidation of the cytokine network that participates in the pathogenesis of KS, many questions remain unanswered. Future challenges will include: further refinements in the aforementioned model systems to more reliably and realistically reflect bona fide KS lesion; clarification of the role of cofactors that are necessary and sufficient to create KS besides HHV-8; identification of the cell of origin of KS (i.e. vascular/lymphatic endothelial cell versus bone marrow-derived cell); the specific contribution of virus-derived or host cell-derived genes that contribute not only to early patch-/plaque-stage lesions, but ultimately to the creation of more aggressive tumor-stage lesions; and the development of better therapeutic reagents that target key molecular mediators to avoid non-specific toxicities or side effects that can be particularly damaging to immunocompromised patients.

**Acknowledgements.** This work was supported in part by Public Health Service Grants CA76951 and CA86435 from the National Institutes of Health.

## References

Ahmed A, Isa MS, Garba HA, Kalayi GD, Muhammad I, Egler LJ (2001) Influence of HIV infection on presentation of Kaposi's sarcoma. Trop Doct 31:42–45

Albini A, Soldi R, Giunciuglio D, Giraudo E, Benelli R, Primo L, Noonan D, Salio M, Camussi G, Rockl W, Bussolino F (1996) The angiogenesis induced by HIV-1 tat protein is mediated by the Flk-1/KDR receptor on vascular endothelial cells. Nat Med 2:1371–1375

Alonso K, Pontiggia P, Medenica R, Rizzo S (1997) Cytokine patterns in adults with AIDS. Immunol Invest 26:341–350

Ariyoshi K, Schim v d L, Cook P, Whitby D, Corrah T, Jaffar S, Cham F, Sabally S, O'Donovan D, Weiss RA, Schulz TF, Whittle H (1998) Kaposi's sarcoma in the Gambia, West Africa is less frequent in human immunodeficiency virus type 2 than in human immunodeficiency virus type 1 infection despite a high prevalence of human herpesvirus 8. J Hum Virol 1:193–199

Arvanitakis L, Geras-Raaka LE, Varma A, Gershengorn MC, Cesarman E (1997) Human herpesvirus KSHV encodes a constitutively active G-protein-coupled receptor linked to cell proliferation. Nature 385:347–350

Bais C, Santomasso B, Coso O, Arvanitakis L, Raaka EG, Gutkind JS, Asch AS, Cesarman E, Gerhengorn MC, Mesri EA (1998) G-protein-coupled receptor of Kaposi's sarcoma-associated herpesvirus is a viral oncogene and angiogenesis activator. Nature 391:86–89

Barillari G, Gendelman R, Gallo RC, Ensoli B (1993) The Tat protein of human immunodeficiency virus type 1, a growth factor for AIDS Kaposi sarcoma and cytokine-activated vascular cells, induces adhesion of the same cell types by using integrin receptors recognizing the RGD amino acid sequence. Proc Natl Acad Sci U S A 90:7941–7945

Beral V, Peterman TA, Berkelman RL, Jaffe HW (1990) Kaposi's sarcoma among persons with AIDS: a sexually transmitted infection? Lancet 335:123–128

Blackbourn DJ, Fujimura S, Kutzkey T, Levy JA (2000) Induction of human herpesvirus-8 gene expression by recombinant interferon gamma. AIDS 14:98–99

Bower M, Fox P, Fife K, Gill J, Nelson M, Gazzard B (1999) Highly active anti-retroviral therapy (HAART) prolongs time to treatment failure in Kaposi's sarcoma. AIDS 13:2105–2111

Buonaguro L, Buonaguro FM, Tornesello ML, Beth-Giraldo E, Del Gaudio E, Ensoli B, Giraldo G (1994) Role of HIV-1 Tat in the pathogenesis of AIDS-associated Kaposi's sarcoma. Antibiot Chemother 46:62–72

Cesarman ER, Nador G, Bai F, Bohenzky RA, Russo JJ, Moore PS, Chang Y, Knowles DM (1996) Kaposi's sarcoma-associated herpesvirus contains G protein-coupled receptor and cyclin D homologs which are expressed in Kaposi's sarcoma and malignant lymphoma. J Virol 70:8218–8223

Chang J, Renne R, Dittmer D, Ganem D (2000) Inflammatory cytokines and the reactivation of Kaposi's sarcoma-associated herpesvirus lytic replication. Virology 266:17–25

Chang Y, Cesarman E, Pessin MS, Lee F, Culpepper J, Knowles DM, Moore PS (1994) Identification of herpesvirus-like DNA sequences in AIDS-associated Kaposi's sarcoma. Science 266:1865–1869

Deeks SG, Hecht FM, Swanson M, Elbeik T, Loftus R, Cohen PT, Grant RM (1999) IIIV RNA and CD4 cell count response to protcase inhibitor therapy in an urban AIDS clinic: rcsponse to both initial and salvage therapy. AIDS 13:F35–F43

Dittmer D, Stoddart C, Renne R, Linquist-Stepps V, Moreno ME, Bare C, McCune JM, Ganem D (1999) Experimental transmission of Kaposi's sarcoma – associated herpesvirus (KSHV/HHV-8) to SCID-hu Thy/Liv mice. J Exp Med 190:1857–1868

Ensoli B, Sirianni MC (1998) Kaposi's sarcoma pathogenesis: a link between immunology and tumor biology. Crit Rev Oncog 9:107–124

Ensoli B, Barillari G, Salahuddin SZ, Gallo RC, Wong-Staal F (1990) Tat protein of HIV-1 stimulates growth of cells derived from Kaposi's sarcoma lesions of AIDS patients. Nature 345:84–86

Ensoli B, Buonaguro L, Barillari G, Fiorelli V, Gendelman R, Morgan RA, Wingfield P, Gallo RC (1993) Release, uptake, and effects of extracellular human immunodeficiency virus type 1 Tat protein on cell growth and viral transactivation. J Virol 67:277–287

Ensoli B, Gendelman R, Markham P, Fiorelli V, Colombini S, Raffeld M, Cafaro A, Chang HK, Brady JN, Gallo RC (1994) Synergy between basic fibroblast growth factor and HIV-1 Tat protein in induction of Kaposi's sarcoma. Nature 371:674–680

Flore O, Rafii S, Ely S, O'Leary JJ, Hyjek EM, Cesarman E (1998) Transformation of primary human endothelial cells by Kaposi's sarcoma-associated herpesvirus. Nature 394:588–592

Foreman KE, Friborg J, Kong W, Woffendin C, Polverini PJ, Nickoloff BJ, Nabel GJ (1997) Propagation of a human herpesvirus from AIDS-associated Kaposi's sarcoma. N Engl J Med 336:163–171

Foreman KE, Friborg J, Chandran B, Katano H, Sata T, Mercader M, Nabel GJ, Nickoloff BJ (2001) Injection of human herpesvirus-8 in human skin engrafted on SCID mice induces Kaposi's sarcoma-like lesions. J Dermatol Sci 26:182–193

Friedman-Kien AE, Lauberstein L, Marmor M, Hymes K, Green J, Ragaz A, Gottlieb J, Muggia F, Demopoulos R, Weintraub M, Williams D (1981) Kaposi's sarcoma and pneumocystis pneumoniae among homosexual men: New York City and California. MMWR Morb Mortal Wkly Rep 30:305–308

Gallo RC (1998a) The enigmas of Kaposi's sarcoma. Science 282:1837–1838

Gallo RC (1998b) Some aspects of the pathogenesis of HIV-1 associated Kaposi's sarcoma. J Natl Cancer Inst Monogr 23:55–57

Ganem D (1995) AIDS: Viruses, cytokines and Kaposi's sarcoma. Curr Biol 5:469–479

Ganju RK, Munshi N, Nair BC, Liu ZY, Gill P, Groopman JE (1998) Human immunodeficiency virus tat modulates the Flk-1/KDR receptor, mitogen-activated protein kinases, and components of focal adhesion in Kaposi's sarcoma cells. J Virol 72:6131–6137

Gao SJ, Kingsley L, Li M, Zheng W, Parravicini C, Ziegler J, Newton R, Rinaldo CR, Saah A, Phair J, Detels R, Chang YA, Moore PS (1996) KSHV antibodies among Americans, Italians, and Ugandans with and without Kaposi's sarcoma. Nat Med 2:925–928

Gaynor RB (1995) Regulation of HIV-1 gene expression by the transactivator protein Tat. Curr Top Microbiol Immunol 193:51–77

Griffiths PD (1995) Interaction between herpesviruses and HIV. Curr Opin Infect Dis 8:479–482

Harrington WJ, Sieczkowski L, Sosa C, Chan-a-Sue S, Cai JP, Cabral L, Wood C (1997) Activation of HHV-8 by HIV-1 tat. Lancet 349:774–775

Herndier BG, Werner A, Arnstein P, Abbey NW, Demartis F, Cohen RL, Shuman MA, Levy JA (1994) Characterization of a human Kaposi's sarcoma cell line that induces angiogenic tumors in animals. AIDS 8:575–581

Hofman FM, Wright AD, Dohadwala MM, Wong-Staal F, Walker SM (1993) Exogenous tat protein activates human endothelial cells. Blood 82:2774–2780

Huang LM, Chao MF, Chen MY, Shih HM, Chiang YP, Chuang CY, Lee CY (2001) Reciprocal regulatory interaction between human herpesvirus 8 and human immunodeficiency virus type 1. J Biol Chem 276:13427–13432

Jacobson LP, Yamashita TE, Detels R, Margolick JB, Chmiel JS, Kingsley LA, Melnick S, Munoz A (1999) Impact of potent antiretroviral therapy on the incidence of Kaposi's sarcoma and non-Hodgkin's lymphomas among HIV-1-infected individuals. Multicenter AIDS Cohort Study. J Acquir Immune Defic Syndr 21 [Suppl 1]:S34–S41

Katano H, Sata T (2000) Human herpesvirus 8-virology, epidemiology and related diseases. Jpn J Infect Dis 53:137–155

Kirshner JR, Staskus K, Haase A, Lagunoff M, Ganem D (1999) Expression of the open reading frame 74 (G-protein-coupled receptor) gene of Kaposi's sarcoma (KS)-associated herpes virus: implications for KS pathogenesis. J Virol 73:6006–6014

Lunardi-Iskandar Y, Gill P, Lam VH, Zeman RA, Michaels F, Mann DL, Reitz MS, Kaplan M, Berneman ZN, Carter D (1995) Isolation and characterization of an immortal neoplastic cell line (KS Y-1) from AIDS-associated Kaposi's sarcoma. J Natl Cancer Inst 87:974–981

Mercader M, Taddeo B, Panella JR, Chandran B, Nickoloff BJ, Foreman KE (2000) Induction of HHV-8 lytic cycle replication by inflammatory cytokines produced by HIV-1-infected T cells. Am J Pathol 156:1961–1971

Mercader M, Nickoloff BJ, Foreman KE (2001) Induction of human immunodeficiency virus 1 replication by human herpesvirus 8. Arch Pathol Lab Med 125:785–789

Monini P, Colombini S, Sturzl M, Goletti D, Cafaro A, Sgadari C, Butto S, Franco M, Leone P, Fais S, Melucci-Vigo G, Chiozzini C, Carlini F, Ascheri G, Cornali E, Zietz C, Ramazzotti E, Ensoli F, Andreoni M, Pezzotti P, Rezza G, Yarchoan R, Gallo RC, Ensoli B (1999) Reactivation and persistence of human herpesvirus-8 infection in B-cells and monocytes by Th-1 cytokines increased in Kaposi's sarcoma. Blood 93:4044–4058

Nakamura S, Sakurada S, Salahuddin SZ, Osada Y, Tanaka NG, Sakamoto N, Sekiguchi M, Gallo RC (1992) Inhibition of development of Kaposi's sarcoma-related lesions by a bacterial cell wall complex. Science 255:1437–1440

Nickoloff BJ, Kunkel SL, Burdick M, Strieter RM (1995) Severe combined immunodeficiency mouse and human psoriatic skin chimeras. Validation of a new animal model. Am J Pathol 146:580–588

Parravicini C, Chandran B, Corbellino M, Berti E, Paulli M, Moore PS, Chang Y (2000) Differential viral protein expression in Kaposi's sarcoma-associated herpesvirus infected diseases. Kaposi's sarcoma, primary effusion lymphoma and multicentric Castleman's disease. Am J Pathol 156:743–749

Polverini PJ, Nickoloff BJ (1995) Role of scatter factor and the c-met protooncogene in the pathogenesis of AIDS-associated Kaposi's sarcoma. Adv Cancer Res 66:235–253

Salahuddin SZ, Nakamura S, Biberfeld P, Kaplan MH, Markham PD, Larsson L, Gallo RC (1988) Angiogenic properties of Kaposi's sarcoma-derived cells after long-term culture in vitro. Science 242:430–433

Sarid R, Flore O, Bohenzky RA, Chang Y, Moore PS (1998) Transcription mapping of the Kaposi's sarcoma-associated herpesvirus (human herpesvirus 8) genome in a body cavity-based lymphoma cell line (BC-1). J Virol 72:1005–1012

Sarid R, Olsen SJ, Moore PS (1999) Kaposi's sarcoma-associated herpesvirus: epidemiology, virology, and molecular biology. Adv Virus Res 52:139–232

Schulz TF (1998) Kaposi's sarcoma-associated herpesvirus (human herpesvirus-8). J Gen Virol 79:1573–1591

Schwarz M, Murphy PM (2001) Kaposi's sarcoma-associated herpesvirus G protein-coupled receptor constitutively activates NF-$\kappa$B and induces proinflammatory cytokine and chemokine production via a C-terminal signaling determinant. J Immunol 167:505–513

Skobe M, Brown LF, Tognazzi K, Ganju RK, Dezube BJ, Alitalo K, Detmar M (1999) Vascular endothelial growth factor-C (VEGF-C) and its receptors KDR and flt-4 are expressed in AIDS-associated Kaposi's sarcoma. J Invest Dermatol 113:1047–1053

Staskus KA, Zhong WD, Gebhard K, Herndier B, Wang H, Renne R, Beneke J, Pudney J, Anderson DJ, Ganem D, Hasse AT (1997) Kaposi's sarcoma-associated herpesvirus gene expression in endothelial (spindle) tumor cells. J Virol 71:715–719

Whitby D, Howard MR, Tenant-Flowers M, Brink NS, Copas A, Boshoff C, Hatzioannou T, Suggett FE, Aldam DM, Denton AS, Miller RF, Weller IVD, Weiss RA, Tedder RS, Schulz TF (1995) Detection of Kaposi sarcoma associated herpesvirus in peripheral blood of HIV-infected individuals and progression to Kaposi's sarcoma. Lancet 346:799–802

Yang TY, Chen SC, Leach MW, Manfra D, Homey B, Wiekowski M, Sullivan L, Jenh CH, Narula SK, Chensue SW, Lira S (2000) Transgenic expression of the chemokine receptor encoded by human herpesvirus 8 induces an angioproliferative disease resembling Kaposi's sarcoma. J Exp Med 191:445–453

# Connective Tissue Tumors

Bernhard Zelger

## Abstract

Connective tissue consists of collagen, elastic fibers and ground substances produced by fibrocytes. These cells are usually spindle-shaped with slender nuclei and bipolar cytoplasmic extensions. Apart from labeling for vimentin and variable reactivity for factor XIIIa and CD34, fibrocytes are immunonegative. Electron microscopy reveals prominent endoplasmic reticulum, but is otherwise indistinct. Lesions with fibrocytic differentiation can be divided into five categories: scars, keloids, dermatofibromas, nodular fasciitis, and superficial fibromatoses are *inflammatory lesions*. Thereby, dermatofibromas and their subcutaneous/deep soft tissue counterpart nodular fasciitis can present with a wide variety of clinicopathologic variants which may be misinterpreted as malignancies. Prurigo nodularis, chondrodermatitis nodularis helicis, acanthoma fissuratum, and knuckle pads are *hyperplasias*; fibroma molle, fibrous papules, connective tissue nevi, and elastofibroma are *hamartomas*; and fibroma of tendon sheath, pleomorphic fibroma, and giant cell tumor of tendon sheath are *benign neoplasms*. Deep fibromatoses, dermatofibrosarcoma protuberans, giant cell fibroblastoma, giant cell angiofibroma, hyalinizing spindle cell tumor with giant rosettes, solitary fibrous tumor, myxofibrosarcoma, low-grade fibromyxoid sarcoma, acral myxoinflammatory fibroblastic sarcoma, and classical fibrosarcoma, are *malignant neoplasms*, that is fibrosarcomas of variable malignant potential. Lesions dominated by myocytes/myofibroblasts, e.g. cutaneous myofibroma/infantile myofibromatosis, or by macrophages, e.g. xanthogranulomas, are not part of this chapter.

Connective tissue (Enzinger and Weiss 1995) consists of collagen, elastic fibers, and ground substances produced by fibrocytes. It forms the "skeleton" of all other tissues. Fibrocytes and activated fibroblasts are derived from the mesoderm. Immunohistochemically, fibrocytes are indistinct, positive for vimentin, with variable reactivity for factor XIIIa in the papillary dermis as

Recent Results in Cancer Research, Vol. 160
© Springer-Verlag Berlin Heidelberg 2002

well as for CD34 in the reticular dermis. Ultrastructurally, cells show prominent endoplasmic reticulum, but are otherwise indistinct.

Connective tissue tumors are part of soft tissue tumors. The WHO classification (Weiss 1994) separates them into fibrous and fibrohistiocytic tumors. This is puzzling for several reasons. First, there is no reason to split fibrocytic lesions into two groups. There is no fibrohistiocyte, i.e. a cell with "overlap" between fibrocytes and macrophages, but there are only lesions characterized by the presence of both of these cell types. Second, there is even no "histiocyte" as, besides Langerhans cells and monocytes and macrophages, many other cells are found in the "tissue" (from the Greek: *to histion*) such as fibrocytes, endothelial cells, neural cells. Similarly, diseases once thought to be derived from "histiocytes" are heterogeneous; these include generalized eruptive histiocytoma, a macrophage disease, histiocytoma, a fibrocytic lesion, and atypical regressive histiocytosis, a CD30$^+$ large cell anaplastic lymphoma. Third, tumor is a descriptive term for lesions larger than 2 cm in diameter, and not a specific type of disease. Most dermatofibromas are only papules or nodules and as such would not be included in this classification. It is obvious that in such terminologic chaos no classification will function. With the attempt to incorporate prognostic significance as done by the WHO when introducing "intermediate" grade lesions the chaos becomes even worse.

In my contribution on connective tissue tumors I group lesions with fibrocytic differentiation according to classic pathology as inflammatory lesions, hyperplasias, hamartomas, and benign and malignant neoplasms. Malformations, cysts as well as deposits and metabolic disorders are of subordinate importance. I do not discuss lesions dominated by myocytes/myofibroblasts as found in cutaneous myofibroma/infantile myofibromatosis, or those with predominance of macrophages such as in xanthogranulomas.

## Inflammatory Lesions

When fibrocytes and their products are predominant in a nodular to diffuse dermatitis and panniculitis, this is known as fibrosing dermatitis and panniculitis (Ackerman et al. 1997). In *(hypertrophic) scars*, fibrocytes and fibrillary collagen are oriented parallel, and venules perpendicular to the skin surface. In *keloids*, fibrocytes are aligned along markedly thickened collagen bundles in a haphazard array within a background of prominent mucin.

In *dermatofibromas*, fibrocytes, and often macrophages, and coarse collagen bundles are distributed in a haphazard array in the reticular dermis, and the epidermis is hyperplastic. Early lesions, when rich in granulation tissue, have been termed *sclerosing hemangiomas* or, when rich in macrophages, (fibrous) "*histiocytomas*", while late lesions are known as *fibroma durum, subepidermal nodular fibrosis* or *sclerosis*. There is enormous variability in these lesions (Calonje and Fletcher 1994), either due to architectural features or cellular and stromal peculiarities or a combination of both (Zelger et al. 2000). Recognition of each of these clinicopathologic variants allows a histopathologist to apply a

**Table 1.** Clinicopathologic variants of dermatofibroma and nodular fasciitis (with main pitfalls)

| | |
|---|---|
| Dermatofibroma variants with mostly architectural peculiarities | Deep penetrating and giant dermatofibroma (dermatofibrosarcoma protuberans), atrophic dermatofibroma (atrophic dermatofibrosarcoma protuberans), aneurysmal/angiomatoid fibrous histiocytoma (Kaposi's sarcoma), hemangiopericytoma-like fibrous histiocytoma (monophasic cellular type of infantile myofibromatosis), palisading cutaneous fibrous histiocytoma (schwannoma) |
| Dermatofibroma variants with mostly high-power peculiarities | Clear cell dermatofibroma (renal cell carcinoma metastasis), granular cell dermatofibroma (granular cell tumor), myofibroblastic dermatofibroma (amianthoid/intranodal myofibroblastoma), sclerotic dermatofibroma (keloid), atypical/pseudosarcomatous fibrous histiocytoma and dermatofibroma with monster cells (atypical fibroxanthoma), hemosiderotic/elusive dermatofibroma (melanoma), cholesterotic dermatofibroma (gout), myxoid dermatofibroma (cutaneous myxoma) |
| Dermatofibroma variants with both architectural and high-power peculiarities | Epithelioid cell histiocytoma (Spitz nevi), cellular benign fibrous histiocytoma (cutaneous leiomyosarcoma), smooth muscle proliferation in dermatofibroma (infantile myofibromatosis), multinucleate cell angiohistiocytoma (Kaposi's sarcoma), cellular neurothekeoma (myxoid neurothekeoma/nerve sheath myxoma), combined dermatofibroma (miscellaneous entities) |
| Nodular fasciitis variants | Parosteal fasciitis, cranial fasciitis, intravascular fasciitis (giant cell tumor of soft parts), proliferative myositis (reticulohistiocytoma), atypical decubital fibroplasia, intradermal nodular fasciitis (cutaneous myxoma), pseudosarcomatous fasciitis (myxofibrosarcoma), proliferative fasciitis (reticulohistiocytoma), infiltrative fasciitis (myxofibrosarcoma), plexiform fibrohistiocytic tumor (plexiform spindle cell nevus), fibrous hamartoma of infancy (neurofibroma), plexiform xanthoma and plexiform xanthomatous tumor (xanthogranuloma) |

confident benign label to lesions which might otherwise elude diagnosis, or tempt him or her to describe "new" entities, and to avoid misdiagnosis as malignancies (Table 1). We must also be fully aware that some fibrosarcomas may closely mimic dermatofibromas; such lesions have incorrectly been described as metastasizing fibrous histiocytomas (Guillou et al. 2000).

*Nodular fasciitis* (Ackerman et al. 1995) is in the subcutis and deeper soft tissue what dermatofibroma represents in the papillary and reticular dermis, i.e. a fibrosing panniculitis. At scanning magnification, lesions are moderately well circumscribed with either a round to oval or an irregular stellate appearance. Some lesions may achieve a plexiform architecture (Zelger et al. 1997). Fibrocytes are plump with large oval nuclei and elongated extensions of cytoplasm ("fibroblasts"). Prominent mucin in spaces between fibrocytes and collagen bundles gives these lesions a characteristic feathery or tissue culture-like appearance. The more loose appearance of nodular fasciitis in the fully developed stage than that of most dermatofibromas is due to the less-restricted growth conditions in the subcutis compared with the dense collagen network in the dermis. Late lesions are similar to fully developed lesions, but with fibroplasia, and sclerosis increasing as granulation tissue, fibrocytes and mucin decrease. According to the life cycle, the location as well as individual peculiarities a wide variety of synonyms have been given to nodular fasciitis (Table 1).

In *superficial fibromatoses* a longstanding fibrosing dermatitis in a particular location may cause shrinkage of the affected tissue and disable the patient. This is known as *Dupuytren's contracture* of the hands, as *Ledderhose's disease* of the feet, penile *Peyronie's disease*, or *cervical and gingival fibromatosis*. Some rare disorders in childhood such as infantile digital fibromatosis and juvenile hyaline fibromatosis are inherited. In contrast to deep fibromatoses ("desmoids") which may frequently recur and rarely metastasize (see fibrosarcomas), all "superficial" lesions show benign behavior.

## Hyperplasias

*Prurigo nodularis* (Ackerman et al. 1997) results from persistent rubbing of skin over a long time. This process mostly occurs in pruritic skin that is grossly normal at the beginning, but may also be superimposed upon other pruritic conditions such as lichen planus, allergic contact dermatitis and mycosis fungoides, to mention but a few examples. Persistent rubbing back and forth over the skin causes everything below to become thickened. When lesions are more scratched than rubbed, the surface becomes eroded to ulcerated and such lesions are known as *"picker's nodules"*. In *chondrodermatitis nodularis helicis* a similar effect is achieved by chronic pressure of the helical cartilage. In contrast to skin, cartilage does not tend to loose elasticity and does not shrink with increasing age (in older people ears seem to grow and become larger than the rest of the body!). In *acanthoma fissuratum* a similar process is due to badly fitting spectacles or self-manipulation in psychiatric patients, and in knuckle pads is due to chronic occupational trauma to the hands of manual workers such as farmers, sailors, workmen, etc, or self-manipulation.

Acral skin on the non-acral side, easily recognized by hair follicles, is a clue to *lichen simplex chronicus*, the histopathologic hallmark of rubbing. Beside epidermal hyperplasia, the connective tissue is also involved: coarse collagen fibers are arrayed in vertical streaks parallel to the rete ridges, as are dilated vessels with plump endothelial cells and slightly thickened walls. The papillary dermis is thickened dislocating the superficial vascular plexus further away from the epidermis than usual. An even more vigorous process will involve the reticular dermis which becomes thickened due to increase of fibrocytes, collagen fibers and mucin. This process is best seen around adnexal structures whose individual tubules and glands are separated from their usual close proximity. In all instances, cessation or reduction of the artificial, occupational or self-mutilating trauma will restore or at least ameliorate the clinical appearance.

## Hamartomas

In *fibroma molle* (syn. *acrochordon* or *skin tag*) an exophytic lesion reveals a core of loose connective tissue with an increased number of fibrocytes, vessels and frequently mature adipocytes. The epidermis is slightly hyperplastic, sometimes with some moderate melanocytic hyperplasia. Multiple fibromata mollia may occur together with *fibrofolliculomas* and *trichodiscomas*, and hamartomas of follicular differentiation in *Birt-Hogg-Dube syndrome.*

*Fibrous papules* (syn. *perifollicular fibroma, melanocytic angiofibroma, angiofibroma*) are another very common hamartoma (Ackerman et al. 1993). Besides follicular components fibrocytes, collagen and vessels make up the bulk of the lesions. The epidermis above the lesions may be slightly hyperplastic with melanocytic hyperplasia. The very same lesions with even greater prominence of stromal components occur in large numbers in *adenoma sebaceum* or *tuberous sclerosis* (*Pringle-Bourneville disease*). In these conditions similar periungual lesions with prominence of interfollicular fibroplasia and near absence of perifollicular fibroplasia are known as *Koenen tumors.* In the male genitalia there is another expression of this hamartoma, so-called *pearly penile papules.* In brief, the papule, irrespective of number and location, is a hamartoma that involves epithelial (hair follicles, epidermis, and melanocytes) and/or non-epithelial (fibrocytes, interfollicular and perifollicular fibrous tissue, and blood vessels) structures.

*Connective tissue nevi* (syn. *collagenoma, elastoma*) may be solitary (mesenchymal nevi of Lewandowsky type) or multiple. They are also found as *shagreen patches* in *tuberous sclerosis* and in *Buschke-Ollendorff syndrome* (syn. *dermatofibrosis lenticularis disseminata*). The latter is a combination of cutaneous connective tissue nevi with asymptomatic bone lesions known as *osteopoikilosis* which may be misinterpreted as osteoplastic metastases from prostatic cancer. Histology reveals an irregular arrangement of the dermis often difficult to appreciate with H&E staining, but better outlined by elastic stains.

In *elastofibroma* (dorsi) a mixture of fibrocytes, collagen, elastic tissue, mature adipocytes, vessels and prominent nerves is found. Most significantly, there are numerous eosinophilic elastic fibers arranged as thick beaded or serrated fibers or in globoid aggregates.

## Benign Neoplasms

*Fibromas* are benign neoplasms with fibrocytic differentiation. The term fibroma has been uncritically used for a variety of other diseases such as fibroma durum and sclerotic fibroma (variants of dermatofibroma), and fibroma molle (a hamartoma). In contrast to these processes, benign fibrocytic neoplasms are well-circumscribed, show clefts between the lesion and the surrounding connective tissue and, thus, are frequently prone to "pop out of the skin" during surgery when these clefts are incised. In contrast to inflammatory and hamartomatous fibrocytic disorders, which are very common, benign neoplasms with fibrocytic differentiation are rare.

In *fibroma of tendon sheath*, a mixture of fibrocytes with mature collagen is seen mostly on the hands and feet. The frequently close connection with tendons has given these lesions their name. They may yet be observed elsewhere. In *pleomorphic fibroma*, characteristic floret-like giant cells are interspersed between fibrocytes, collagen and prominent mucin. In *giant cell tumor of tendon sheath*, bizarre giant cells of foreign body type, frequently numerous siderophages and sheets of lipophages are found. The stroma between the monomorphous sheets of fibrocytes may be variably fibrotic to sclerotic and not infrequently shows pseudovascular clefts.

## Malignant Neoplasms

*Fibrosarcomas* are neoplasms of fibrocytic differentiation capable of killing the patient by their local destructive or metastatic potential. A variety of entities with variable biologic behavior fall into this category. At the low grade end there are *deep fibromatoses* ("desmoids") (Rock et al. 1984), which may occur in extraabdominal (60% of cases, following trauma or surgery), abdominal (25%, post partum in cesarean scars) or intraabdominal (15%, frequently associated with *Gardner's syndrome*) location. Asymmetry, a nodular to fascicular growth and irregular "infiltrative" margins are characteristic. Cellularity, atypia and mitotic activity vary both within and between individual tumors as do mucin, fibrosis and sclerosis ("keloidal hyalinization"). At the high-grade end there is "classical" fibrosarcoma, a highly cellular neoplasm with characteristic herringbone-like fascicles. More than 60% of patients develop metastases in lymph nodes and internal organs and do not survive 5 years after diagnosis. Fortunately, such lesions are rare, in particular in the skin.

*Dermatofibrosarcoma protuberans* (Fletcher 1995) is the most common fibrosarcoma of the skin. With inadequately wide excision (<3 to 5 cm) recurrences due to discontinuous growth are characteristic. Histology reveals an irregular lace-like to multilayered infiltration of the subcutis by slender fibrocytes and fine collagen fibers. Lesions are positive for CD34. According to the variable clinicopathologic presentation there are numerous subtypes: pigmented (Bednar), atrophic, myxoid, myoid, fibrosarcomatous, with giant rosettes, and mixed subtypes.

There is a spectrum of similar fibrocytic malignancies which are CD34 positive. This is best established for *giant cell fibroblastoma* (Shmookler et al. 1989), an entity characterized by pseudovascular "angiectoid" clefts lined by bizarre giant cells. Overlap with dermatofibrosarcoma protuberans is well established: on one hand, there are cases with combined features, and on the other, recurrences of giant cell fibroblastoma as dermatofibrosarcoma protuberans or vice versa. Similar overlap is true for *giant cell angiofibroma* (Dei Tos et al. 1995), an entity characterized by a "patternless" stroma with prominent vascularity, mucin, and bizarre giant cells akin to those in giant cell fibroblastoma, and *hyalinizing spindle cell tumor with giant rosettes* (Lane et al. 1997; Zamecnik 2001), a fibromatosis-like spindle cell neoplasm with giant hyalinized rosettes resembling palisaded granulomas. A well-defined lobulated lesion characterized by a "patternless" pattern is also seen in *solitary fibrous tumor* (Okamura et al. 1997). "Patternless" is a term indicating the marked variation in cellularity, the variable presence of mucin and collagen, sometimes almost with "keloidal hyalinization" as in desmoids, and the frequent presence of a hemangiopericytoma-like vascular pattern. Lesions are composed of spindle-shaped fibrocytes with little indistinct palely eosinophilic cytoplasm, but there are also more plump cells with round to oval nuclei, moderate atypia and mitoses. Necrosis is rare, but may occur. In the author's experience all these neoplasms are variants of low-grade fibrosarcoma.

Some dermatofibrosarcoma protuberans may show progression to *myxofibrosarcoma* (myxoid malignant fibrous histiocytoma). Myxofibrosarcoma (Mentzel et al. 1996) is another form of fibrosarcoma usually seen in the subcutis or deep soft tissue. A multinodular myxoid neoplasm of irregular silhouette consists of thin-walled curvilinear vessels, and hyperchromatic spindle and stellate fibrocytes with poorly defined, sometimes vacuolated cytoplasm. The small, bubbly vacuoles contain mucin sensitive to hyaluronic acid (pseudolipoblasts). The cellularity and degree of atypia parallel the histologic grade. In high-grade lesions, areas of the tumor show a pattern identical to the non-specific reaction pattern of pleomorphic malignant fibrous histiocytoma (Fletcher 1992). *Juxtaarticular myxoma* seems, at least in some cases, to be a low-grade variant of myxofibrosarcoma. Similarly, some lesions with greater prominence of a whorled stromal fibrosis have been separated from myxofibrosarcoma as *low-grade fibromyxoid sarcoma* (Evans 1993) or, in acral location, as *acral myxoinflammatory fibroblastic sarcoma* (Meis-Kindblom and Kindblom 1998). Immunohistochemically, most of these neoplasms are negative except for vimentin.

## References

Ackerman AB, DeViragh PA, Chongchitnant N (1993) Neoplasms with follicular differentiation. Lea and Febiger, Philadelphia

Ackerman AB, Cavegan BM, Robinson MJ, Abad-Casintahan MFA (1995) Ackerman's resolving quandaries in dermatology, pathology and dermatopathology. Promethean Medical Press, Philadelphia

Ackerman AB, Chongchitnant N, Sanchez J, Guo Y, Bennin B, Reichel M, Randall MB (1997) Histologic diagnosis of inflammatory skin disorders. An algorithmic method based on pattern analysis, 2nd edn. Williams and Wilkins, Baltimore

Calonje E, Fletcher CDM (1994) Cutaneous fibrohistiocytic tumors: an update. Adv Anat Pathol 1:2–15

Dei Tos A, Seregard S, Calonje E, Chan JKC, Fletcher CDM (1995) Giant cell angiofibroma. A distinctive orbital tumor in adults. Am J Surg Pathol 19:1286–1293

Enzinger FM, Weiss SW (1995) Soft tissue tumors, 3rd edn. Mosby, St Louis

Evans HL (1993) Low-grade fibromyxoid sarcoma. A report of 12 cases. Am J Surg Pathol 17:595–600

Fletcher CDM (1992) Pleomorphic malignant fibrous histiocytoma: fact or fiction? A critical reappraisal based on 159 tumors diagnosed as pleomorphic sarcoma. Am J Surg Pathol 16:213–228

Fletcher CDM (1995) Diagnostic pathology of tumors. Churchill Livingstone, Edinburgh

Guillou L, Gebhard S, Salmeron M, Coindre JM (2000) Metastasizing fibrous histiocytoma of the skin: a clinicopathologic and immunohistochemical analysis of three cases. Mod Pathol 13:654–660

Lane KL, Shannon RJ, Weiss SW (1997) Hyalinizing spindle cell tumor with giant rosettes: a distinctive tumor closely resembling low-grade fibromyxoid sarcoma. Am J Surg Pathol 21:1481–1488

Meis-Kindblom JM, Kindblom LG (1998) Acral myxoinflammatory fibroblastic sarcoma. A low grade tumor of the hands and feet. Am J Surg Pathol 22:911–924

Mentzel T, Calonje E, Wadden C, et al (1996) Myxofibrosarcoma: clinicopathologic analysis of 75 cases with emphasis on the low-grade variant. Am J Surg Pathol 20:391–405

Okamura JM, Barr RJ, Battifora H (1997) Solitary fibrous tumor of the skin. Am J Dermatopathol 19:515–518

Rock MG, Pritchard DJ, Reiman HM (1984) Extraabdominal desmoid tumors. J Bone Joint Surg 66A:1369–1374

Shmookler BM, Enzinger F, Weiss SW (1989) Giant cell fibroblastoma: a juvenile form of dermatofibrosarcoma protuberans. Cancer 15:2154–2161

Weiss SW (1994) Histological typing of soft tissue tumours. In: Sobin LH (ed) International histological classification of tumours, Fascicle 3, 2nd edn. Springer, Berlin Heidelberg New York

Zamecnik M (2001) Fibrosarcomatous dermatofibrosarcoma protuberans with giant rosettes. Am J Surg Pathol 23:41–45

Zelger B, Weinlich G, Steiner H, Zelger BG, Egarter-Vigl E (1997) Dermal and subcutaneous variants of plexiform fibrohistiocytic tumor. Am J Surg Pathol 21:235–241

Zelger BG, Sidoroff A, Zelger B (2000) Combined dermatofibroma: co-existence of two or more variant patterns in a single lesion. Histopathology 36:529–539

# Psychosocial Aspects 7

# How to Identify Patients in Need of Psychological Intervention

Gerhard Strittmatter, Marlene Tilkorn, and Reinhard Mawick

## Abstract

The identification of skin cancer patients in need of psychosocial intervention is a necessary prerequisite to relieving their distress and specifically supporting their coping strategies. The influence of early support even on prognosis has been shown in melanoma patients. Only a few patients ask for support themselves. The workload of doctors and nurses limits their ability to identify patients in need of support. Conducting interviews during daily hospital routine is time-consuming and cannot be implemented adequately. The screening of psychosocial risk patients needs to be based on standardized instruments. They should be easy to implement during the every-day routine. The Hornheide questionnaire with 27 items, the short form of the questionnaire with 9 items, and the Hornheide Screening Instrument (HSI) with 7 interview questions have been developed to achieve this aim in skin cancer patients. The Hornheide questionnaire offers a differentiated analysis of distress, and facilitates an accurate intervention according to the individual distress of the patient. The short form does not provide a differentiated analysis of distress. Its advantage is the speedy identification of patients at psychosocial risk. The HSI is for use during the anamnestic interview. In correlation with reduction of hospitalization time the HSI is most practicable for routine clinical implementation.

## Introduction

An important part of psychooncological care of tumor patients is treatment-integrated psychosocial support in the acute stage of treatment. In this period, the basic strategies for coping with cancer and its treatment are developed. The aim is to encourage the active cooperation of the patients from the beginning, to mobilize their resources and to improve their quality of life. The main question is how to identify patients in need of psychosocial

Recent Results in Cancer Research, Vol. 160
© Springer-Verlag Berlin Heidelberg 2002

intervention in time and with reliability. These questions are important for three reasons:

1. It is part of the concept of psychooncology that the emotional condition of patients and their coping strategies are taken into consideration during the whole treatment.
2. It is a matter of ethics to offer the necessary psychological support to highly distressed patients. However, very few ask for support themselves. To assist all is impossible, even wrong, and to wait until somebody is obviously driven to despair is equally wrong since in the latter case precious time is lost while the patient wastes energy which is needed urgently to cope.
3. The random prospective longitudinal study in melanoma patients by Fawzy et al. (1993) indicated that early structured psychoeducational intervention which strengthens effective coping and reduces emotional distress can have a positive influence on the rate of relapse and survival time. The aim is to support effective coping strategies and mobilize resources by realistic assessment of the emotional status ("don't minimize, mobilize!").

The workload of doctors and nurses limits their ability to identify patients in need of support (Hardman et al. 1989; Razavi et al. 1990). Conducting interviews during daily hospital routine is time-consuming and cannot be implemented adequately with a great number of patients (Watson 1992). Specific instruments for the identification of cancer patients in need of support have not been published. The screening instrument developed by Weisman et al. (1980) in the framework of "Project Omega" simply cannot be applied to the German situation due to cultural differences. Existing questionnaires are often too long, somatic items are misleading, and not relevant for cancer patients because of psychiatric symptoms. Cancer patients should not be seen from a psychopathological point of view because they are normal individuals who happen to be suffering from deep distress (Moorey and Greer 1989). There are a few studies in which standardized instruments have been used to assess the psychological morbidity of cancer patients. These include the Hospital Anxiety and Depression (HAD) scale (Zigmond and Snaith 1983), the Mental Adjustment to Cancer (MAC) scale (Greer and Watson 1987; Watson et al. 1988) and the Brief Symptom Inventory (BSI) (Derogatis and Meliseratos 1983). Herrmann and coworkers (1994) have presented a German version of the HAD scale for implementation in routine medical care. Watson and coworkers (1994) developed a short form of the MAC scale ("Mini-MAC") for the speedy assessment of coping styles.

Although these instruments record important clinical symptoms and significant coping strategies, they are not specific instruments for the clarification of the support requirements in psychooncology. They can only differentiate partly (see Brandberg et al. 1992) and leave relevant variables out of the picture (see Grassi et al. 1993). The screening of psychological risk patients must be based on standardized instruments with known validity and reliability to assess the distress of the patients correctly (Moorey and Greer

1989). At the same time the necessary instruments must be easy to handle in the clinical setting in order to be implemented (Iscoe et al. 1991).

The following research project serves as valid and reliable clarification of this question of indication. Three instruments were developed: the Hornheide Questionnaire (HF) with 27 items, the short form of the questionnaire (HFK) with 7 items and the Hornheide Screening Instrument (HSI) with 7 interview questions (Strittmatter et al. 2000).

## Hornheide Questionnaire

The Hornheide Questionnaire was implemented for the differentiated self-assessment of distress in patients with facial and skin cancer. It is a practicable questionnaire for the postoperative assessment of distress and for the identification of patients in need of support (Strittmatter 1997; Strittmatter et al. 1998; Tilkorn et al. 1990). It consists of 27 items in eight dimensions. Problems are recorded and the intensity of distress they cause with the help of a five-step ordinal rating scale. The dimensions proved by factor analysis are: physical functioning, emotional functioning, cancer-related fears, tension and restlessness, self-confidence (body image), social support, medical support, occupational and financial problems. The Hornheide Questionnaire is based on a problem-oriented, functional perception of diagnosis. It offers a differentiated analysis of distress and facilitates an accurate intervention according to the particular distress of the patient.

The identification of patients at psychosocial risk results from the sum of the patient's subjective self-assessment and expert-defined cut-off points. The criterion identification of psychosocial risk patients by specific cut-off points corresponds with the measure of Greer and coworkers (Greer et al. 1992; Moorey and Greer 1989; Moorey et al. 1994) for offering psychological therapy to those patients beyond specific cut-off points. It is also identical to the definition of psychological morbidity (Greer et al. 1992) using the statistical criterion "standard deviation +1" in a survey of a sample of hospital patients, later to be included in the study.

A systematic clinical study in a consecutive sample of 846 skin cancer patients confirmed the high reliability of the questionnaire (Cronbach Alpha 0.8980) as well as the statistical control in a sample of 132 skin cancer patients. Its content validity could be proven by the well-documented development steps of the questionnaire according to statistical and clinical criteria (Strittmatter 1997). The validity of the questionnaire has proved its worth in a study with two different samples of melanoma patients in Freiburg ($n = 223$) and Innsbruck ($n = 215$). It shows that the questionnaire originally developed for inpatients is a valid and economical screening instrument for the assessment of the support requirement in melanoma outpatients (Rumpold et al. 2000). The questionnaire has been implemented in different studies in German-speaking countries for the same purpose (Augustin et al. 1997; Rumpold et al. 2000; Söllner et al. 1997, 1998; Zschocke et al. 1996).

## Short Form of the Hornheide Questionnaire

To reduce the effort in terms of time and energy for patients and coworkers, the short form was developed with the most selective items of the Hornheide Questionnaire (Strittmatter 1997). It is able to speedily identify patients at psychosocial risk and consists of nine items. The existence of problems is recorded and the intensity of distress they cause with the help of a five-step ordinal rating scale. The selection of patients in need of support – in analogy to the normal version of the questionnaire – results from the sum of the patient's subjective self-assessment and expert-defined cut-off point.

The evaluation of the short-form questionnaire was carried out on a consecutive sample of 122 skin cancer patients. The results proved the short-form questionnaire to be a valid and reliable self-assessment instrument (Cronbach Alpha 0.8077). In comparison with the normal version of the Hornheide Questionnaire the short form identifies 7.2% more patients as patients at psychosocial risk. All in all, the short-form questionnaire represents a compromise between higher practicability (saving time and energy for patients and coworkers) and lack of information within certain limits (caused by item reduction). In comparison with the normal version, the short form renounces differentiated assessment of distress. Its advantage lies in the speedy identification of patients at risk. The short-form questionnaire has been implemented in different clinical studies to indicate support requirements of cancer patients. In a study in different oncological outpatient departments in several German Federal States, 1200 outpatients with different sites and types of cancer were assessed with the short-form questionnaire (Heymanns et al. 2000). This version is currently being implemented in hospitalized patients in the context of a pilot study "Surgical Oncology" at Kiel Christian-Albrechts-University in the Department of General and Thorax Surgery.

## Development of the Hornheide Screening Instrument

The Hornheide Questionnaire and the short form are instruments for postoperative implementation. Preoperative use would be an additional burden because of the nature of some questions (worries about the progress of the tumor or worries about social, occupational and financial consequences). Hospitalization time is being reduced more and more. Therefore patients do not have a chance to receive treatment-integrated support unless new criteria are found to solve the question of indication for counseling and support. The authors had the task of finding a possible method of identifying patients at psychosocial risk in the context of the anamnestic interview without presenting a questionnaire. The development of the instrument was carried out in a study involving the checking demographic variables, objective criteria, expert assessment by the interviewer and self-assessment by the patient as criteria for the identification of patients in need of support (Strittmatter et al. 2000).

## Material and Method

A group of 122 patients (60 male, 62 female, average age 56.2 years) from a consecutive sample with defined skin cancers (48.2% malignant melanoma, 28.7% basal cell cancer, 9% squamous cell cancer, 13.9% other types of skin cancer) were recorded using a catalogue of different criteria on the first hospitalization day. The valid Hornheide Questionnaire was administered four days later for the identification of support requirements. By discriminant analysis (SPSS 8.0) the discriminant function as the best statistical model to explain the need for support (dependent variable) was calculated. The criteria of the catalogue serve as independent variables.

The catalogue consists of four parts:

1. Seven objective criteria record treatment-relevant data: imminent large facial operation, possible extended functional impairment, planned amputation, first extended metastases, history of long-term use of psychiatric drugs, history of psychiatric or psychotherapeutic interventions, treatment delay.
2. Three demographic criteria: unemployment, family status and distance from hospital to home.
3. Five observer-rated measures contain questions about the patient's nonverbal behavior (body language), about the discrepancy between self-assessment and observer assessment, about denial of problems by the patient and about the discrepancy between findings and feelings.
4. Finally, 15 interview questions concerning emotional and physical well-being, operation anxiety, social support, cancer-related concerns of the family, other concerns, tension and restlessness, quality of information about disease and treatment.

For methodological reasons (better control of interfering variables), the interviews and the expert assessment were carried out by three trained members of the psychosocial team.

## Results

Of the 122 patients, 39 (32%) were in need of support according to the criteria of the Hornheide Questionnaire. The discriminant analysis showed the following results:

1. The sociodemographic variables did not have discriminant function. They were not useful indication criteria.
2. The discriminant function of the observer-rated measures was insufficient to identify support requirements.

3. The objective criteria were inadequate to identify the entire need. Analysis of the accuracy of classification showed that only 23.7% of patients at psychosocial risk were identified by the objective criteria, while 76.3% were falsely classified as low-risk patients.

4. The discriminant function based on the 15 interview questions showed a high accuracy of identification. The percent of "grouped" cases correctly classified was 72.7%.

   - After excluding those items related to specific treatment (surgery, radiotherapy) and to the relationship with the medical staff and items proving too vague in the situation of the interview (such as the question about mood) seven interview questions remained. Independent of diagnosis and treatment these questions were suitable in the context of the anamnestic interview.

   Compared with all other item combinations, this combination of seven interview questions and their total score achieved the best result. All in all, 85.7% of grouped cases were correctly classified. The discriminant function based on these seven interview items and their total score was of great value for this purpose ($F$-value 0.756, canonical correlation 0.656, Wilks' lambda 0.569, chi-squares 63.632, d.f. 8, significance 0.000). A distinct difference between the mean values of supported and nonsupported patient groups could be demonstrated. Tests for significance of the differences between the mean value of the single variables showed that all mean value differences were significant.

5. Combinations of interview items with selected objective criteria do not provide better accuracy in well-selected patients.

## Hornheide Screening Instrument

Based on the results of the discriminant analysis, the Hornheide Screening Instrument consisting of seven interview questions (see Fig. 1) achieved the highest proportion of correctly identified patients (85.7%). Cronbach alpha of the instrument was 0.6147 (standardized item alpha 0.7382).

## Discussion

Under the present difficult economic conditions of health care, the hospitalization time of cancer patients is being reduced more and more. The Hornheide Screening Instrument presents a practicable and effective method of identifying patients at psychosocial risk on the first day of hospitalization. In the context of the anamnestic interview, the doctor or psychologist asks the questions and ticks the corresponding answers. The patient does not have to fill in a questionnaire. The evaluation results from the discriminant function with the help of the SPSS program or by filling in the ticked values into the discriminant function.

**Hornheide Screening Instrument**

Interview questions

1. How did you feel physically during the past three days?

| pretty good 0 | medium 1 | pretty bad 2 |
| --- | --- | --- |

2. How did you feel emotionally during the past three days?

| pretty good 0 | medium 1 | pretty bad 2 |
| --- | --- | --- |

3. Is there anything apart from the present illness that worries you?

| yes 2 | no 0 |
| --- | --- |

4. Do you have somebody with whom you can talk about your concerns and anxiety?

| yes 0 | no 2 |
| --- | --- |

5. Is your stay in hospital a particular burden to someone in your family?

| yes 2 | no 0 |
| --- | --- |

6. During the day are you able to relax and find inner peace?

| yes 0 | no 2 |
| --- | --- |

7. How well informed are you about your illness and treatment?

| pretty good 0 | medium 1 | pretty bad 2 |
| --- | --- | --- |

Sum:

| 0 | 1 | 2 | 3 | 4 | 5 | 6 | 7 |
| --- | --- | --- | --- | --- | --- | --- | --- |
|   | 8 | 9 | 10 | 11 | 12 | 13 | 14 |

**Doctor in charge**      Name of patient

Ward:     Diagnosis:

Interviewer:     Date:

**Evaluation**

Patient in need of support     yes     no

**Interventions**

Date     Interventions     Coworkers

**Fig. 1.**

The screening instrument introduced above is of great importance for the quality assurance of treatment-integrated support and counseling. At the earliest possible time patients who urgently need psychosocial intervention will be identified.

The decisive step of the study described above is the detection of the items allowing the identification from the very first day without causing distress to the interviewee. The instrument can be easily implemented. It is transferable to other types of cancer because it does not contain any skin cancer-specific questions. Practicability testing of the screening instrument as part of daily hospital routine has shown that the instrument is well received by the doctors in charge. The interview items are easily integrated into the anamnestic interview. The patients view the questions positively. Other validation studies with different types of tumors are planned.

## References


Augustin M, Zschocke I, Dieterle W, Schöpf E, Muthny F (1997) Bedarf und Motivation zu psychosozialen Interventionen bei Patienten mit malignen Hauttumoren. Z Hautkr 72:333–338

Brandberg Y, Bolund C, Sigurdardottir V, Sjöden PO, Sullivan M (1992) Anxiety and depressive symptoms at different stages of malignant melanoma. Psychooncology 1:71–78

Derogatis LR, Melisaratos N (1983) The Brief Symptom Inventory (BSI): an introductory report. Psychol Med 13:595–605

Fawzy IF, Fawzy NW, Hyun C, Elashoff R, Guthrie D, Fahey JL, Morton DL (1993) Malignant melanoma. Effects of an early structured psychiatric intervention, coping, and affective state on recurrence and survival 6 years later. Arch Gen Psychiatry 50:681–690

Grassi L, Rosti G, Lasalvia A, Marangolo M (1993) Psychosocial variables associated with mental adjustment to cancer. Psychooncology 2:11–20

Greer S, Watson M (1987) Mental adjustment to cancer: its measurement and prognostic importance. Cancer Surv 6:439–453

Greer S, Moorey S, Baruch JDR, Watson M, Robertson BM, Mason A, Rowden L, Law MG, Bliss JM (1992) Adjuvant psychological therapy for patients with cancer: a prospective randomised trial. BMJ 304:675–681

Hardman A, Maguire P, Crowther D (1989) The recognition of psychiatry morbidity on an oncology ward. J Psychosom Res 33:235–239

Herrmann C, Buss U, Lingen R, Kreuzer H (1994) Erfassung von Angst und Depressivität in der medizinischen Routineversorgung. Dtsch Med Wochenschr 119:1283–1286

Heymanns J, Breuer F, Hinrichs HF, Ruhmland B, Strittmatter G, Reichelt R (2000) Detecting psychosocial needs in ambulatory cancer patients during chemotherapy. J Cancer Res Clin Oncol [Suppl] 126 :R9

Iscoe N, Williams JI, Szalai JP, Osoba D (1991) Prediction of psychosocial distress in patients with cancer. In: Osoba D (ed) Effect of cancer on quality of life. CRC Press, Boca Raton, pp 41–59

Moorey S, Greer S (1989) Psychological therapy for patients with cancer: a new approach. Heinemann Medical Books, Oxford

Moorey S, Greer S, Watson M, Baruch JD, Robertson BM, Mason A, Rowden L, Tunmore R, Law MG, Bliss JM (1994) Adjuvant psychological therapy for patients with cancer: outcome at one year. Psychooncology 3:39–46

Razavi D, Delvaux N, Farvacques C, Robaye E (1990) Screening for adjustment disorders and major depressive disorders in cancer in-patients. Br J Psychiatry 156:79–83

Rumpold G, Augustin M, Zschocke I, Strittmatter G, Söllner W (2000) Die Validität des Hornheider Fragebogens zur psychosozialen Unterstützung bei Tumorpatienten: Eine Untersuchung an zwei repräsentativen ambulanten Stichproben von Melanompatienten. Psychother Psychosom Med Psychol 51:25–33

Söllner W, Zingg-Schir M, Rumpold G, Fritsch P (1997) Attitude toward alternative therapy, compliance with standard treatment, and need for emotional support in patients with melanoma. Arch Dermatol 133:316–321

Söllner W, Augustin M, Zschocke I (1998) Melanompatienten: Psychosoziale Belastung, Krankheitsverarbeitung und soziale Unterstützung. Ein systematisches Review. Psychother Psychosom Med Psychol 48:338–348

Strittmatter G (1997) Indikation zur Intervention in der Psychoonkologie. Psychosoziale Belastungen und Ermittlung der Betreuungsbedürftigkeit stationärer Hauttumorpatienten. Waxmann, Münster

Strittmatter G, Mawick R, Tilkorn M (1998) Psychosozialer Betreuungsbedarf bei Gesichts- und Hauttumorpatienten. Psychother Psychosom Med Psychol 48:349–357

Strittmatter G, Mawick R, Tilkorn M (2000) Entwicklung und klinischer Einsatz von Screening-Instrumenten zur Identifikation betreuungsbedürftiger Tumorpatienten. In: Bullinger M, Siegrist J, Ravens-Sieberer U (eds) Lebensqualitätsforschung aus medizinpsychologischer und -soziologischer Perspektive. Hogrefe, Göttingern, pp 59–75 (Jahrbuch der Medizinischen Psychologie, vol 18)

Tilkorn M, Mawick R, Sommerfeld S, Strittmatter G (1990) Lebensqualität von Patienten mit bösartigen Gesichts- und Hauttumoren. Entwicklung eines Fragebogens und erste Ergebnisse einer Studie. Rehabilitation 29:134–139

Watson M (1992) Screening for psychological morbidity. In: Zittoun R (ed) Quality of life of cancer patients. A review. International congress of psychosocial oncology, Beaune, France, 12–14 Oct 1992, Levallois-Perret (France), Editorial Assistance, pp 151–153

Watson M, Greer S, Young J, Inayat Q, Burgess C, Robertson B (1988) Development of a questionnaire measure of adjustment to cancer: the MAC scale. Psychol Med 18:203–209

Watson M, Law M, dos Santos M, Greer S, Baruch J, Bliss JM (1994) The Mini-Mac: further development of the mental adjustment to cancer scale. Psychooncology 3:153

Weisman AD, Wordon JW, Sobel HJ (1980) Psychosocial screening and intervention with cancer patients. Research Report. Funded by National Cancer Institute, Grant no. CA-19797, 1977–1980. General Hospital, Boston

Zigmond AS, Snaith RP (1983) Hospital anxiety and depression scale. Acta Psychiatr Scand 67:361–370

Zschocke I, Augustin M, Stein B, Deußen-Wernicke T, Muthny FA (1996) Vergleichende Betrachtung psychosozialer Belastungsfaktoren bei stationären Patienten mit verschiedenen Haut-Tumoren. In: Brähler E, Schumacher J (eds) Psychologie und Soziologie in der Medizin. Psychosozial Verlag, Gießen, p 213

# Psychotherapeutic Interventions in Melanoma Patients

Wolfgang Söllner, Renate Gross, and Susanne Maislinger

## Abstract

*Objectives:* The need for and the effectiveness of psychotherapy in the treatment of patients with skin cancer have been shown. However, only insufficient data are available to answer the questions as to what kind of psychotherapy is useful and how psychotherapeutic interventions should be designed. *Methods:* During the past 7 years we performed crisis intervention, focal therapy and longer-lasting psychodynamically orientated psychotherapy within a consultation liaison service with the Department of Dermatology of Innsbruck University Hospital. We investigated the type of interventions using qualitative content analysis of the written records of weekly supervisory sessions. *Results:* Standard methods of psychotherapy are often not appropriate for the confrontation of tumor-related fears in melanoma patients. Modifications of psychotherapeutic interventions and more structured support are necessary to meet overwhelming negative emotions caused by the existential threat of the disease. Therefore, we turned to using expressive-supportive methods combining psychodynamic psychotherapy with relaxation, imaginative methods, and structured picture drawing. *Conclusions:* Psychotherapists treating skin cancer patients should receive special education in such methods. To better cope with distressing emotions and to avoid burn-out and withdrawal from severely ill or dying patients, psychotherapists should take part in peer supervision regularly.

## Introduction

The usual psychotherapeutic techniques are often not appropriate for cancer patients in general and for skin cancer patients in particular for several reasons:

Recent Results in Cancer Research, Vol. 160
© Springer-Verlag Berlin Heidelberg 2002

1. Tumor-related fears are an obvious and current topic in psychotherapy of cancer patients. Melanoma patients very often suffer intense fear regarding tumor progression, because even with early detection and a thin melanoma, prognosis may be uncertain over the long term and other tiny moles might become malignant and life threatening (Brandberg et al. 1992; Kelly et al. 1995). Moreover, in skin cancer patients, the visibility of the cancer or the scar reminds patients of the cancer disease even though prognosis might be good. Patients with a melanoma located in an area of the body that is usually not covered by clothes suffer pronounced distress (Söllner et al. 1998).
2. In contrast to the danger they have to face, cancer patients often do not feel physically ill at the beginning of the disease, at least until the onset of oncological treatment. In non-progressive disease, the sequelae of the operation as well as side effects of chemotherapy, immune therapy or radiation may impair patients more than the disease itself.
3. During certain stages of the disease as well as treatment, denial is an important coping mechanism and may influence motivation for psychotherapy and the course of such therapy. Especially in the months after diagnosis, denial occurs frequently and makes psychotherapeutic intervention difficult or even impossible (Levine and Ziegler 1975; Kneier and Temoshok 1984; Söllner et al. 1999).
4. Skin cancer affects the organ that mediates interpersonal contact. This influences social contact and may lead to social withdrawal and increases tabooing of cancer (Cassileth et al. 1983; Söllner et al. 1999). A special issue for many melanoma patients is the fact that the sun, which usually is experienced as a source of warmth and delight, becomes an evil and a danger.
5. One of the most important differences in psychotherapeutic work between cancer patients and patients who are not physically ill is the fact that time perspectives may be limited due to the illness. Supportive care of the patient and his or her loved ones during the phase of palliative treatment and the process of dying may include psychotherapeutic strategies. Patients who have received psychotherapy during the earlier phases of cancer disease are often accompanied by their psychotherapist during the last stage of life.
   Psychotherapeutic interventions and techniques must consider these characteristics of cancer disease and the specific patterns of coping with the illness.

Several authors have developed modifications of psychotherapeutic interventions with cancer patients (Greer et al. 1992; Spiegel and Classen 1999). However, only a small number of publications deal with specific modifications of psychotherapy in skin cancer patients, and melanoma patients in particular. F.I. Fawzy and coworkers (1990, 1993) developed a structured short-time group intervention for patients with early-stage melanoma. This intervention was predominantly psychoeducational and focused on stress management, enhancement of active coping strategies, and health education (e.g. sun protection). N.W. Fawzy (1995) developed a psychoeducational intervention for individual melanoma patients to be conducted by trained cancer nurses. No specific modifications of more intensive and longer-lasting psychotherapy with skin cancer patients have yet been described. In our daily practice of consultation-liaison (CL) psychosomatics we therefore developed such modified psychotherapeutic interventions.

## Methods

Since 1994 we have been conducting a psychotherapeutic CL service at the Department of Dermatology of Innsbruck University Hospital. More than half of the patients treated in this CL service have been melanoma patients. Usually we contact the patients during their hospital stay after excision of the primary tumor. Patients referred by the oncologists are mostly those with a poor prognosis or with disfiguring operations. In one or more diagnostic interviews we assess psychosocial distress, individual coping strategies and the perceived emotional and practical support from the patient's social network. We offer further psychotherapeutic support to the following groups of patients: those suffering significant distress, those with coping behavior characterized by helplessness, patients with poor social support, and patients who want psychotherapy themselves. Psychotherapeutic interventions are started during the hospital stay, and, if indicated, are continued in our psychotherapeutic outpatient department. The psychotherapy we provide is based on psychodynamic principles.

A treatment plan for each patient is worked out in our weekly CL conference. Additionally, the process of psychotherapy is supervised by experienced psychotherapists in weekly team sessions. Particularly, we discuss modifications of established psychotherapeutic interventions and their consequences for the therapeutic relationship, and we produce written records of these discussions. These records are evaluated with the help of content analysis (Mayring 1985). We present the results of this analysis and demonstrate modifications of psychotherapeutic techniques and peculiarities of the therapeutic relationship between patient and therapist using case vignettes.

## Results

### Types of Intervention

Psychotherapeutic interventions can be classified into three types: crisis intervention, short-term focal therapy, and long-term psychotherapy. The most prevalent types of psychotherapeutic work were crisis-intervention and short-term emotional support. In most cases, this was performed during the hospital stay, and during typical periods of the course of the disease: the period following diagnosis of the melanoma, recurrence or detection of metastases, and the period of palliative care. It consisted of one to ten sessions, often including a close relative of the patient. Short-term focused psychotherapy often followed crisis intervention and was performed in our psychotherapeutic clinic after the patient had been discharged. Usually, it consisted of 20 to 40 sessions. Relatives of the patients were included only rarely in some sessions. Long-term psychotherapy (regular weekly sessions over a period of more than 1 year) was performed only in a few cases. It was based on the psychodynamic theoretical approach.

## Modification of Psychotherapeutic Techniques

The type of psychotherapeutic intervention not only influenced the focus but also the amount of activity of the psychotherapist in dealing with the concerns and fears of the patients. Focusing on the actual situation of the patients (including distressing treatment procedures) during crisis intervention and short-term psychotherapy, the therapists actively addressed the patients' individual and social resources. They assessed the kind of emotional and behavioral strategies patients had developed to cope with previous crisis situations and asked how patients mobilized and perceived emotional and practical support from significant others. Close relatives were invited to take part in some of the sessions to help them to better cope with the situation and to strengthen the social support of the patient. Active coping strategies such as information seeking, diversion, hedonism and others were supported by the therapist. Sometimes the psychotherapist actively sought to improve doctor-patient communication by discussions with oncologists or with the ward team or by proposing joint sessions with the treating physician, the patient and his or her relatives.

In the first years of our CL service, we learned from our experience that unstructured therapy sessions and frankly addressing the patients emotions often resulted in intensification of the fears in the patient and, subsequently, in resistance to psychotherapy. We therefore started to use or intensify anxiety-reducing techniques. Besides increasing the supportive activity of the psychotherapist, as pointed out above, we developed a more structured procedure for the therapy sessions. We introduced relaxation techniques, guided imagery and also proposed tasks for the time between sessions such as drawing pictures. These techniques are supportive on the one hand and enhance the expression of emotions on the other without provoking uncontrolled regression. After some initial sessions the patient can be instructed how to use relaxation or imagery during medical therapy procedures or to become calm when sleepless. Moreover, these techniques allow body-image disturbances to be addressed in a more direct way than purely verbal methods. Guided imagery and the method of structured picture drawing are described in more detail in the following two case vignettes.

## Relaxation and Guided Imagery

Mrs. A, aged 42 years, was referred to the CL psychotherapist from the dermatological ward at her own request. She had recently been told of the diagnosis of several widespread metastases of a malignant melanoma that had originally been treated 12 years previously. Her whole social system, especially her husband, but also the treating oncologists, were shocked by the current situation. Everybody's helplessness became obvious to her. Her wish for psychotherapy at first aimed to support during the medical treatment (chemotherapy and immunotherapy). Therefore guided imagery seemed to be a suitable method. The beginning of the intervention was characterized by the application of a relaxation technique, focusing mainly on breathing, after which she was guided into her imaginative picture, which she had been able to select herself previously. In the second half of the session the theme of the imagination and her emotions and thoughts relating to it could be talked about. Two of those guided imaginations are described in the following.

In one of the early sessions she felt as if she were in a big park in Great Britain which she knew from her last holiday. She was sitting under a huge tree, with a very wide trunk she could lean on, and its branches covering her like a roof. Green was the predominant color and feeling free and secure was the most important emotion. No other person appeared in this picture, although her husband and her children had been the most important people in her life for the last two decades. She remembered this holiday as the time she had most enjoyed for years. Although having three children, she had decided to travel alone with a friend. In the following months of therapy this topic came up even more, in the sense that affection and responsibility for her children were very important on the one hand, but on the other hand life had also become more precious for herself alone. The picture of this guided imagination is the place where she tried to go to in her mind during the following first course of chemotherapy. Through this she could recall the feelings of security and freedom, which were able to provide a little relief.

In one of the next sessions she expressed the wish to have a walk in nature as the topic of the guided imagination. During this session she became anxious and nervous and wanted to finish it early. In her imagination she was lying in the grass enjoying a summer day when suddenly a snake approached her noiselessly. Fear was coming up very quickly in this situation, similar to the noiseless way in which the cancer disease came up in her life. This session can be seen as the decisive step towards the important topics in the further psychotherapeutic work with Mrs. A. Being symbolized in the picture of the imagination first, it was easier for her to face her feelings and to verbalize to some extent her worries and fears, which at first glance seemed to be too horrifying to talk about at all. This experience led her to decide to continue psychotherapy and she attended weekly therapeutic sessions. Step by step, the method of guided imagination became less important in the following months as it was now possible for her to verbalize crucial topics directly. Psychotherapy with her continued until her death 1½ years later.

## Structured Picture Drawing

Mr. B, aged 55 years, was referred to the CL service by his oncologist because of high level of anxiety and panic attacks after surgical removal of a superficial spreading melanoma on his back with a depth of 1.5 mm. He lived with his mother, and his partner was a nurse 10 years his junior. He avoided speaking about his feelings and expressed himself in a rather "technical" way. We offered weekly psychotherapeutic sessions and asked him to draw three pictures between sessions. He was to feel free in his choice of themes, material, and colors. However, one picture was required to focus on a theme in his past, one on his present situation, and one on the future. He was informed that the esthetic value of the drawings was of no importance (some patients are encouraged to draw with the less dominant hand to avoid such an effect) and that the drawing would be discussed in the following therapy session.

In the first sessions he brought pictures with colored lines and symbols. He completely avoided drawing any figures or people. He was not only afraid of not fulfilling the expectations of the therapist, but imagined that any naturalistic scene would provoke intense feelings of fear and despair. He sought to keep control over his emotions by avoiding verbalization of tumor-related fears. After gaining more confidence in a couple of therapy sessions, he drew a picture about an opera ("Evangeliman") which he had watched some years previously with his aunt. When asked to verbalize his spontaneous ideas concerning this picture, he remembered that the "Evangeliman" committed a crime and set his house on fire, but denied his failures. As a consequence, he had to suffer terribly. Later on he explained that this aunt had suffered and died from a gynecological cancer and had "rotted from inside". For the first time, he was able to express his fears of infirmity and dying. As the theme relating to the present he drew the Grand Canyon which he had visited recently. When asked where he would place himself in this picture, he answered "right down at the bottom of the canyon" which he painted very dark and misty with condors circling above. With a big rock painted in red lying on the ground of the canyon, he associated danger and the feeling that a heavy stone was lying on his chest. At the bottom of the canyon, however, he had drawn some small green trees. Confronted with the antagonism that in the sunless and frightening dark of the canyon's bottom something vivid was growing, he reacted with astonishment and began to see the narrow canyon not only as a danger but also as a shelter where the condors could not do him harm.

In the following 40 therapy sessions fears and wishes first emerged in his pictures and he could detect and verbalize them with the help of his associations and the cautious interpretations of the therapist. The pictures of the first 20 sessions dealt with fears about dying, and the disintegration of his body and his self. While in the beginning this fear was diffuse and destructive, during the process of interpreting and integrating the progressive and sheltering parts of his pictures he began to have a closer look at his fears and remembered frightening and conflict-laden experiences in his childhood.

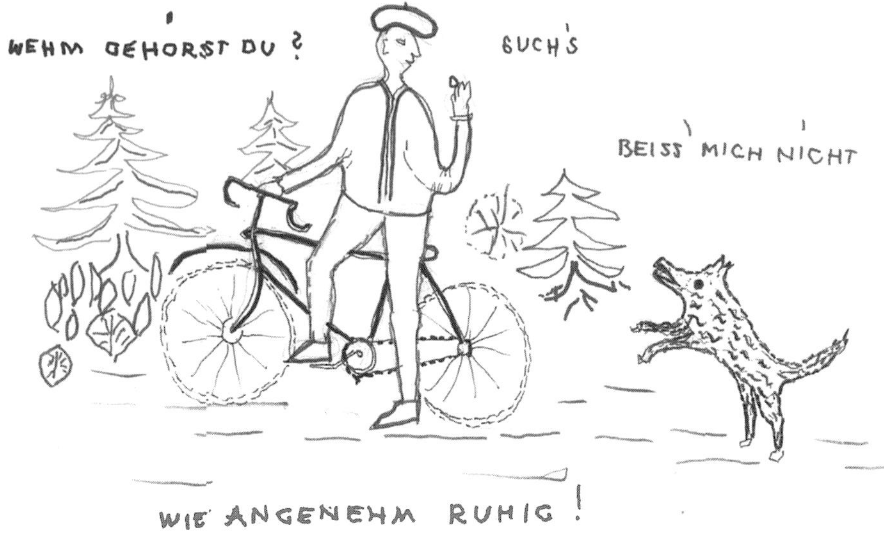


**Fig. 1.** Picture brought by Mr. B, a 55-year-old patient suffering from melanoma, to his last session of focused psychodynamic therapy with structured picture drawing

The last picture about the present showed an excursion with a bicycle which he had undertaken some days before (Fig. 1). A wild brown and black mottled German shepherd dog threatened him when he passed a farmhouse. He experienced intense fear. Nevertheless, he stopped, got off his bicycle, and turned towards the dog. The animal calmed down as Mr. B began to talk calmly to the dog. Asked for his associations, he looked at the drawing and suddenly said with deep emotion: "The dog is my melanoma. I learned not to run away but to stop, to confront it and talk with it. Then it becomes less frightening for me."

## Conclusions

As a consequence of our experience, modifications of psychotherapeutic interventions and more structured support have proved to be necessary to avoid higher levels of regression and overwhelming negative emotions such as anxiety, fear and helplessness in melanoma patients. Relaxation techniques, guided imagery and picture drawing guided by the therapist are an appropriate way to address patients' emotions, and can be used in crisis intervention as well as in short-term or longer-lasting psychotherapy. Psychotherapists treating cancer patients should receive special education in such methods. Psychotherapy with melanoma patients who are encountering an existential threat also causes a significant emotional burden and fear related to death and dying in the psychotherapists themselves. In further research, therapists' countertransference should be studied in more detail. In order to cope with distressing emotions better and to avoid burn-out and withdrawal from severely ill or dying patients, psychotherapists should take part in peer supervision regularly.

## References


Brandberg Y, Bolund C, Sigurdardottir V (1992) Anxiety and depressive symptoms at different stages of malignant melanoma. Psychooncology 1:71–78

Cassileth BR, Lusk E, Tenaglia AN (1983) Patients' perceptions of the cosmetic impact of melanoma resection. Plastic Reconstr Surg 71:73–75

Fawzy FI, Cousins N, Fawzy NW, Kemeny ME, Elashoff R, Morton DL (1990) A structured psychiatric intervention for cancer patients. I. Changes over time in methods of coping and affective disturbance. Arch Gen Psychiatry 47:720–725

Fawzy FI, Fawzy NW, Hyun CS, Elashoff R, Guthrie D, Fahey JL, Morton DL (1993) Malignant melanoma. Effects of an early structured psychiatric intervention, coping, and affective state on recurrence and survival 6 years later. Arch Gen Psychiatry 50:681–689

Fawzy NW (1995) A psychoeducational nursing intervention to enhance coping and affective state in newly diagnosed malignant melanoma patients. Cancer Nurs 18:427–438

Greer S, Moorey S, Baruch JD, Watson M, Robertson BM, Mason A, Rowden L, Law MG, Bliss JM (1992) Adjuvant psychological therapy for patients with cancer: a prospective randomised trial. BMJ 304:675–680

Kelly B, Raphael B, Smithers M, Swanson C, Reid C, McLeod R, Thomson D, Walpole E (1995) Psychological responses to malignant melanoma. An investigation of traumatic stress reactions to life-threatening illness. Gen Hosp Psychiatry 17:126–134

Kneier AW, Temoshok L (1984) Repressive coping reactions in patients with malignant melanoma as compared to cardiovascular disease patients. Psychosom Med 28:145–155

Levine J, Ziegler E (1975) Denial and self-image in stroke, lung cancer and heart disease patients. J Consult Clin Psychol 43:751–757

Mayring P (1985) Qualitative Inhaltsanalyse. In: Jüttemann G (ed) Qualitative Forschung in der Psychologie: Grundlagen, Verfahrensweisen, Anwendungsfelder. Beltz, Weinheim, pp 187–211

Söllner W, Zingg-Schir M, Rumpold G, Mairinger G, Fritsch P (1998) Need for supportive counselling – the professionals' versus the patients' perspective: a survey in a representative sample of 236 melanoma patients. Psychother Psychosom 67:94–104

Söllner W, Zschocke I, Zingg-Schir M, Rumpold G, Stein B, Augustin M (1999) Interactive patterns of social support and individual coping strategies in melanoma patients and their correlations with adjustment to illness. Psychosomatics 40:239–250

Spiegel D, Classen C (1999) Group therapy for cancer patients. A research-based handbook of psychosocial care. Basic Behavioral Sciences, Basic Books, New York

# Subject Index

**A**
ABCD rule   126
Abnormalities   275
– chromosomal   275
Acid   240, 317
– 5-aminolevulinic (ALA)   240, 317
Acral lentiginous melanoma (ALM)   95
Acral myxoinflammatory fibroblastic
    sarcoma   349
Actinic keratoses   240
Adenovirus   180
– recombinant   180
ALA   (see 5-aminolevulinic acid)
ALM   (see Acral lentiginous melanoma)
America Society for Testing
    and Materials   42
American Association of Textile Chemists
    and Colorists   42
5-aminolevulinic acid (ALA)   240, 317
Amplification   95
Analysis   126, 296, 299, 303
– molecular analysis   296, 299, 303
– pattern analysis   126
Anamnestic interview   353
Angiofibroma   348, 349
– giant cell   348, 349
ANN   (see Artificial neural networks)
Antiangiogenic treatment   152
Antibody   317
– anti-CD25   317
Anti-CD25 antibody   317
Anti-Tac(Fv)-PE38   317
Antitumor immunity   173
Apoptosis   246
Argentina   3
Artificial intelligence   129
Artificial neural networks (ANN)   128

Atypia   78
– grading of   78
Atypical Spitz tumor   75
Australia   3, 113
Australian/New Zealand Standard   26
Austria   5
Autologous melanoma cells   175
Autologous tumor cells   175
Awareness   71

**B**
Bacterial superantigen   276
Basal cell carcinoma (BCC)   170, 219, 240,
    246, 259–265
– current treatments   261–263
– new treatment modalities   263–265
BCC   (see Basal cell carcinoma)
B-cell lymphoma   289, 294, 296
– marginal zone   289, 294, 296
– of the leg   294
– primary cutaneous   294
bcl-2 protein   297
Bexarotene   321–327
Bexarotene gel   313
Biological UV dosimeters   59
Biopsy   151, 153
– sentinel node   151, 153
B-K mole syndrome   100
Blastoma   348
– fibroblastoma   348
Blood tests   210
– for diagnosis of metastases   210
Body-image disturbances   365
Bone marrow transplantation   314
Borrelia burgdorferi   297
Borrelia infection   272
Bowen's disease   240

Broad-band UVB   314
Bulky melanoma metastases   156
Burn-out   369

C
Cancer   7–11, 246, 355, 363
– coping with   363–369
– nonmelanoma skin cancer   246
– skin cancer   7–11, 355
Cancer nurse   364
Cancerogenesis   253
– skin   253
Carcinoma   10, 219, 240, 246, 259–265
– basal cell (BCC)   219, 240, 246, 259–265
– squamous cell   10
Care   363, 365
– palliative   365
– supportive   363
Carmustine   312
CD4+ T-cells   248
CD8+ T-cell Priming   172
CD8+ T-cells   248
CD95 ligand   246
CD95 receptor   246
CD95-CD95L interactions   249
Cell carcinoma   10, 170, 219, 240, 246,
   259–265
– basal (BCC)   170, 219, 240, 246, 259–
   265
– squamous   10, 170
Cell cycle regulation   276
Cell growth factor   276
Cell tumor   349
– hyalinizing spindle   349
Cell vaccination   165–168
– dendritic   165–168
Cells   171, 172, 175, 248
– allogeneic melanoma cells   175
– autologous tumor cells   175
– CD4+ T-cells   248
– CD8+ T-cells   248
– cytotoxic T-cells (CTL)   171, 172
– dendritic cells   172
Cellular senescence   276
Center-cell lymphoma   294, 297
– follicle   294, 297
CGH   (see Comparative genomic
   hybridization)
Changing incidence   113
Chemical additives   33
Chemical sunscreens   53
Chemotherapy   311
– topically applied   311
Chlorambucil   313
Chromosomal aberration   92
Chromosomal abnormalities   275

Chromosomes   76, 80, 92, 97
– chromosome   10   80
– chromosome   11p   92, 97
– chromosome   9   76
– chromosome   9p21   76
CIE   (see Commission Internationale
   de l'Eclairage)
Classification   295, 303
– EORTC   295
– of cutaneous lymphomas   303
– of primary cutaneous B-cell
   lymphomas   295
– WHO   295
Clinical findings   294
Clothing   16–23, 35, 49, 51, 56–62, 72
– standard test method   51
– UV-protective clothing   38, 39
Color   62
Commission Internationale de l'Eclairage
   (CIE)   49
Common acquired nevus   77
Communication   365
– doctor-patient   365
Comparative genomic hybridization
   (CGH)   92
Comparison of UPF and SPF   52, 53
Complexes   178
– DNA-liposome   178
Computer-assisted diagnosis   128
Concentric eosinophilic fibrosis   78
Conditions   271
– preneoplastic   271
Congenital nevus   75, 82
– intermediate-sized   82
– small-sized   82
Connective tissue nevus   347
Consultation-liaison service   362, 364
Consumer Products Safety Commission   43
Coping with cancer   363–369
Corticosteroids   313
– topical   313
Crisis intervention   362–369
Crosti's lymphoma   297
Cryosurgery   262
CTL   (see Cytotoxic T-cell)
Curettage   261, 262
Cutaneous B-cell lymphoma   294
– primary   294
Cutaneous lymphoma   303
– classification   303
– diagnosis   303
– immunohistochemistry   303
– molecular analysis   303
– staging   303
Cutaneous melanoma   205, 206
– epidemiology   206

Cutaneous T-cell lymphoma    271, 310,
    321–327
Cytogenetic studies    277
Cytogenetics    92
– molecular    92
Cytokine gene transfer    172
Cytokine profile    276
Cytokine treatment    263
– intralesional    263
– perilesional    263
Cytokines    170, 311, 335
Cytotoxic lymphoma    284
Cytotoxic T-cell (CTL)    171, 172, 178

**D**
De novo melanocytic dysplasia    79
Deep fibromatosis    348
Delayed lymph node dissection
    (DLND)    153
Dendritic cell vaccination    165–168
Dendritic cells    172
Denial    363–369
Denileukin diftitox    313, 317, 321–327
Derivatives    241
– hematoporphyrin    241
Dermatofibroma    344, 345
Dermatofibrosarcoma protuberans    348
Dermatological imaging    129
Dermatological oncology    158
Dermatoscopy    126
Dermoscopy    126
Desmoid fibromatosis    348
Diagnosis    78, 128, 210, 303
– blood tests    210
– computer-assisted    128
– of cutaneous lymphoma    303
– of dysplastic nevus    78
– of metastases    210
Diagnostic reagents    86
Diftitox    313, 317, 321–327
– denileukin    313, 317, 321–327
Digital epiluminescence microscopy    128
Digitized ELM    125
Diseases    240
– Bowen's disease    240
Dissection    151, 153
– lymph node    151, 153
Distress    363, 364
Distribution    219
– topographical    219
Disturbances    365
– body-image    365
DLND    (see Delayed lymph node
    dissection)
DLR biofilm    59
DNA    93, 180

– plasmid    180
DNA-liposome complexes    178
Doctor-patient communication    365
Drugs    317
– multiagent systemic    317
Dying    363
Dysplasia    78, 79
– de novo melanocytic    79
– epithelioid    78
– lentiginous    78
Dysplastic melanocytic nevus    100
Dysplastic nevi share    128
Dysplastic nevus    75, 78
– diagnosis    78
– major criteria    78
Dysplastic nevus syndrome    76

**E**
Elastofibroma    347
Elective lymph node dissection    151
Elective regional lymph node dissection
    153
Electrodessication    262
ELM    125
– digitized    125
Environmental factors    275
EORTC    (see European Organization
    Research and Treatment of Cancer)
Epidemiology    206
– of cutaneous melanoma    206
Epiluminescence microscopy    125, 128
– digital    128
Epithelial malignancy    251–257
Epithelioid dysplasia    78
European Organization for Research
    and Treatment of Cancer (EORTC)    295
– classification    295
Examinations    208, 211
– RT-PCR    211
– technical    208
Excision    261
Extracorporeal photochemotherapy    311
Extrafacial lentigo maligna melanoma
    (LMM)    80
Extranodal non-Hodgkin's lymphoma    310

**F**
Fabric    16–23, 50, 56–60, 62
– color    20
– construction    18, 19
– nonsynthetic    18
– synthetic    18
– thickness    19
– type    18
– weight    19
Fabric care    66

Fabric preparation   44
Factor   222, 275, 276
- cell growth   276
- environmental   275
- prognostic   222
Familial multiple atypical mole melanoma
    syndrome   76
Fears   362, 363, 367
- tumor-related   362, 363, 367
Federal Trade Commission   43
Fiber   62
Fibroblastic sarcoma   349
- acral myxoinflammatory   349
Fibroblastoma   348
- giant cell   348
Fibroma   344–349
- angiofibroma   348, 349
- dermatofibroma   344, 345
- elastofibroma   347
Fibroma molle   347
Fibromatosis   346, 348
- deep   348
- desmoid   348
- superficial   346
Fibroplasia   78
- lamellar   78
Fibrosarcoma   348, 349
- dermatofibrosarcoma protuberans   348
Fibrosis   78
- concentric eosinophilic   78
Fibrous histiocytoma   344, 345
Fibrous papule   347
Flaps   226
- local   226
5-Fluorouracil   262
Follicle center-cell lymphoma   294, 297
- histopathology   297
- prognosis   297
Follow-up   205
- of melanoma patients   205
Follow-up strategies   208
- for malignant melanoma   208
France   5
Full-thickness skin grafts   225

G
Garments   64
Gene expression   85
Gene gun   172, 180
Gene rearrangement   279
- $J_H$   297
Gene therapy   178
- in situ   178
Gene transfer   172
- cytokine   172
Genes   76, 77

- CDKN2A   77
- p16   76
- p53   76
Genetic immunization   170, 178
Genetic instability   101
Genomic instability   276
Germany   6
Giant cell angiofibroma   348, 349
Giant cell fibroblastoma   348
Giant cells   80
- star-burst   80
Giant congenital nevus   82
GM-CSF-secreting tumor vaccine   174
Guided imagery   366–369
Guidelines   205

H
Head   225
Health education   364
Helicobacter pylori   272
Heliotherapy   314
Hematoporphyrin derivatives   241
Herpes virus   332–334
- human   332–334
Heterozygosity   101
- loss of (LOH)   101
Histiocytoma   344, 345
- fibrous   344, 345
Histological mapping   219
Histology   80, 296, 299
- large B-cell lymphoma of the leg   299
- marginal zone B-cell lymphoma   296
- of lentigo maligna (LM)   80
Histopathological classification   92
- of melanocytic tumors   92
Histopathological subtype   219
Histopathology   93
HIV-1   334–337
HMB-45   81
Hornheide questionnaire   353
Hornheide Screening Instrument   353
HRAS mutation   97
Human herpes virus   332–334
Human papillomavirus infection   254
Hyalinizing spindle cell tumor with giant
    rosettes   349
Hybridization   92
- comparative genomic hybridization
    (CGH)   92
Hypericin   317
Hyperthermia   152

I
IFN   (see Interferon)
IFN-$\alpha$   (see Interferon $\alpha$)
IL-12   173

IL-7   173
ILP   (see Isolated perfusion)
Imagery   366–369
–  guided   366–369
Imaging   129
–  dermatological   129
Imiquimod   264
Immune privilege   249
Immune response   195–200
Immune surveillance   249
Immunity   173
–  antitumor   173
Immunization   170, 178
–  genetic   170, 178
Immunocytokine   195, 193
Immunocytoma   296
Immunohistochemistry   303
–  cutaneous lymphoma   303
Immunohistology   294, 296, 299
–  large B-cell lymphoma of the leg   299
–  marginal zone B-cell lymphoma   296
Immunosuppressive treatment   253
Immunotherapy   195–200
In situ gene therapy   178
Infection   254, 272
–  Borrelia   272
–  human papillomavirus   254
Inflammation   272
Informed   71
Injection   176, 177
–  intratumoral   176, 177
Instability   101, 276
–  genetic   101
–  genomic   276
–  microsatellite   101
Interactions   249
–  CD95-CD95L interactions   249
Interchromosomal   14;18 transloca-
   tion   297
Interferon (IFN)   155, 158, 246, 247, 321–
   327
–  intralesional   247
–  pegylated (PEG-IFN)   158
Interferon $\alpha$ (IFN-$\alpha$)   85, 171, 246, 247, 313
Interferon $\gamma$   313
Interleukin-12   318
Intermediate-sized congenital nevus   82
International Society for Cutaneous Lym-
   phomas (ISCL)   273
Intervention   360, 362
–  crisis intervention   362–369
–  psychosocial   360
–  psychotherapeutic   362–369
Interview   353
–  anamnestic   353
Interview questions   358

Intralesional cytokine treatment   263
Intralesional interferon   247
In-transit melanoma metastases   154
In-transit metastases   152
Intratumoral injection   176, 177
In-vitro testing   56–58
–  UPF   56–58
In-vivo testing   58–59
–  SPF   16, 17, 67
ISCL   (see International Society for Cuta-
   neous Lymphomas)
Isolated limb perfusion   152
Isolated perfusion (ILP)   154
ISO-MET   64
Italy   5

J
$J_H$ gene rearrangement   297

K
Kaposi's sarkoma   331
Keloid   344
Keratoses   240
–  actinic   240
Keratosis   9
–  solar   9

L
Labeling   46
Labsphere   63
Lamellar fibroplasia   78
Large B-cell lymphoma of the leg   294, 299
–  histology   299
–  immunohistology   299
–  molecular analysis   299
–  prognosis   299
Laser beam microdissection   294
Laundering   66
Leg   294, 299
–  large B-cell lymphoma   294, 299
Lentiginous dysplasia   78
Lentigo maligna (LM)   75, 80
–  histology   80
Lentigo maligna melanoma (LMM)   80, 81
–  extrafacial   80
Leukin-2   318
Ligands   246
–  CD95   246
LM   (see Lentigo maligna)
LMM   (see Lentigo maligna melanoma)
Local flaps   226
LOH   (see Loss of heterozygosity)
Loss of heterozygosity (LOH)   101
Lymph node dissection   151, 153
–  delayed (DLND)   153
–  elective   151

– elective regional   153
– selective   151, 153
Lymphoma   271, 284, 285, 289, 290, 294, 296
– B-cell   289
– Crosti's   297
– cutaneous   303
– cutaneous T-cell   271, 310, 321–327
– cytotoxic   284
– extranodal non-Hodgkin's   310
– follicle center-cell   294, 297
– large B-cell   294, 299
– marginal zone B-cell   289, 294–299, 303, 310, 321–327
– NK   285
– primary cutaneous B-cell   294
– pseudolymphoma   290
– secondary cutaneous   249
– skin-associated lymphoid tissue (SALT)   296
– T-cell   284

**M**
Malignancy   251–257
– epithelial   251–257
Malignant melanoma   75, 100, 170, 207, 208
– follow-up strategies   208
– prognosis   207
– risk   75
– technical examinations   208
Mapping   219
– histological   219
MAR1/Melan A   211
Margin   152
Margin strip method   220
Marginal zone B-cell lymphoma   289, 294, 296
– histology   296
– immunohistology   296
– molecular analysis   296
– prognosis   296
Mechlorethamine   312
MED   (see Minimal erythema dose)
Melan-A   81
Melanocytic tumors   92
– histopathological classification   92
Melanocytosis   82
– neurocutaneous   82
Melanoma   10, 80, 86, 92, 95, 100, 113, 125, 128, 134, 151, 158, 170, 185–190, 205, 335
– acral lentiginous melanoma (ALM)   95
– cutaneous   205
– extrafacial lentigo maligna (LMM)   80
– malignant   100, 170

– superficial spreading melanoma (SSM)   95
– surgery   151
Melanoma cells   175
– autologous   175
Melanoma control   114
Melanoma immunotherapy   195–200
Melanoma metastases   154
– in-transit   154
Melanoma metastases   156
– bulky   156
Melanoma patients   205
Melphalan   152, 154
Metastases   134, 152–156, 210
– bulky melanoma   156
– diagnosis   210
– in-transit   152
– melanoma   154
Methods   220
– margin strip   220
– Mohs   220
– Munich   220
Methotrexate   313
Microdissection   102, 294, 297
– laser beam   294
Micrographic surgery   219
Microsatellite instability   101
Microsatellites   101
Microscopy   125, 128
– digital epiluminescence   128
– epiluminescence   125
Minimmal erythema dose (MED)   56–60
Mohs method   220
Mole syndrome   100
Molecular analysis   294, 296, 299, 303
– cutaneous lymphoma   303
– large B-cell lymphoma of the leg   299
– marginal zone B-cell lymphoma   296
Molecular cytogenetics   92
Mortality   113
– of melanoma   113
Multiagent systemic drugs   317
Multiple atypical nevus   76
Munich method   220
Mutation   97
– HRAS   97
Mycosis fungoides   310

**N**
Need of support   357
Neoplasia   272
Neoplastic T-cell   310
Neurocutaneous melanocytosis   82
Nevus   75–78, 82, 92, 100, 347
– architectural disorder   76
– atypical Spitz nevus   75

- common acquired  77
- congenital  75, 82
- connective tissue  347
- cytologic atypia  76
- dysplastic  75, 78
- dysplastic melanocytic  100
- giant congenital  82
- intermediate-sized congenital  82
- multiple atypical  76
- small-sized congenital  82
- Spitz nevus  92
NK activity  173
NK lymphoma  285
Non-Hodgkin's lymphoma  310
- extranodal  310
Nonmelanoma skin cancer  246
Nurse  364
- cancer nurse  364

O
Oligonucleotide array  85
Oncology  158, 354
- dermatological  158
- psychooncology  354
Optical brightening agent  22, 23
Organ transplant patients  251–257
- skin cancer  252
Oxygen  242
- singlet  242

P
p16 gene  76
p53 gene  76
Palliative care  365
- palliative treatment  363
Papillomavirus infection  254
- human  254
Papule  347
- fibrous  347
Parapsoriasis en plaques  271
Pathogenesis  274, 297
Patients  251–257, 353, 365
- doctor-patient communication  365
- organ transplant  251–257
- psychosocial risk  353
Pattern analysis  126
PCR  (see Polymerase chain reaction)
PDT  (see Photodynamic therapy)
Pegylated interferon (PEG-IFN)  158
Pentostatin  313
Perfusion  152
- isolated limb  152
Perilesional cytokine treatment  263
Pharmacogenomics  86
Phase  81
- vertical growth  81

Photoaging  22
Photochemotherapy  311
- extracorporeal  311
Photodynamic therapy (PDT)  240, 263,
  317
Photon radiation  317
- total body  317
Photoprotection  16–23, 49–53, 70–72
- chemical sunscreens  53
- clothes  49
- fabrics  50
Photosensitive disorders  16–18, 22
Photosensitizer  240
Photostability  22
Plasmid DNA  180
Point mutation  76
- UV light-induced  76
Polymerase chain reaction (PCR)  101, 310
Polysulphone films  59
Positron emission tomography  210
Preneoplastic conditions  271
Prevention  71
Primary cutaneous B-cell lymphomas  294,
  295
- classification  295
Primary prevention  117
Profile  276
- cytokine  276
Prognosis  207, 296–299
- follicle center-cell lymphoma  297
- large B-cell lymphoma of the leg  299
- malignant melanoma  207
- marginal zone B-cell lymphoma  296
Prognostic factors  222
Protection against UV  51, 52
- color  51
- porosity  52
- stretch  51
- weave  51
- weight  51
Proteins  210, 297
- bcl-2  297
- protein S100  210
Protoporphyrin IX  241
Pseudolymphoma  290
Psychooncology  354
Psychosocial intervention  360
Psychosocial risk  355
Psychosocial risk patients  353
- screening of  353
Psychosocial support  353
Psychotherapy  362–369
- psychotherapeutic intervention
  362–369
- psychotherapeutic techniques  365
- short-term psychotherapy  365

Public education   70–72
Public health approach   114

**Q**
Quality assurance   360
Quality control   129
Questionnaire   353
– Hornheide   353

**R**
Radiation   254
– ultraviolet   254
Radiotherapy   234–238, 262
– of skin tumors   234–238
Reagents   86
– diagnostic   86
Receptors   246
– CD95   246
Recombinant adenovirus   180
Recombinant vaccinia virus   195–200
Reconstructive surgery   225
– in the face   225
Recurrence rates   219
Recurrences   156
Regulation   276
– cell cycle   276
Relaxation   362, 366–369
Resection margin   151
Reticulohistiocytoma of the dorsum   297
Retroviral vector   177
RFT5-SMPT-dgA   317
RT-PCR examinations   211

**S**
SALT lymphoma   (see Skin-associated
   lymphoid tissue lymphoma)
Sarcoma   331, 349
– acral myxoinflammatory fibroblastic
   349
– fibrosarcoma   348, 349
– Kaposi's   331
Seal of Recommendation   67
Secondary cutaneous lymphoma   294
Selective lymph node dissection   151, 153
Senescence   276
– cellular   276
Sentinel lymph nodes   134
Sentinel node biopsy   151, 153
Sézary syndrome   310
Sign   81
– the swallow's nest   81
Singlet oxygen   242
Skin   310
Skin cancer   7–11, 71, 165, 246, 252, 256,
   355
– in organ transplant patients   252, 256

– nonmelanoma   246
– treatment   165
Skin Cancer Foundation   67
Skin cancerogenesis   253
– in organ transplant patients   253
Skin grafts   225
– full-thickness   225
Skin tumor   234–238, 256
– radiotherapy   234–238
Skin-associated lymphoid tissue (SALT)
   lymphoma   296
Small-sized congenital nevus   82
Social network   364
Social support   364, 365
Solar exposure   49
Solar keratosis   9
Solar ultraviolet radiation   49
Spain   6
Spectral irradiance   57
Spectrophotometers   56, 57
Spectrophotometric measurement   17, 56,
   57
SPF   (see Sun-protection factor)
Spindle cell tumor   349
– hyalinizing   349
Spitz nevus   92
Squamous cell carcinoma   10, 170
SSM   (see Superficial spreading melanoma)
Staging   303
– cutaneous lymphoma   303
Standard test method for clothes   51
Standards (UV-protective clothing)   16–23,
   35, 56–60
– AATCC   23
– AS/NZS   18, 23
– CEN   23, 56
Star-burst giant cells   80
Stem cell transplantation   314
Stress management   363
Stretch   32
Structured picture drawing   362, 367–369
Studies   277
– cytogenetic   277
Subclinical tumour extension   219
Substantial protection   49
Subtype   219
– histopathological   219
Sun   363
Sun protection   15–23, 70–72
Sun protection factor (SPF)   16, 17, 50–52,
   57
Sun protective clothing   26
Sunburn   16
Sunscreen   9, 53
– chemical   53
Sunscreen use   10

Superantigen   276
- bacterial   276
Superficial fibromatosis   346
Superficial spreading melanoma (SSM)   95
Supervision   362, 369
Support requirements   354
Supportive care   363
Surgery   151, 219, 225, 261, 262
- Cryosurgery   262
- melanoma   151
- micrographic   219
- reconstructive   225
Surgical repair   225
Surrogate marker   86
Switzerland   6
Syndrome   76, 100, 310
- B-K mole syndrome   100
- dysplastic nevus   76
- familial multiple atypical mole
  melanoma   76
- Sézary syndrome   310
Systemic drugs   317
- multiagent   317

T
TAT   331–339
T-cell lymphoma   271, 284, 310, 321–327
- cutaneous   271, 310, 321–327
T-cell receptor   185–188, 190–193
T-cells   248, 310
- CD4$^+$ T-cell   248
- CD8$^+$ T-cell   248
- neoplastic   310
- tumor infiltrating (TIL)   185, 186, 191–
  193
Technical examinations   208
- in maligna melanoma   208
Telecommunication   129
Testing for photoprotection   49, 50
- in vitro test (UPF)   49, 50
- in vivo technique (SPF)   49, 50
Textile chain   66
Textile materials   35
Textiles   16–23, 56–60
Therapeutic procedures   219
Therapy   240, 263, 317
- photodynamic (PDT)   240, 263, 317
Tinosorb   52, 53
- rinsing solution   53
- washing powder   52
Tissue nevus   347
- connective   347
Titan dioxide   20–23
TNF   (see Tumour necrosis factor)
Tomography   210
- positron emission   210

Topical corticosteroids   313
Topically applied chemotherapy   311
Topographical distribution   219
Total body photon radiation   317
Total skin electron beam   311
Transplantation   314
- bone marrow   314
- stem cell   314
Treatment   253, 263, 363
- immunosuppressive   253
- intralesional cytokine   263
- palliative   363
- perilesional cytokine   263
Tumor   75, 92
- melanocytic   92
Tumor cells   175
- autologous   175
Tumor extension   219
- subclinical   219
Tumor infiltrating T-cell (TIL)   185, 186,
  191–193
Tumor necrosis factor (TNF)   152, 155
Tumor progression   363
Tumor vaccine   174
- GM-CSF-secreting   174
Tumor-related fears   362, 363, 367
Tyrosinase   211

U
Ultraviolet protection factor (UPF)   16–23,
  27, 28, 35, 49–53, 56–62
- clothing   35, 38, 39
- in vitro   56–68
- in vivo   58–59
Ultraviolet radiation   70–72, 254
United Kingdom   4
UPF   (see Ultraviolet protection factor)
UPF rating scheme   28
UPF swing tags   30
US Food and Drug Administration   42
USA   5
UV   16–23, 56–60
- absorbers   20–23
- absorption   20, 57
- dosimetry   56–60
- exposure   16
- protection   16–23
- scattering   57
- source   56
- transmission   17–19, 56–60
UV absorber   62
UV exposure   71
UV index (UVI)   71
UV light-induced point mutation   76
UV meter   64
UV protection   7–11

UV protection factor   (see Ultraviolet
   protection factor)
UV transmittance   62
– clothing   62
UV transmittance testing   45
UVA   16, 17, 20
UVB   16, 58, 59
UVI   (see UV Index)
UV-protective clothing   35, 38, 39
UVR transmittance   49

**V**
Vaccination   165–168
– dendritic cell   165–169

Vaccine   171, 174
– tumor vaccine   174
Vector   177
– retroviral   177
Vertical growth phase   81
Virus   275, 332–337
– HIV-1   334–337
– human herpes   332–334

**W**
Weather bulletin   71
Wetting   32
World Health Organization (WHO)   295

Printing (Computer to Film): Saladruck Berlin
Binding: Stürtz AG, Würzburg